Clinical Drug Trials and Tribulations

DRUGS AND THE PHARMACEUTICAL SCIENCES

A Series of Textbooks and Monographs

ADDITIONAL VOLUMES IN PREPARATION

Modern Pharmaceutics: Fourth Edition, Revised and Expanded, *edited by Gilbert S. Banker and Christopher T. Rhodes*

Clinical Drug Trials and Tribulations

Second Edition, Revised and Expanded

edited by

Allen Cato
Lynda Sutton

Cato Research Ltd.
Durham, North Carolina

Allen Cato III

Cato Research Ltd.
San Diego, California

MARCEL DEKKER, INC.   NEW YORK • BASEL

ISBN: 0-8247-0314-6

This book is printed on acid-free paper.

Headquarters
Marcel Dekker, Inc.
270 Madison Avenue, New York, NY 10016
tel: 212-696-9000; fax: 212-685-4540

Eastern Hemisphere Distribution
Marcel Dekker AG
Hutgasse 4, Postfach 812, CH-4001 Basel, Switzerland
tel: 41-61-261-8482; fax: 41-61-261-8896

World Wide Web
http://www.dekker.com

The publisher offers discounts on this book when ordered in bulk quantities. For more information, write to Special Sales/Professional Marketing at the headquarters address above.

Current printing (last digit):
10 9 8 7 6 5 4 3 2 1

PRINTED IN THE UNITED STATES OF AMERICA

To my wife, Adrian; my three sons, Allen III, Mike, and Dan; and my eight grandchildren. Thank you for your love, support, and understanding of my many absences from our family life while out in the fascinating pursuit of clinical drug development. This book is also dedicated to all patients—past, present, and future—who volunteer to participate in clinical drug trials. Without them, no drug could ever be shown to be safe or efficacious. These individuals are the silent heroes behind every advancement in drug therapy.

Allen Cato

To my mentor, best friend, partner, and co-founder of Cato Research, Allen, who has taught me to think rationally about drug development rather than check boxes; to Dr. Joy Cavagnaro, who has taught me how to think "backwards" relative to planning drug development programs; to my mother, who, as an accomplished writer, instilled in me at an early age the need to rewrite every paragraph at least five times; and to my father, whose constant support and encouragement allowed me to attempt and achieve tasks that others said were impossible.

Lynda Sutton

To my family, friends, colleagues, and all whose lives may be improved by the development of new therapies. Thanks also to my mentors at the University of North Carolina and in the pharmaceutical industry from whom I learned the science of pharmacokinetics and how to apply these diverse principles to drug development. In particular, I thank my father for emphasizing to me that, in addition to all the scientific disciplines involved, common sense and creativity are also necessary components of proficient drug development.

Allen Cato III

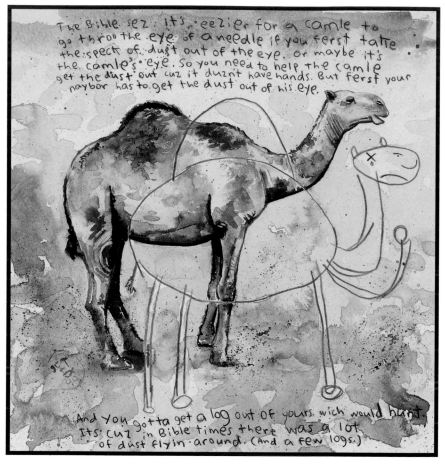

And again I say unto you, It is easier for a camel to go through the eye of a needle, than for a rich man to enter into the kingdom of God.

Matthew 19:24

Preface

The drug development industry continues to be a highly charged, fascinating, and ever-evolving field. The industry has changed significantly in the 14 years since the first edition of *Clinical Drug Trials and Tribulations* was published, and this second edition of this book addresses those changes and continues to explore the problems and challenges that individuals in this industry experience daily.

The information presented is directed both at the fortunate individuals already involved in drug development and at those adventuresome sorts who are considering entering the field. We hope this book will provide readers with insights into this exciting arena and begin to explain the complicated process of developing a promising new drug.

Although this book has some elements of a "how-to" publication, it really is meant to address the "whys" of development, such as why certain decisions are made in the development of a new chemical entity and the consequences of those decisions. Certainly, the one rule of clinical drug development seems to be that things never turn out as designed or expected. The number of difficult decisions that must be made during the course of clinical drug development seems endless, as are the daily tribulations and challenges that have never before been encountered. We explore these issues by discussing topics such as international regulation and deregulation, venture capital investment, the Investigational New Drug application process, informed consent, and changes in manufacturing. These areas are affecting the way nonclinical and clinical studies are conducted today, and examining them brings to light many of the intriguing tribulations of clinical trials.

   No book is ever written alone, and we are thankful to the many individuals involved in the production of this one. First, we want to thank all the chapter authors, who contributed their time, energy, and expertise to this effort despite busy work schedules. In addition, we acknowledge the efforts of the individuals who assisted with the issuance of the first edition, in particular Linda Cocchetto, Robert Sutton, and Paul Stang. We also thank Barbara Proujan, Tricia Eimers, and Paula Brown for their work on this project. And lastly, thanks to Trish Nolan. Without her perseverance, the second edition as presented now would not exist. Our everlasting gratitude goes to all of these dedicated, hard-working people. Although we're sure they could write about their own tribulations in producing this volume, together we have produced a book that will provide further insight into this challenging field.

Allen Cato
Lynda Sutton
Allen Cato III

Contents

Contributors

David F. Bernstein, Ph.D.   Cato Research Ltd., Corona del Mar, California

Peggy J. Berry, B.S., R.A.C.   Department of Regulatory Affairs, Dey Laboratories, Napa, California

Rocco L. Brunelle, M.S.   Eli Lilly and Company, Indianapolis, Indiana

Angela Cahill   Bethesda, Maryland

Allen Cato, M.D., Ph.D.   Cato Research Ltd., Durham, North Carolina

Allen Cato III, Ph.D.   Cato Research Ltd., San Diego, California

Daniel C. Cato, M.S.   Cato Research Ltd., Durham, North Carolina

David M. Cocchetto, Ph.D.   United States Regulatory Affairs, GlaxoSmith-Kline, Research Triangle Park, North Carolina

Dale H. Cowan, M.D., J.D., F.A.C.P.   Community Oncology Group, Cleveland Clinic Foundation, Cleveland, Ohio

Joseph A. DiMasi, Ph.D.   Tufts Center for the Study of Drug Development, Tufts University, Boston, Massachusetts

David S. Duch, Ph.D.   Cato Research Ltd., Durham, North Carolina

Robert M. Ferris, Ph.D.   Retired, Charlotte, North Carolina

Cheryl K. Fiedler, Pharm.D.   SCIREX Corporation, Hartford, Connecticut

Jean M. Findlay, M.D., F.A.A.P.   Regional Pediatric Associates, Durham, North Carolina

Marion J. Finkel, M.D.   Pharmaceutical and Regulatory Consultant, Morristown, New Jersey

Diana E. Fordyce, Ph.D., R.A.C.   Department of Regulatory Affairs, Cato Research Ltd., Durham, North Carolina

Richard Granneman, Ph.D.   Abbott Laboratories, Abbott Park, Illinois

Marlene E. Haffner, M.D., M.P.H.   United States Food and Drug Administration, Rockville, Maryland

David L. Horwitz, M.D., Ph.D.   LifeScan (a Johnson & Johnson Company), Milpitas, California

Nelson S. Irey, M.D.†   Armed Forces Institute of Pathology, Washington, D.C.

Todd S. Keiller, M.B.A.   Healthcare Business Development, Inc., Hopkinton, Massachusetts

Louis A. Morris, Ph.D.   Louis A. Morris & Associates, Dix Hills, New York

F. Richard Nichol, Ph.D.   Nichol Clinical Technologies Corporation, Newport Beach, California

Myron B. Peterson, M.D., Ph.D., F.A.A.P.   Cato Research Ltd., Washington, D.C.

Paul J. Reitemeier, Ph.D.   National Center for Ethics, Veterans Health Administration, White River Junction, Vermont, and Department of Medicine, Dartmouth Medical School, Hanover, New Hampshire

---

† Deceased

Peter H. Rheinstein, M.D., J.D., F.A.A.F.P., F.C.L.M.   Department of Medical and Clinical Affairs, Cell Works Inc., Baltimore, Maryland

H. Russell Searight, Ph.D.   Department of Community and Family Medicine, St. Louis University School of Medicine, St. Louis, Missouri

Jay Philip Siegel, M.D., F.A.C.P.   Center for Biologics Evaluation and Research, United States Food and Drug Administration, Rockville, Maryland

Lynda Sutton, B.S.   Cato Research Ltd., Durham, North Carolina

David B. Thomas, M.A.   Department of Clinical and Regulatory Affairs, Roche Molecular Systems, Inc., Pleasanton, California

W. Leigh Thompson, M.D., Ph.D., Sc.D., F.A.C.P., F.C.C.M.*   Eli Lilly and Company, Indianapolis, Indiana

Susan L. Watts, Ph.D.   Department of Regulatory Affairs and Quality Assurance, Family Health International, Research Triangle Park, North Carolina

Karen D. Weiss, M.D.   Office of Therapeutics Research and Review, Center for Biologics Evaluation and Research, United States Food and Drug Administration, Rockville, Maryland

Michael G. Wilson, M.S.   Michael G. Wilson and Company, Inc., New Palestine, Indiana

---

* Retired

Clinical Drug Trials and Tribulations

1

Current Challenges and Future Directions of Drug Development

Allen Cato
Cato Research Ltd., Durham, North Carolina

Lynda Sutton
Cato Research Ltd., Durham, North Carolina

Allen Cato III
Cato Research Ltd., San Diego, California

It may be easier for a camel to pass through the eye of a needle than it is for a new chemical entity to reach the marketplace. Drug development is a long and costly process fraught with tribulation. The tortuous pathway traveled by a new drug from synthesis to sale requires the constant percolation of data through rigorous clinical and regulatory filters. This process is complex, and success cannot be guaranteed. The ability to always predict which drug will have all the qualities necessary to gain regulatory approval and to be marketed remains as elusive as a camel in a needle's eye.

New drugs do make it from discovery to the market, but only at the approximate rate of one in every 10,000 new molecules synthesized. It is a long, costly, and extremely risky process involving a steady progression through multiple stages, with treacherous decision points along the way. Most of all, it is a process involving the constant percolating of data through rigorous filters strewn with tribulations and complicated by the difficulty of making decisions that affect human health when all the facts are not known.

Despite the daunting challenge of bringing a new drug from discovery to market, new medicines continue to be developed that may have a significant effect on our health. You may wonder, "What has medicine done for mankind lately?" In the United States, the adult life expectancy increased by nearly

30 years over the last century, primarily because of the availability and management of vaccines and immunization schedules, antibiotics, and sanitation measures. As evidenced by the following statistics from the Centers for Disease Control (CDC) (1), the development of vaccines has had a major impact on our health:

> Smallpox killed an average of more than 1500 people per year between 1900 and 1904; it is now eradicated worldwide, and children are no longer vaccinated against the disease.
>
> Polio struck more than 16,000 people annually in the early 1950s; today, it has been eliminated from the Western Hemisphere.

During the past 50 years, vaccines also have been responsible for drastically reducing the morbidity and mortality from measles, *Haemophilus influenzae* type b (Hib), diphtheria, pertussis, tetanus (DPT, typically administered together), hepatitis B, and chicken pox. In addition to improved health, substantial economic benefits have been realized. For example, the CDC estimates that the United States recoups its investment in the eradication of smallpox every 26 days. Despite the obvious advances of modern medicine, many patients still have infectious, chronic, or genetic diseases and will benefit from the research of today finding the effective treatments of tomorrow. Pharmaceutical research targeting the top 12 major medical needs exceeds $645 billion annually in direct medical expense and lost productivity. The diseases included in this figure are Alzheimer's disease, arthritis, asthma, cancer, congestive heart failure, coronary heart disease, depression, diabetes, hypertensive disease, osteoporosis, schizophrenia, and stroke (2). Just as it did 50 years ago, innovation continues today to bring us new knowledge through genetic research, molecular biology, and enhanced computer technology. This is the promising future of drug development.

However, developing the vaccines or any of the drugs potentially used to treat the indications listed above is a substantial undertaking. To comprehend clearly the magnitude of the drug-development process, it is useful to consider the many different areas involved. Figure 1 depicts some of the key disciplines contributing to the process. Information from each of these areas feeds into a common funnel with a filter, where multiple decisions must be made progressively regarding the compound's survival, or lack thereof.

Figures 2 and 3 illustrate the process broken down into preclinical and clinical segments. Keep in mind, however, that the process is a dynamic one. The various disciplines listed are constantly interacting, and the entire flow of data requires constant feedback and fine tuning. For example, a compound's toxicity, however slight, may be considered to outweigh its pharmacological effect. This information would be given by the toxicologist to the chemist, who would make other compounds with slight modifications, attempting to retain the pharmacological effect while decreasing or eliminating the toxic effect.

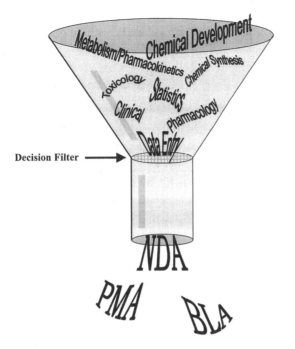

Figure 1 Overall drug development.

Once a compound has been synthesized in the lab and tested in animals, an Investigational New Drug (IND) application is submitted to the U.S. Food and Drug Administration (FDA), requesting permission to initiate clinical studies of the drug in humans. The IND summarizes the preclinical work and includes the first clinical protocol. It is not until the drug has been experimentally tested in humans under controlled conditions (after Phase III) that the company may file an application to market the drug (a New Drug Application [NDA] if filed with the FDA, or a Marketing Authorization Application [MAA] if filed in Europe). The application summarizes all preclinical (safety and efficacy in animals), clinical (safety and efficacy in humans), and manufacturing data known about the drug, and requests permission to market this new drug.

Figure 4 illustrates the attrition ratio of a new chemical entity as it works its way from synthesis through preclinical development to IND, and subsequently through clinical development to NDA. An attrition ratio of 10,000:1 (not considered good betting odds by most people) is the bad news. The good news is that 95% of all drugs for which an NDA is submitted are ultimately approved for marketing.

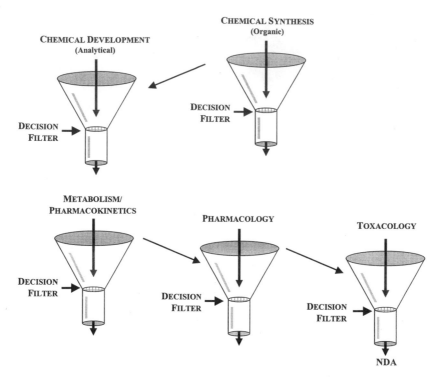

Figure 2 Preclinical drug development.

The tribulations involved in getting a compound through all the decision funnels is a costly process, as seen in Fig. 5. The cost per new drug approved is growing steadily every year. On average, the cost in 1987 was $231 million per approved drug, but by 1998 that figure had increased to $500 to $600 million or more (3). As figures demonstrate, the costs are approximately split between preclinical and clinical development. This average cost represents the expenses in maintaining a full preclinical and clinical research unit for each new drug approved. It perhaps makes it easier to understand why large pharmaceutical companies are sometimes reluctant to pursue development of new drugs likely to have a sales potential of less than several hundred million dollars per year (see Chapter 13 on orphan drugs for a more thorough discussion). This reluctance on the part of large companies leaves opportunities for smaller companies to develop new drugs with smaller potential earnings. If successful, these smaller companies may then grow into large pharmaceutical companies and provide additional treatments that otherwise might have never been made available to patients in need.

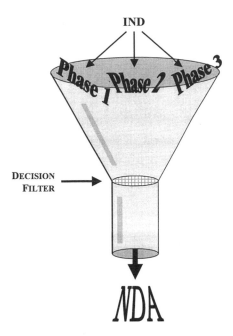

Figure 3 Clinical drug development.

Drug development is not only a costly process, it is time-consuming as well (Fig. 6). Although all pharmaceutical companies and many doctors and patients would like to see the FDA approval times reduced, it is obvious that if approval times were substantially reduced, it would still require many years for the development of a new chemical entity. In fact, the average time of review by the FDA has decreased over the past few years, but the actual time to market has remained about the same because the clinical development time has increased (3,4).

The lengthy time required for drug development markedly reduces the patent life remaining after drug approval for marketing (Table 1). The shrinking patent protection afforded newly marketed drugs is one reason patent applications are usually not filed with the first synthesis of a new compound. Pharmacological and toxicological testing is usually performed before a patent is filed; it usually takes a year or two before the patent is accepted and officially issued. Therefore, the remaining patent life is still slightly greater than the original patent life minus the total developmental time (Fig. 6). The delay in patent filing helps explain why pharmaceutical companies are somewhat secretive about their preclinical research process. The danger in delaying filing for a patent is the risk that another

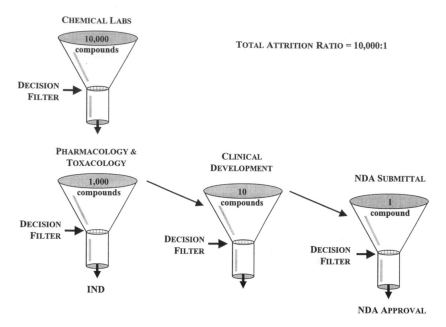

Figure 4 Attrition rate for overall drug development (average).

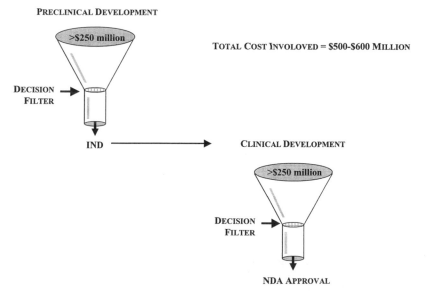

Figure 5 Average cost of overall drug development.

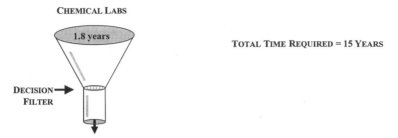

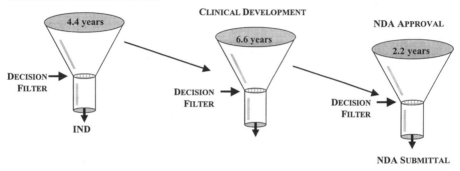

Figure 6 Average time required for overall drug development.

Table 1 Average Effective Patent Life (from NDA approval date)

Year	Patent life without extension	Patent life with Waxman-Hatch extension
1966	13.6 years	NA
1979	9.5 years	NA
1984	9.2 years	11.1 years
1987	10.4 years	12.2 years
1995	7.8 years	11.1 years

NA = not applicable—before Waxman-Hatch enacted.

Total patent life (from patent approval date)	20 years
Before June 8, 1995	17 years
After June 8, 1995	20 years

company or individual may discover the same treatment modality and be the first to file the patent.

Having looked at an overview of the drug development process, it is appropriate to explain how the decision filter works. In preclinical testing of a drug, a toxicological screen is performed with the intent of demonstrating not only a safe dose, but also the toxic effects. In general, doses of drug that will induce significant toxicity are administered to animals. Some types of toxicity are more acceptable than others; for example, if animals were to die unexpectedly and sporadically throughout several dose ranges without less severe, prodromal preceding toxicities, administration to humans would be prohibitive. There would be no way to assure that the same phenomenon (e.g., unexpected death) would not occur in humans.

How, then, are such judgments made regarding "acceptable" potential toxicities? As an example, a great need exists for new antipsychotic compounds. One such compound was shown to induce lipidosis in the rat after 3 months' exposure, though no such effects were seen in the dog (Table 2). Lipidosis is the deposition of fat in cells, and if carried to an extreme, can kill the cell. In particular, lipidosis-induced vacuoles in the rat were noted in the spleen, liver, and lymphocytes. Because the anticipated dose in humans was 5–10 mg/kg per day, this finding in rats at 12–100 mg/kg per day was a cause of concern. The compound looked promising if the lipidosis problem could be solved. To help with the decision, a review of the literature was performed. As shown in Table 3, only one marketed compound known to have caused lipidosis in rats also had a similar effect in humans. Thioridazine (Mellaril), a widely used compound in humans, was used as a positive control (Table 2). In addition, many other compounds have been shown to induce lipidosis in rats but not in humans (5). These agents, like our compound, are mostly for central nervous system diseases. A decision had to be made to proceed to humans or to stop developing the compound. What would you do?

The actual decision made in this case was to proceed to clinical trials. The reasoning was as follows:

Table 2 Preclinical Toxicology (Anticipated dose in humans: 5–10 mg/kg/day)

Species	Drug	Dose (mg/kg/day)	Time (months)	Effect
Rat	Inv. drug	12–100	3	Lipidosis
Rat	Mellaril	24	3	Lipidosis
Dog	Inv. drug	20	3	No effect
Dog	Inv. drug	40	3	Increased liver weight

Table 3 Drugs Known to Induce Lipidosis

Drug	Therapeutic action
In animals	
Imipramine (Troframil)	Antidepressant
Fenfluramine (Pondimin)	Anorectic
Thioridazine (Mellaril)	Antipsychotic
Chlorcyclizine (Fedrazil)	Antihistamine
Zimelidine	Antidepressant
In humans and animals	
Chloroquine (Plaquenil)	Antimalarial

1. Other marketed compounds are known to induce lipidosis and lymphocyte vacuolization in laboratory animals, but not in humans.
2. A peripheral marker is available. Although the drug may induce fatty vacuolization in the liver, a liver biopsy is not needed to detect it because the process, should it occur, would likely be detected in the lymphocytes.
3. The cytoplasmic vacuolization observed in animals was found to be reversible when the drug was discontinued. Should lipidosis occur during clinical trials, subjects or patients should undergo a full recovery when the drug is discontinued.

The drug was subsequently tested in humans at dosages as high as 500 mg/day for up to 6 weeks. Blood was routinely drawn for careful examination of the lymphocytes and liver chemistries; no toxic effects were discerned. The compound ultimately failed the decision filter, however, because of its lack of efficacy.

I. PHASES OF CLINICAL DRUG DEVELOPMENT

The case described represents just one of many decisions that must be made before beginning clinical trials. Clinical drug trials are described as Phases I–V. The first trials in humans that test the drug for safety are considered Phase I. These studies usually employ normal volunteers, and may expose about 50 individuals to the drug. For known toxic compounds such as anticancer agents, only patients with the targeted illness would be used.

The first studies to define efficacy are considered Phase II. These studies are typically conducted to determine the best dosage regimen for the Phase III efficacy studies. In general, 100–300 patients would be entered into various controlled clinical trials during this phase. Phase III, considered an extension of Phases I and II, exposes a larger number of patients (e.g., 1000–3000) to the test drug under controlled trials to further delineate the safety and efficacy profile of the drug. For example, special studies in the pediatric or elderly population may be performed during Phase III (although the studies themselves may be Phase I-type studies). After a successful Phase III program, an NDA may be filed with the appropriate regulatory agency.

Phase IV studies may be done for two different reasons. Marketing-oriented trials may extend the recommended duration of treatment, or they may be primarily instructive in nature to help familiarize more practitioners with the drug's efficacy and side effects. Phase IV trials may be required by the FDA as a condition of approval to extend the knowledge of the pharmacological effects of a drug while allowing simultaneous availability to patients. Phase V studies may extend the indications of a drug to an entirely different disease state. For example, propranolol (Inderal) was first marketed for the management of angina pectoris caused by coronary atherosclerosis. Indications were later extended to management of hypertension, reduction of mortality after myocardial infarction, adjunctive therapy for pheochromocytoma, management of hypertrophic subaortic stenosis, and prophylaxis of migraine headaches.

II. COMPONENTS OF THE CLINICAL TRIAL

Before discussing some of the problems that can arise during clinical trials, a brief review of some of the basic components constituting a clinical trial is in order. Figure 7 illustrates the study periods providing the framework for any clinical trial.

Prestudy activities include design and setup of the study, and poststudy activities include data entry, analysis, and report generation. Inclusion and exclusion criteria are determined early in the clinical development process, during the screening period. Before entry into the study, baseline determinations are made to which all subsequent changes will be compared. The heart of a trial is the treatment phase, which consists of drug safety modules and auxiliary modules (Fig. 8), many of which will repeat measurements made at the time of the initial screening or baseline. For Phase II and Phase III trials, specific parameters of efficacy will be assessed. The posttreatment period is the stage at which final measurements are made for safety; it is also the time to assess the effect of withdrawal of drug relative to elimination of the disease state or a return toward the baseline state.

Complex problems reach the decision filter at every stage of drug development, even in the early clinical pharmacology phase (Fig. 9). To delineate the pharmacokinetics of the compound in humans, it is common during Phase I to

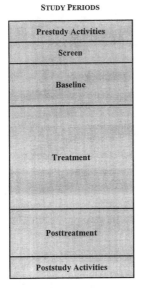

Figure 7 Primary clinical data modules in clinical trials.

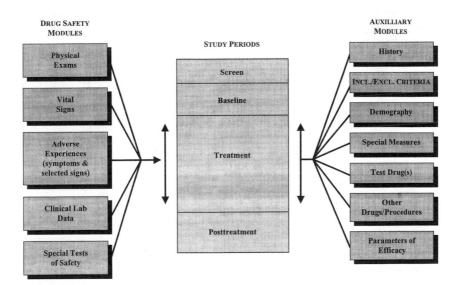

Figure 8 Primary clinical data modules in clinical trials.

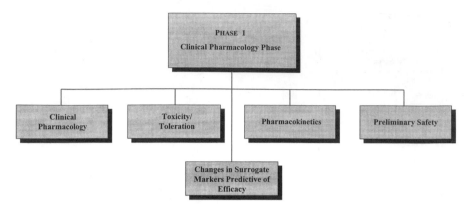

Figure 9 Investigational drug development.

measure blood concentrations of the test drug as dosage is increased. Sometimes the pharmacokinetic data of a study can illuminate problems inherent within the study. A case in point is the development of a drug in which three similar Phase III studies were conducted. In one of the studies, no patients in the active group had measurable concentrations. The placebo group's samples were then analyzed and it was discovered that the randomization scheme was reversed for this study. A second case in point is a Phase I bioequivalence study in which two patients with similar initials each had a single sample that drastically deviated from their expected profile. When the concentrations were transposed to each other's profile, they seemed to make sense, pharmacokinetically. Reanalysis confirmed the concentrations. The Phase I unit, which used bar-coded wristbands, emphatically denied that there could have been a mixup. A battery of tests was conducted on the remaining samples and proved that the samples had been switched. Several pages of the pharmacokinetic report discussed this issue, and, convincingly, the bioequivalence analysis was then conducted on the samples belonging to the appropriate subjects. The products were bioequivalent. Without moving the data to their appropriate places, the products were not bioequivalent.

A final case in point relates a problem that occurred during Phase I testing of an antidepressant compound. It illustrates that no matter how prepared you think you are, the unexpected or unanticipated can happen. The incident took place during a double-blind, placebo-controlled, dosage-titration trial in normal volunteers. Both plasma and urine samples were being collected for quantitative analysis of drug levels. Results demonstrated detectable levels of drug in all of the volunteers at the lowest dosage given. However, at the highest dosage administered, much to everyone's surprise, drug was not detected in some of the volunteers. Many possible explanations exist, including the following:

1. *The drug is inhibiting its own absorption at higher dosages.* Even if this phenomenon were true, detectable levels should exist in all volunteers.
2. *The assay was not working properly.* The appropriate amount of drug was recorded from spiked samples randomly distributed throughout the test samples; this procedure made assay problems less likely.
3. *The drug is inducing its own metabolism.* Even so, although levels of drug at higher dosages might be lower, they should not be undetectable.
4. *Some volunteers failed to ingest drug.* The test site used elaborate procedures to ensure that volunteers ingested the test drug. This type of problem was endemic when prisoners were commonly used as volunteers. They would swallow the drug, then go to the bathroom and induce vomiting.
5. *Placebo and active drug are mixed.* Such a situation could arise either before dosing (packaging error), or after dosing (sampling or labeling error after blood and urine are collected). If blood and urine specimens were mislabeled, some instances might occur in which detectable drug existed in blood but not in urine, or vice versa. In no instance, however, did this situation occur. Because blood and urine samples were collected from the placebo volunteers to keep the study double-blind, those specimens were analyzed. In some cases, drug was detected, with both urine and blood samples correlating positively or negatively. Finally, drug was analyzed that had been packaged for backup volunteers in case of dropouts. An absence of drug was demonstrated in some of the ''active'' volunteers, and drug was detected in some of the ''placebo'' volunteers.

Because an elaborate system of checks and crosschecks was in place to guard against the possibility of drug mispackaging, it was impossible to think about such a wholesale mixup. After considerable inquiry, an almost impossible reason surfaced. A disgruntled employee had deliberately sabotaged the packaging by intentionally mixing drug and placebo.

A packaging error such as the one described is extremely costly. In this case, the study had to be repeated, with the following consequences:

1. Volunteers had to be reexposed to the test drug and associated procedures.
2. The cost of doing the Phase I trial doubled.
3. The development of the drug was delayed for 3 months.

A new drug can potentially reach sales of hundreds of millions of dollars in its first year. The ultimate dollar cost of a 3-months' delay is obvious, in addition to the fact that patients are denied the use of the drug for 3 months. The

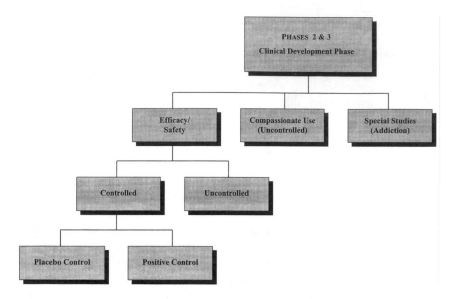

Figure 10 Investigational drug development.

situation above in the Phase I trial describes a tribulation that can occur at any point in clinical drug development. However, many issues specific to Phases II and III also must be anticipated. As seen in Fig. 10, different types of efficacy studies may be undertaken (see Chapter 6). Special studies, such as tests for addictive potential or studies allowing compassionate use of the drug (see Chapter 9), occur during these phases.

As already shown in Fig. 8, information regarding safety is collected in every study. An attempt is always made to determine any adverse events that may be caused by the drug. The process is especially difficult in patients, because illness itself is defined by a grouping of adverse events. The critical question when any adverse event occurs during a clinical trial is, ''Why did it occur?'' Did the event occur spontaneously, or as a result of an underlying disease, or as a result of a procedure conducted? Or was it caused by the drug?

What data are needed to answer those questions? Figure 11 depicts points along the course of a clinical trial at which data must be gathered to make an assessment. Figure 12 lists some of the numerous information points required before an accurate judgment can be made.

If Figures 11 and 12 seem unnecessarily complex and unduly detailed relative to the assessment of causality for an adverse event, consider the study of an antidepressant. A probe was made at baseline just before initiation of treatment

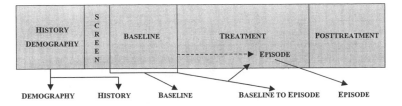

Figure 11   Information required for reporting adverse experiences.

(see Fig. 11) to determine the clinical status of the depressed individuals who were about to enter into the study. As seen in Table 4, an impressive background of complaints existed before any drug medication. In a 6-week study, multiple probes will be performed to detect adverse events. Consider, then, if headache is reported as an episode during treatment (Fig. 11), it will be extremely difficult to assign causality relative to baseline when more than half the patients reported headache at baseline.

The symptoms listed in Table 4 afflict all of us from time to time, but assessments of causality for more serious events should not require the detailed data reporting depicted in Fig. 12, right? Wrong! Table 5 lists serious adverse events not present at baseline but occurring during placebo treatment. If these events had taken place during active therapy, it would have been very difficult to avoid assigning causality to the drug (see Chapter 14).

Any type of adverse event must then flow through the decision filter. The tribulations associated with assessing causality can be multiplied if case report forms (CRFs) are improperly designed. Poorly designed CRFs during Phase II will compound and multiply the problems encountered in Phase III. Proper design of CRFs at the start of clinical trials will create a firm foundation for passing through the multiple decision filters on the way to new drug approval.

A type of tribulation that occurs more in Phase II, and particularly in Phase III trials, involves adherence to the drug regimen. Drug adherence is loosely described as the number of dosages actually taken by a patient compared with the number prescribed. Alas, as with most things in life, further reflection reveals a far more complex subject. Were dosage administrations properly spaced, were they taken with meals (if required) or without food (if required), were they taken with forbidden concomitant medications? With larger Phase III outpatient studies, the variability of adherence is exaggerated. Adherence is further hindered by prolonged or complex prescriptions. It can destroy the statistical validity of an otherwise carefully controlled trial.

Consider the extreme example of a 71-year-old patient who was admitted to the intensive care unit after being found unconscious at home. Because of his

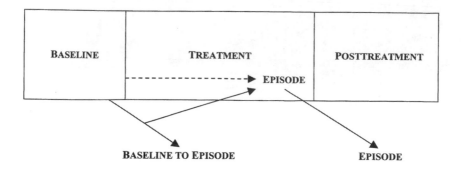

BASELINE   **TREATMENT**   **POSTTREATMENT**

EPISODE

BASELINE TO EPISODE   **EPISODE**

Serious adverse events (SAEs)
    Intensity
    Status at start of episode
    Causal relationship

Test agent administration
    Dose start or number of days taken
    Route of administration
    Dosage
    Min
    Max
    At onset
    Stopped temporarily?
    Permanently discontinued?
    Date

Concomitant medications
    Max dosage
    Dosage—start of episode

Nondrug therapy

Intercurrent illness/complication(s)

(Detailed sequence of events)
    Time or time range from start of test agent
    (including hours/minutes, if required)

Test agent dosage and dosage changes
    SAEs
    Name
    Countermeasures
    Outcome
    Other medications
    Test procedures/results
    Comments
    Death—autopsy/biopsy, etc.

SAEs summary
    SAE name(s)
    Date of onset
    Max intensity
    Seriousness
    Test agent dosage
    Countermeasures
    Dechallenge
    Rechallenge
    Outcome
    Causal relationship

Narrative summary-investigation

Sponsor's evaluation

Figure 12   Information required for assessing adverse experiences.

Table 4 Observed Adverse Events at Baseline

Event	Percent of patients
Insomnia	92
Tiredness/fatigue	74
Anorexia	59
Headache	54

deteriorating condition, he had been prescribed 13 different medications at one time or another, but no one had ascertained whether he had adhered to his dosage regimen. The ambulance staff found 46 bottles containing 10,685 tablets for 13 different medications in his room (6)!

III. THE FUTURE

Although the search for new chemical entities or natural product extracts to treat diseases is likely to continue for years to come, changes are underway that will have a profound impact on how we diagnose and treat disease. The identification of various active entities such as cytokines and delineation of their functions has already led to a new class of molecular therapies. This process is going to take a quantum leap forward now that the entire genetic code of a human being is accessible on the Internet.

One new area generating interest and huge investment is called pharmaco-genomics—an attempt to identify therapy targeted to an individual's specific genetic composition. The desired result would enhance efficacy, or minimize toxicity, or both. A consequence of deciphering the human genetic code is the increasing number of blood tests that can reveal disease-gene mutations and pre-

Table 5 Serious Adverse Events
Not Present at Baseline and Occurring
During Therapy with Placebo

Marked EKG changes
Grossly abnormal EEG
Acute renal failure
Seizures
Sudden death

dict with varying degrees of certainty the chances of progressing to a disease state. However, with this new technology, new tribulations immediately appear: Do you want to know that when you are 40 or 50 years of age you may be diagnosed with Huntington's disease, a degenerative brain disorder for which no treatment currently exists?

A huge knowledge gap exists between knowing a gene's structure and understanding its function. Some functions are currently known, however, and some of these genes are the reason for the enthusiasm many hold for gene transfer, creating a permanent or semipermanent change in the human body. Many tribulations face gene transfer such as getting the gene into a cellular nucleus, having it express the necessary protein, and having the DNA remain long enough for it to do its job. Probably the first successes will be with genes that are needed only for a short time, such as those expressing for angiogenesis. Likely within a few years (not decades), advanced coronary arterial disease will be treated with gene coding. Rather than, or perhaps in concert with, coronary arterial bypass grafting, there will be an ability to grow new vessels to supply oxygen to arterial tissue that continues to be viable.

Although gene transfer may be the wave of the future, its safety and efficacy must still be satisfied through the drug development process. Regulatory scrutiny has already exceeded its previous bounds, but there continue to be areas that can reduce the time and cost of drug development. Technologically trailing only slightly behind gene transfer is electronic data capture and real-time data analysis. Once this technology is implemented, data capture and analysis times for all studies can be greatly reduced, creating substantial cost savings. The sheer tonnage of data required to pass just the clinical decision filter (Fig. 13) is enormous. If each case report form has an average of 200 data characters, with 25 pages of CRFs per patient, the total data bits required for a conservatively sized NDA of 2000 patients or volunteers would be 10 million. Information technology will help manage these data in efficient and less expensive ways.

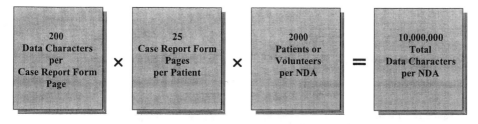

Figure 13 Quantity of clinical data characters required for an NDA.

IV. CONCLUSION

Guiding a new chemical entity through the tribulations involved in the drug testing and approval process is a task that is exciting and rewarding as well as long
and complex. Advances in gene transfer, electronic data capture, and real-time
data analysis all promise to increase our chances of success. Ultimately, however,
it is through dedication, skill, and lots of luck that the drug development process
is successful and we can provide a new medication to the people who need it to
fight the pain and suffering of illness. At those times, the camel truly has made
its way home through the eye of a needle.

REFERENCES

1. Impact of vaccines universally recommended for children—United States, 1900–
    1999. MMWR Morb Mortal Wkly Rep 1999 Apr 2; 48(12):243–248.
2. The Pharmaceutical Research and Manufacturers of America. Pharmaceutical Indus-
    try Profile 2000. Washington DC, 2000.
3. Tufts Center for the Study of Drug Development. Outlook 2000. Boston, 2000.
4. Spilker BA. The drug development and approval process. In: New Medicines in
    Development [PhRMA Web site], September 18, 2000. Available at: http://
    www.phrma.org/searchcures/newmeds/devapprovprocess.phtml. Accessed October
    1, 2000.
5. Lullmann H, Lullmann-Rauch R, Wasserman O. Lipidosis induced by amphiphilic
    cationic drugs. Biochem Pharmacol 1978; 27:1103–1108.
6. Smith SE, Stead KC. Non-compliance or misprescribing? Lancet 1974; 1:937.

2
Preclinical Drug Discovery and Development

David S. Duch
Cato Research Ltd., Durham, North Carolina

Robert M. Ferris
Retired, Charlotte, North Carolina

I. INTRODUCTION

The major change that has occurred in the drug development process over the last 15–20 years has been the introduction of significant advances in new technologies that expedite the design, screening, and identification of new chemical entities. A brief review of these technologies, together with a review of the various approaches used in the discovery of new chemical entities, is presented to update the readers and encourage their deeper involvement in areas pertinent to their interests. The use of these technologies has forced the drug discovery process to evolve into a rapid, integrated, and usually very targeted process. In addition, changes in regulatory requirements, as well as the introduction of International Conference on Harmonization (ICH) Guidelines, have led to new concepts for the timely and cost-efficient development of drugs for registration in world markets. The authors' experiences in interpreting these guidelines and applying them to the drug development process are presented for the readers' consideration.

II. DRUG DISCOVERY

A. Source of Molecules Used in Drug Discovery Process

Anyone interested in drug discovery must first address the issue of the source of molecules that will ultimately provide the new drugs. Some of the oldest sources

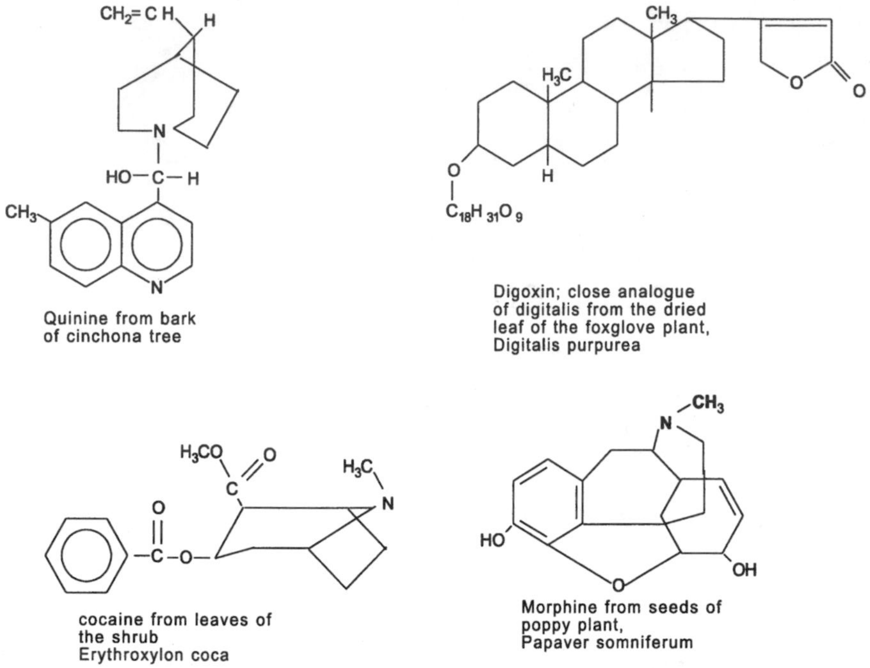

CH₂=CH, H

HO—C—H

CH₃

N

Quinine from bark
of cinchona tree

CH₃

H₃C

O

$C_{18}H_{31}O_9$

H

Digoxin; close analogue
of digitalis from the dried
leaf of the foxglove plant,
Digitalis purpurea

H₃CO

O

C

O

C—O—

H₃C

N

cocaine from leaves of
the shrub
Erythroxylon coca

CH₃

N

HO

OH

O

Morphine from seeds of
poppy plant,
Papaver somniferum

Figure 1   Structures of natural products.

of drugs have come from plants and their analogs, microbial broths containing various metabolites of microorganisms, animal cells and their extracts, animal and marine toxins, and, more recently, genetic engineering (Fig. 1).

Recent advances in technologies such as combinatorial chemistry and computer-assisted design have markedly increased the ability of the chemist to supply new chemical entities for study. However, diversity of molecules is not easily obtainable, even with the advent of these new advances in technology. In fact, high-throughput screening techniques have made the process of screening molecules so rapid that the diversity of structures available for screening has dwindled to the point that the search for natural products with their inherent diversity is now taking on additional importance.

B.   Methods Used in the Drug Discovery Process

1.   General Screening

Many previous drug discovery programs were based on the random screening of large numbers of chemically diverse compounds through one or more biological assays in hopes of finding a therapeutically useful property. These biological assays consisted of in vitro assays (e.g., enzymes or binding assays), assays in isolated tissues, and in vivo animal models. However, it is probably fair to say that few pharmaceutical companies are presently synthesizing compounds with the intent of putting them through a general screening program. Most compounds are now made with a specific therapeutic target in mind. It should be recognized that many innovative leads for new drug development have come from the general screening process. It is expected that, as the quest for diversity in new molecules intensifies, the demand for general screening will increase in order to identify the novel pharmacological properties of these agents.

2. Targeted Screening

Many pharmaceutical companies test compounds in assays specifically selected to reveal the therapeutic activity of interest. Such a process is usually referred to as *targeted screening*. For example, large-scale, cell-based assays have been developed to screen for potential antitumor agents (1). As an outgrowth of earlier antitumor screening methods, the National Cancer Institute has developed a disease-oriented approach to drug discovery that uses a total of 60 human tumor cell lines derived from eight cancer types (lung, colon, breast, melanoma, kidney, ovary, brain, and leukemia). The initial design proposed that leads demonstrating disease specificity would be selected for further testing based on disease type specificity in the assay, unique structure, potency, and demonstration of a unique pattern of cellular cytotoxicity or cytostasis, since this pattern could indicate a unique mechanism of action or intracellular target. Computerized programs have been developed to prioritize and enhance the diversity of compounds entered into the screen as well as to analyze the data obtained in relation to the other compounds in the database. Results obtained using this cell-based assay have recently been reviewed (2).

An alternative approach to the evaluation and selection of antitumor agents based on targeted screening has been developed by Von Hoff (3). This assay determines the response of the individual patient's tumor to specific antitumor agents and has been used both to screen for new agents, as well as to determine tumor types against which an agent will be active.

Evaluation of the activity of different molecules on a specific enzyme or receptor, for example, on dopaminergic D2 receptors, in search of a novel antipsychotic agent is an additional example of targeted screening. This approach is generally more cost-effective and more rapid than a general screening program (4). Targeted screening can improve specificity, efficacy, and duration of action, while minimizing side effects. However, compounds having activity against other targets would not be selected using this limited approach. Since compounds made for one purpose frequently demonstrate pharmacological properties in other areas

(5), it can be argued that it is probably prudent to subject a compound library periodically to some form of general screening.

3. Molecular Modification

Identification of a lead structure rarely yields a compound that possesses all the properties needed for full clinical development. Most of the time, the compound has to be modified to improve potency, reduce side effects, increase bioavailablilty, decrease metabolism, decrease toxicity, or alter its properties in some other favorable way to make the compound a viable therapeutic agent. This process is called *lead structure optimization.* Maxwell has divided this process into two classes, enlightened or unenlightened opportunism (5). An example of enlightened opportunism is that of discovering new pharmacological properties at an early stage and developing better agents than the original with this activity (Fig. 2).

For example, cisplatin, an important chemotherapeutic agent, has doselimiting nephrotoxicity and neurotoxicity. Additional studies yielded an analog, carboplatin, that had mylosuppression as the limiting toxicity. Further synthesis yielded oxaliplatin and later DWA 2114R, which have sensory neuropathy and neutropenia, respectively, as the limiting toxicities. Additional examples of enlightened opportunism can be found in a review article by Maxwell (5).

Enlightened opportunism is in contrast to unenlightened opportunism, where, at a late stage in the development of a compound, one attempts to make

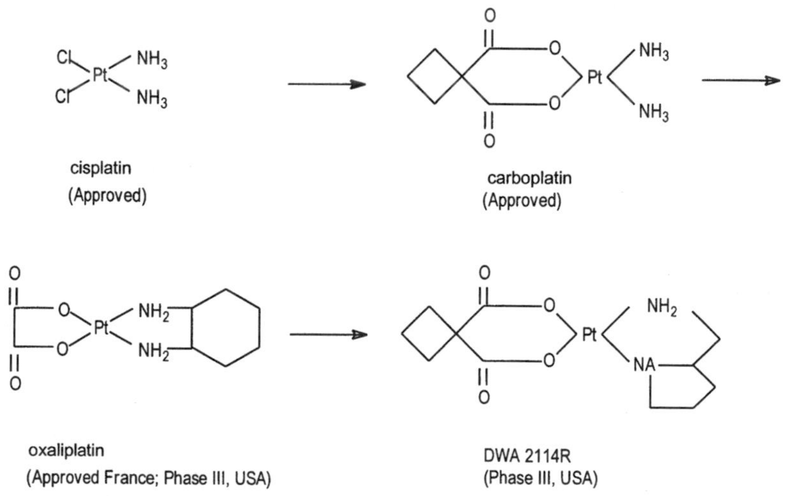

Figure 2 Examples of enlightened opportunism.

yet another close chemical variation in a therapeutic area where multiple agents already exist. Unenlightened opportunism is often referred to as the me-too approach. An example of this approach can be seen in the development of the tricyclic antidepressants, illustrated in Fig. 3.

In addition to the example given above, enlightened opportunism may also take the form of combining the important structural features of two or more classes of compounds into one molecule in an attempt to achieve a superior therapeutic agent (5).

A third type of enlightened opportunism can come from the early utilization of new knowledge developed in biochemistry, physiology, and other biological sciences (5). An example would be the recent impetus give to drug discovery by initiation of the genome project.

4. Rational Drug Design

Rational drug design, the basic research approach to drug discovery, is based on the premise that a thorough knowledge of the biochemical and physiological mechanisms that are responsible for the normal functioning of a particular organ system will allow an understanding of any pathophysiology of the same system. This understanding will in turn permit drugs to be designed that will affect the

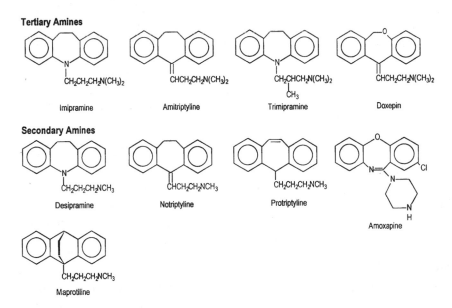

Figure 3 Tricyclic antidepressants.

altered target (e.g., enzyme, receptor, or cell) and correct the deficiency. Such a rationale has led to very targeted screening approaches such as receptor-oriented drug research, reversible and irreversible enzyme inhibitors, inhibitors of voltage- and receptor-operated ion channels, and inhibitors of transporter systems (6). For example, the synthesis of nucleoside analogs as chemotherapeutic agents has been based on the concept that these analogs will inhibit nucleic acid synthesis, which will in turn result in disruption of cell replication, and ultimately, cell death (7). Fluorouracil, cytosine arabinoside, and 6-mercaptopurine are examples of drugs rationally designed for cancer chemotherapy. Some early inhibitors of mono- amine oxidase, dihydrofolate reductase, and angiotensin converting enzyme were derived from rational concepts (6). For interesting reviews of this subject, see Maxwell (5) and Kubinyi (6).

5.   Clinical Observations

Many innovative drugs have originated from the astute observations of physicians who recognized that what appeared to be apparent side effects of drugs were actually novel therapeutic properties. The discovery of the diuretic and glucose- lowering activities of the antibacterial sulfonilamides, which were developed into three distinct classes of sulfonamide drugs (i.e., antibacterials, diuretics, and hy- poglycemics), is often cited as an example (6). Consider as well, the antidepres- sant effects of the tuberculostat, iproniazid; the anxiolytic properties of the neuro- leptic, buspiron; and the antirheumatic effects of the antibacterial, penicillamine (5,6). This source of drug discovery has slowed markedly in recent years, possibly because of the imposition of regulatory guidelines needed to ensure the safety of drug development (5).

An interesting case description and analysis of research that led to innova- tive therapeutic agents since World War II can be found in the book, *Drug Dis- covery, A Casebook and Analysis,* by Maxwell and Eckhardt (8).

C.   Influence of Recent Developments in Technology on Present and Future Discovery Processes

The above approaches to drug discovery always have and will continue to be the basic guidelines by which new drugs are discovered. However, during the last decade, major changes have occurred in the development of new technologies that have in turn revolutionized our approach to drug design and discovery. These new technologies have had enormous impact on the strategies and costs of drug development today, and they will continue to play an increasingly dominant role in drug development processes in the future. In the section that follows, several of these new technologies will be discussed with the intent of introducing the readers to the basic concepts involved in each area and then, hopefully, serving as an impetus to encourage them to delve further into those areas of particular interest.

1. Compound Libraries and Combinatorial Chemistry

As mentioned earlier in this chapter, the major pharmaceutical companies are interested in accumulating large numbers of compounds with a great diversification of chemical structures for use in establishing new leads for drug development. These chemical libraries can be prepared synthetically or biosynthetically and screened for pharmacological activity in a variety of different formats (e.g., libraries of soluble molecules; libraries of molecules tethered to resin beads, silica chips, or other solid supports; or recombinant peptide libraries on bacteriophage and other biological display vectors) (9). Some companies exchange small collections of compounds to increase the different classes of agents available for screening, and collections of compounds or plant extracts are available from independent brokers (10).

These libraries are valuable resources, because they may contain the new protypes for new therapeutic classes of drugs (11). Each year, new biological targets are discovered; therefore, these libraries are constantly being rescreened year after year in novel assays. The systematic and repetitive, covalent connection of a set of different building blocks of varying structures to each other in order to yield a large array of diverse molecular entities is referred to as *combinatorial chemistry* (9). The primary strategies of combinatorial chemistry are to make a large number of chemical variants all at one time, to test them for biological activity, and to isolate and identify the most promising compounds for further development (12). These chemical libraries contain so many compounds that special methods of cataloging, storage, and retrieval are required to use the library effectively. Two general methods of synthesis are used to create combinatorial libraries. The first is split synthesis, in which compounds are assembled on surfaces of beads or particles (12). In a split-and-combine technique, either specific mixtures or individual compounds are synthesized on single beads. In a series of steps, the beads are divided into several groups, and a new building block is added. The different groups of beads are then recombined and separated again into new groups. The next building block is added, and the process continues until the desired combinatorial library has been assembled. Each bead in the library holds multiple copies of a single library member (12). Split synthesis is generally used to produce small quantities of a relatively large number of compounds, requires a solid support, and permits assays to be performed on pools of compounds.

The second method for creating combinatorial libraries is parallel synthesis. In this process, which is usually automated, compounds are synthesized in separate vessels (most recently microtiter plates, but solid support can be used) without remixing. Parallel synthesis yields larger quantities of a relatively small number of compounds, and can be done on either solid or liquid support. Assays can be done on individual compounds (12). Excellent reviews of this subject have been published (13–16).

2.   Combinatorial Chemistry and High-Throughput Screening

The number of potential drug targets that could emerge from molecular biology research such as the Human Genome Project, as well as the demands for improved or novel therapies for cancer, cardiovascular, and neurological diseases have created the need for the synthesis and rapid testing of large numbers of compounds. These demands are being filled through the development of combinatorial chemistry combined with high-throughput screening. These techniques have been and continue to be developed and used throughout the pharmaceutical industry. Although these techniques have not yet yielded drugs that have been approved for marketing, several candidates have been discovered using these techniques and are currently being tested in clinical trials. The status of combinatorial chemistry within the pharmaceutical industry has recently been reviewed (17).

It has been proposed that combinatorial chemistry will allow access to the constantly increasing number of new targets, will speed up the drug discovery process, will markedly increase success rates from the classic 1 in 10,000, and will enable rapid, continuous analoging and optimization of active compounds to drug candidates. The development of combinatorial chemistry has led to the need for assay systems capable of determining the activity of large numbers of compounds. Numerous high-throughput assay systems have been developed, although a large number of these screens remain proprietary and are not generally accessible. The development of high-throughput screening has been aided by the significant advances in automation and robotics. These systems allow the continuous analysis of combinatorial libraries with a wide variety of targets. Combinatorial chemistry has evolved rapidly from its early focus on the generation of large numbers of molecules to a powerful combinatorial design technology for the generation and optimization of pharmaceutical leads to produce drug candidates (18). Among the techniques that have been used in high-throughput screens are mass ligand binding, yeast cell-based assays using reporter genes, and scintillation proximity assays (13–16). In addition, techniques that incorporate both compound creation and screening of large libraries in one process have also been described (19,20).

3.   Bioinformatics

The immense growth in biotechnology, together with the marked expansion of information technology, has lead to the formation of a new concept called *bioinformatics* (21). The impetus for this birth probably came from the development of rapid DNA sequencing methods that emerged in the mid-1970s (22). One of the most significant advances in data acquisition has come from the proliferation of Internet resources devoted to the life sciences. The Internet can serve as a starting point for a data search (21,22). The data are comprehensive, up to date, validated, and rapidly accessible (21). The Internet provides integrated information retrieval, homology searching, exon identification, and mapping data (22). Bioinformatics is playing an important role in the drug development process and is vital for integration of the much less collated and systematized data that exist for drug absorption, toxicity, excretion, metabolism, and distribution. Computer resources now play an integral part in high-throughput screening techniques, lead optimization and lead discovery, the use of robotics in synthesis and screening, the design of ligands, and in molecular modeling. Bioinformatics will revolutionize the process of drug discovery and development in the near future.

4. Chirality

Today, preclinical development of new chemical entities must take into account, at very early stages, the issue of whether the molecule possesses any chiral centers. If so, the enantiomers should be resolved, and their efficacy, toxicity, and safety should be assessed. The results of these studies will help determine whether to develop an individual enantiomer or the racemate. The decision to develop a racemate or an enantiomer should be made only after a thorough understanding of the pharmacological, toxicological, and pharmacokinetic properties of the substance. Although not all-inclusive, the following examples illustrate typical situations in which a racemate might be developed (23):

The enantiomers have been shown to have pharmacological and toxicological profiles similar to the racemate.

The enantiomers are rapidly interconverted in vitro and/or in vivo so that administration of a single enantiomer offers no advantage.

One enantiomer of the racemate is shown to be pharmacologically inactive, and the racemate is demonstrated to be safe and effective.

Synthesis or isolation of the preferred enantiomer is not practical.

Individual enantiomers exhibit different pharmacological profiles, and the racemate produces a superior therapeutic effect relative to either enantiomer alone.

The decision to market one enantiomer or the racemate should be made on a case-by-case basis after considering all available data.

5. X-Ray Crystallography

The goal of rational drug discovery and development is the enhancement of the activity of a ligand to obtain a clinically useful agent. The development of therapeutic entities from lead compounds requires the systematic modification of the chemical structure of the lead compounds to optimize the activity desired. One of the techniques that has been used in this process is x-ray crystallography. A knowledge of the three-dimensional structure of the pharmacologically relevant receptor-ligand complexes at the level of resolution achieved by using x-ray crystallography has the potential to speed the discovery and development of lead compounds into clinically effective drugs. Through these techniques, the specific interactions that are important in the molecular recognition and binding of the ligand to its macromolecular target can be ascertained. In addition, the development of the technology for obtaining large amounts of the target macromolecule, such as recombinant DNA technology and the technology for the analysis of the ligand–macromolecular interactions, has aided the rapid development of new chemical entities for clinical evaluation.

X-ray crystallography has been instrumental in the design of inhibitors active in the renin–angiotensin system (24) and in the design of lipophilic inhibitors of the enzyme thymidylate synthase (25). However, the development of inhibitors of human immunodeficiency virus (HIV) protease can be considered as one of the best examples of the extensive use of x-ray crystallography for the structure-assisted design of inhibitory molecules. The identification of the HIV protease as a member of the aspartate protease family facilitated the design of inhibitors of this enzyme, since earlier studies using x-ray crystallography had been carried out on aspartate proteases such as renin. Detailed reviews on the structure and function of HIV protease and its inhibitors have recently been published (26,27). Since the publication of the first crystallographic structure of an inhibitor complexed to the protease appeared, hundreds of structures of such complexes have been solved in dozens of laboratories. These studies have led to the clinical development and use of several protease inhibitors as therapy for HIV infection.

6. Quantitative Structure–Activity Relationships

Intermolecular forces are important in the interaction of drugs with their targets. Parameters such as lipophilicity, polarizability, and electronic and steric parameters have been used to describe the intermolecular forces of the drug–receptor interaction and the transport and distribution of drugs in a quantitative manner and to correlate them with biological activities. Many types of biological data, such as affinity data, rate constants, inhibition constants, and pharmacokinetic parameters, can be described by quantitative structure–activity relationships (QSAR).

The most widely used QSAR analysis has been the Hansch analysis (28), an extra thermodynamic, linear free energy-related analysis, which describes the affinity of ligands or other biological activities in terms of physicochemical parameters, such as lipophilicity. A second, though less widely used, approach was described by Free and Wilson (29). This is an additivity model, which is based on a strict additivity concept of group contributions to biological activities. Studies stemming from attempts to map a receptor surface from the results of Hansch analyses led to the development of three-dimensional QSAR. An extensive review of the development and advances in QSAR has recently been published (30).

7. Monoclonal Antibodies

The pioneering work of Milstein (31) initiated the development of monoclonal antibodies as a therapeutic entity. Normal immune responses of B lymphocytes are polyclonal in nature and yield a heterogeneous mixture of antibodies. In order to produce monoclonal antibodies, murine antibody-producing cells were immortalized by fusion with plasma cell tumors incapable of producing immunoglobulin but capable of supporting antibody synthesis and secretion. Subsequent cloning of the hybridomas yielded clones that are capable of producing large amounts of homogeneous murine antibody that react with a single epitope.

However, the use of murine antibodies in humans is restricted because of the immunogenic nature of the immunoglobulins. Repeated use of murine antibodies elicits an anti-immunoglobulin response known as the human antimouse antibody (HAMA) response. In addition, other limitations to the use of antibodies have been observed and have been overcome in part through the use of genetic engineering to humanize the murine antibodies (32). The redesign of murine antibodies using these techniques has resulted in the formation of antibodies that elicit a considerably reduced immune response relative to the murine antibody.

Although monoclonal antibodies have been most widely used for the diagnosis and treatment of cancer, they are also being evaluated as therapies in other areas as well. For example, abciximab (c7E3 Fab) is a chimeric human-murine monoclonal antibody Fab fragment that binds to the platelet glycoprotein IIb/IIIa receptor and inhibits platelet aggregation. The addition of abciximab to standard aspirin and heparin therapy reduced the incidence of ischemic complications during the initial postoperative period in high-risk patients who were undergoing percutaneous coronary angioplasty or directional atherectomy. Abciximab also reduced the incidence of clinical restenosis when compared with placebo during a 6-month follow-up of these patients (33).

Monoclonal antibodies have been widely used for the diagnosis, localization, and treatment of cancer (34). Their advantages include a relative selectivity for tumor tissue coupled with a relative lack of toxicity. However, their ability to affect tumors is minimal unless aided by other mechanisms, the amount of antibody delivered to tumors is low, and the diffusion of antibody through tumors is often poor. The development of a HAMA response is also limiting. To aid in the antitumor effectiveness of monoclonal antibodies, antitumor drugs such as doxorubicin, toxins such as the ricin A chain, and radionuclides have been conjugated to the antibodies (34). In addition, unconjugated antibodies can mediate complement-dependent cytotoxicity and antibody-dependent cellular cytotoxicity. For example, the effect of the monoclonal antibody 17–1A, a monoclonal antibody against colorectal cancer, has been evaluated in patients with Dukes' Stage C colorectal cancer who had undergone curative surgery and were free of manifest residual tumor. After a median follow-up of 5 years, antibody treatment reduced the overall death rate by 27%. Effectiveness was most pronounced in patients who had distant metastasis as the first sign of relapse, and toxic effects were infrequent (35).

8.   Gene Therapy

Human gene transfer is a therapeutic approach in which the genome of human somatic cells, but not germline cells, is modified for the purpose of treating disease. It has also been used to generate a population of marked cells for the purpose of tracing the origins of recurrent tumors. A large number of gene therapy protocols have been designed to treat cancer, HIV infection, and diseases caused by a gene defect, such as cystic fibrosis, familial hypercholesterolemia, and severe combined immunodeficiency caused by adenosine deaminase deficiency (36,37).

The transfer of genes to the target cells has been accomplished through the use of viral vectors or nonviral delivery. Nonviral delivery systems include in-vivo delivery using plasmid–liposome complexes, direct injection of naked DNA, and transfection of target cells ex vivo. The viral vectors that have been the most widely studied include retroviruses, adenoviruses and adeno-associated viruses; however, the use of herpes virus for delivery to the central nervous system (CNS) and vaccinia virus vectors have also been investigated (38,39).

Each of these means of transfer has advantages and disadvantages. Gene delivery using either liposomes or naked DNA has no involvement of viruses and thus could not replicate or recombine to form infectious agents, Moreover, use of these methods of delivery would cause fewer inflammatory or immune responses and can be used to transfer genetic material of unlimited size. These advantages are offset by the inefficiency of transfer and the temporary expression of the transferred gene. The viral vectors have a greater efficiency of gene transfer. Retroviral vectors require dividing cells for integration of the genetic material whereas adenoviruses and adeno-associated viruses do not require cellular proliferation. Retroviruses and adeno-associated viruses, but not adenoviruses, result in a stable incorporation of the genetic material into the genome of the target cell. With adenoviruses or liposomes as vectors, the transferred genetic material remains epichromosomal, and consequently, there is only short-term expression of the transferred gene. Therefore, to maintain persistent expression, frequent administration would be required. Since adenovirus is immunogenic, repeated use of this vector could be limited by an immune response. A potential advantage of adeno-associated virus is that it has never been shown to have any pathogenic effect in humans.

As of the end of 1995, more than 40 clinical trials involving the transfer of genes to humans have been reported (36, #13648). The majority of these trials utilized a retroviral vector and involved treatment of neoplastic disease. However, trials for the treatment of cystic fibrosis, familial hypercholesterolemia, and adenosine deaminase deficiency have also been initiated. The results so far indicate that human gene transfer is indeed a viable form of disease therapy.

9. Genomics

One of the goals of the Human Genome Project is to determine the sequences of the 100,000 genes in the human genome. In general, the approach has been to sequence sections of cDNA from libraries created from RNA of various tissues to obtain ''expressed sequence tags.'' Since the source cDNA libraries from various human tissues are normalized to remove housekeeping genes, the frequency that certain cDNAs appear in the various tissue-specific databases will be a reflection of their expression levels. Using the present techniques, the sequencing rate is relatively slow. However, new sequencing techniques are being developed that will be more rapid, efficient, accurate, and cost-effective (40).

High-throughput methods using DNA arrays for the monitoring of gene expression patterns in a highly parallel fashion have been developed (41,42). DNA arrays of genomic fragments, cDNA clones, or oligonucleotides are also allowing genome-wide genetic mapping, the cloning of members of gene families within and across species, the scanning for mutations in genes, and the definitions of networks of genes controlled by particular transcription factors (43).

Genomics will provide a large number of potential targets. However, one of the challenges inherent in the use of these targets for drug development is the identification of targets that cause a specific disease rather than those that just correlate with the disease. It has been reported (44) that the most important diseases for which treatment is needed number between 100 and 150. Many of these diseases are caused, at least in part, by genetic factors. On the basis of multigene involvement in many genetic diseases as well as other assumptions, it was concluded that there was a potential for 3000 to 10,000 new and interesting drug targets. Since targets for which therapies presently exist number only slightly over 400, the potential targets for which there are no drugs far outnumbers those for which there are (44).

III. DRUG DEVELOPMENT

Once a compound has met the criteria to justify calling it the ''lead molecule'' of choice, it undergoes more advanced studies aimed at determining its potency

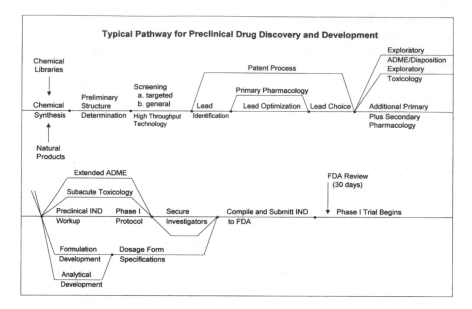

Figure 4 Typical pathway for new drug discovery and development up to Phase I trials in humans.

in vivo in the appropriate animal models. Some indication of oral bioavailability is obtained, together with preliminary data, to indicate whether the primary activity resides in the parent molecule or a metabolite. The therapeutic ratio is determined, and an indication of the toxicity profile of the compound is obtained. These studies are always designed with a focus on the primary indication intended for humans. This type of orientation is necessary to obtain the data needed to fulfill the regulatory requirements for the Investigational New Drug Application (IND).

Figure 4 illustrates a new drug development plan of the preclinical strategies necessary for creating the preclinical data package for submission of an IND to regulatory authorities.

A. Pharmacology

At the present time, regulatory agencies do not define precise requirements for submission of pharmacological data for an IND, New Drug Application (NDA), CTX, or Marketing Authorization Application (MAA). The following recommendations have been suggested as appropriate procedures to be followed for submissions to the United States, United Kingdom, and European authorities. In the

following sections, the actual guidelines dealing with submission of pharmacological data to regulatory agencies in the United States, United Kingdom, and
Europe are presented as close as possible to that stated in the regulatory guidelines. The comments immediately following a specific guideline are the authors'
interpretation of how these guidelines should be executed. This interpretation is
based on personal experience and information gained from many years of work
in these areas.

Each of the regulatory agencies requires that the pharmacological properties of the compound be presented in three separate sections: (1) primary pharmacology, which should discuss activity related to the proposed therapeutic use; (2)
secondary pharmacology, which should describe other activities; and (3) drug
interactions, which is required when relevant.

1. Primary Pharmacology

The primary pharmacology is concerned with defining the pharmacological actions relevant to the proposed therapeutic use. The term *pharmacological actions*
encompasses all potential therapeutic actions as well as conventional pharmacological activities.

Listed below are the actual guidelines that deal with the requirements necessary for adequate presentation of the primary pharmacology of a new chemical
entity (NCE).

> *Where possible, it is desirable to present data that establish the mechanism
> of the principal pharmacological action.*

Frequently, it is not possible to fully explain the mechanism of action of
a particular compound. This is particularly true for CNS-active compounds. At
other times, it may be simple to explain the mechanism of action of a compound
(i.e., antidepressant activity achieved through inhibition of monoamine oxidase,
or antihypertensive activity resulting from beta-receptor blockade). It should be
kept in mind that this guideline is not meant to delay the filing of an IND while
the researcher attempts to elucidate the mechanism of action of a compound. It
is simply a request to do what is reasonable without undue delays in filing.

> *The validity of models used should be established where practicable.*

Validity means that accepted models, either so established in the literature
or through appropriate defensible studies conducted in one's own laboratories,
should be used. Nevertheless, there are always inherent dangers in being totally
confident that any animal model will be predictive of a drug's efficacy in humans.
For example, the reversal of tetrabenazine-induced sedation and ptosis in mice
has been routinely used in some laboratories as a reliable and predictive test for
antidepressant activity in humans. However, it was soon discovered that, while

the test was predictive for antidepressants of the noradrenergic class, it failed to detect antidepressants working through serotonergic mechanisms. That is, it detected amitriptyline, but not fluoxitine. Thus, if one relied solely on the antitetrabenazine test for selecting antidepressant drugs, key discoveries in serotonerigic area, such as prozac, would be missed.

As another example, in vivo antitumor studies were most frequently carried out using tumors implanted subcutaneously or intraperitoneally. Although these models gave useful information regarding the in vivo activity of a drug candidate, they lacked many of the intrinsic characteristics of the tumors in humans. Even when human tumors were used, tumors grown subcutaneously lacked the natural microenvironment of the original tumor; the implanted tumors had, in most cases, been passaged for many generations either in culture or in animals and were therefore subject to change or selection during this period of time; the host animals lacked an efficient immune system; and metastatic disease was rarely a factor. These problems were addressed, to some extent, through intravenous administration or orthotopic implantation of tumor cells. The importance of the tumor microenvironment to the response to chemotherapy has been studied using both murine tumors and human tumor xenografts (45,46). Murine or human colon carcinomas were implanted subcutaneously or into different visceral organs and the response of the tumors to either 5-fluorouracil or doxorubicin, were determined. Marked differences in response to chemotherapy were observed. For example, subcutaneous tumors were sensitive to doxorubicin whereas lung or liver metastases were not. In contrast, sensitivity to 5-fluorouracil was less dependent on sites of tumor growth. Tumors growing in liver were resistant to both drugs. These results indicated that tumors implanted subcutaneously, the model most widely used for antitumor drug development, appeared to be an inappropriate and overly sensitive model for chemotherapy in humans.

Many of the limitations of the tumor models have been overcome through the establishment of transgenic models of tumor development (47). More than two dozen tumor types have been modeled. As one example, transgenic models of prostate cancer have been developed that possess many of the characteristics of the disease in humans (48). Mice develop spontaneous autochtonous disease that progresses through mild to severe hyperplasia and ultimately to metastatic disease and therefore would provide a more suitable model for testing both chemopreventive or therapeutic drug candidates.

An alternative method for producing disease specific models uses homologous recombination of a gene construct in cultured embryonic stem cells to produce a cell line having a precise gene replacement that can be used to create animals transmitting the gene replacement through the germline. The goal of these methods is to make a null mutation, known as a knockout, and replace the specific gene of interest with one that is inactive or altered. Models of a wide variety of human disorders have been constructed using this technique (49). These models have been used to study the pathology, as well as to evaluate potential therapies, of these diseases. For example, knockout mice have been used to determine the effectiveness of the very-low-density lipoprotein receptor gene as a therapeutic gene for the treatment of hypercholesterolemia (50) and to evaluate the chemopreventative effects of omega-3 polyunsaturated fatty acids on intestinal adenomatous polyposis (51). A number of Internet sites are dedicated to transgenic and knockout strains (52).

Some limitations to the extrapolation of animal data for the prediction of the human response include the following (53):

> There may be pharmacokinetic differences between test animals and humans.
> Idiosyncratic adverse events in humans, the mechanism of which are poorly understood, are not normally demonstrable in animals by standard investigation.
> Underlying pathological conditions or drugs may exacerbate underlying diseases in humans which do not exist in healthy animals.
> Relationships that might exist between the drug and its metabolites on the one hand, and an underlying disease on the other, that cannot adequately be investigated or predicted from studies which have been conducted in animals.
> Species differences in anatomy and physiological functions.
> Species differences in tolerance and enzyme induction.
> Adverse drug events that can only be communicated verbally by the patient are not normally recognized in animals.
> Some evidence of pharmacological activity should be demonstrated by the proposed clinical routes of administration.
> Comparison with other standard drug substances of the same therapeutic class is desirable.

Comparison of the data for the compound under development to a standard or reference drug is highly desirable and is an encouraged and recommended practice. However, there are examples where comparison with standards could be very time-consuming and could delay the filing of an IND. Once again, one must use the best managerial and scientific judgment in order to arrive at a reasonable course of action.

Results should be expressed in quantitative terms (e.g., dose- and time-related effects).

These data will ultimately have to be correlated with pharmacokinetic and toxicological data. In fact, it is advisable to do joint pharmacodynamic and pharmacokinetic studies when feasible.

2. Secondary Pharmacology

A general pharmacological profile, that is, secondary pharmacology, of a new chemical entity is also required, with special attention to any effects additional to the primary pharmacological action. The aim of the secondary pharmacological studies should be to establish the effects on the major physiological systems by using a variety of experimental models. More extensive investigation is required if the doses producing secondary effects approach those producing the primary pharmacological (therapeutic) effect. Both in vitro and in vivo data should be presented. Good scientific judgment is required to determine the nature and extent of these studies.

Studies conducted to define the secondary pharmacology should be classified under the following headings:

Neuropharmacology
Cardiovascular/Respiratory
Gastrointestinal
Genitourinary
Endocrine
Antiinflammatory
Immunoactive
Chemotherapeutic
Enzyme effects
Other

3. Drug Interactions

Interaction of the drug substance with other compounds, when relevant to the proposed therapeutic usage, should be investigated. These interactions are primarily concerned with drug–drug interactions, but could also include interaction with excipients. Recently, the Food and Drug Administration (FDA) has frequently required metabolism studies (P450 studies) to be conducted as part of the submission package. For additional information, see Sec. III. C.

B. Toxicology Studies

1. In Vivo Versus In Vitro Studies

Toxicological evaluation of a drug candidate has traditionally been carried out in-vivo, usually in mice, rats, dogs, or monkeys. However, there has been an increased effort to develop and use in vitro models for toxicological, as well as pharmacokinetic, evaluation during the development process. The use of in vitro systems has been stimulated by the rapid scientific advances that have been made with regard to the structural and functional multiplicity of mammalian drug-metabolizing enzymes and the genetic and environmental factors that affect their expression. The role of these enzymes in drug metabolism and detoxification and the increased availability of human tissues have also stimulated the development of in-vitro systems, as has the actions of animal rights activists against the use of animals for drug development and toxicological studies.

The in-vitro systems that are being used in drug discovery and development have been classified empirically into three categories: validated screens, value-added screens, and ad-hoc mechanistic screens (54). With regard to the validated in-vitro screens, the in-vitro methods have been shown to reflect activity observed in vivo, the mechanism of action is well understood, and the models have become highly standardized. The level of confidence in the predictability of these models is high, and they can be used to make a decision concerning the selection or advancement of a candidate drug. Examples of validated assays are the genotox-icity screens and the LAL assays for measuring the presence of endotoxin (55,56).

The value-added screens are used in conjunction with traditional in-vivo studies to facilitate the decision process with respect to lead candidate selection and advancement. A large number of the in vitro screens, which have become an integral part of the drug development process, fall into this category; however, the incomplete standardization of these assays do not allow their use alone in making decisions regarding candidate selection or advancement. The in vitro assays described in Sec. III.C include a number of in vitro assays that are used in this way. The use of Caco-2 human colon adenocarcinoma cells in culture to study intestinal transport, metabolism, and toxicity, as well as the use of the human tumor cloning assay to determine the potential benefits of antitumor drugs in individual patients, also fall into this category (3,57,58).

In vitro systems have also been used to study in an ad-hoc fashion mechanisms of cellular damage and toxicity in a system lacking the complex in vivo interactions. Although mechanisms of drug toxicity are often quite complex, the mechanistic studies in vitro can frequently facilitate the prediction of the relevance of preclinical toxicology data to human therapeutic use. However, these types of studies are rarely performed early in the development of a drug candidate (54).

In the United States, the minimum absorption, distribution, metabolism and elimination (ADME) requirements for an IND reflect an emphasis on safety evaluation. ADME data should support toxicology studies by showing evidence for absorption. In addition to the development of an analytical method for measuring unchanged drug, toxicokinetic studies in two species, conducted according to Good Laboratory Practices (GLP) regulations, are required. Toxicokinetics is defined as the generation of pharmacokinetic data, either as an integral component in the conduct of nonclinical toxicity studies or in specially designed supportive studies, in order to assess systemic exposure. The primary objective is to describe the systemic exposure achieved in animals and its relationship to dose level and the time course of the toxicity study. FDA guidelines for the conduct of toxicokinetic studies have been published (59).

The primary species used in preclinical disposition studies are the rat and the dog, since these are the species generally used for the initial toxicology studies. However, if the metabolic profiles for a compound in rat and dog differ quantitatively from those observed in humans, it may be necessary to determine the major routes of biotransformation in other species to select those that will be relevant models for assessing potential long-term toxicity in humans.

Initial toxicology studies performed before administration to humans, that is, acute and subacute studies in two species, are designed to characterize potential toxic effects and should be of sufficient duration to allow the clinician to undertake tolerance studies in humans. In addition, other exploratory or dose-range finding toxicity studies may also be done in conjunction with other preclinical studies in the initial stages of compound evaluation. A regulatory review of preclinical drug development has been recently presented (60).

The development of a typical drug for chronic/intermediate or sustained administration would proceed as follows:

> A new drug candidate is generally tested acutely in at least two mammalian species, usually rat and dog. If there are sufficient data available to suggest that another species more closely represents humans than these two species, then it should be used instead (e.g., monkey.)
>
> The route of administration should be the route intended for use in humans. In practice, intraperitoneal, oral, and at times, intravenous routes are all usually tested in the initial single, dose-rising, acute toxicity test.
>
> The purpose of the acute, single, dose-rising study is to define the adverse effect profile of the drug and to achieve an extrapolated estimate of the LD_{50} of the agent. These studies are usually done in rat and mouse.

Once the data have been obtained for the acute, dose-rising study, the single-dose (acute) toxicity study can be designed.

> *The single-dose (acute) toxicity for a pharmaceutical should be evaluated in two mammalian species (usually rats and dogs) prior to the first human exposure. A dose-escalation study is an acceptable alternative to the single-dose study.*

These studies, in male and female animals (usually groups of 10–30 rats and 2–4 dogs per sex and dose), usually last from 1 to 2 weeks. Animals in the acute toxicity studies (usually groups of 10–30 rats and 2–4 dogs per sex and dose) are observed for one to two weeks following dosing. Acute toxicity studies will support clinical trials ranging from a single dose to dosing of up to 2 weeks in duration.

A repeated-dose toxicity study in two species (one non-rodent) for a minimum of 1, 3, or 6 months would support human clinical trials for up to 1, 3, or 6 months' duration, respectively.

C. Pharmacokinetic and ADME Studies

As part of the drug discovery and development process, pharmacokinetic and ADME studies have become an integral step in the early evaluation of drug candidates. Absorption, half-life, and metabolism are being measured early in the development of a drug candidate in order to exclude those compounds that are poorly absorbed or rapidly metabolized or eliminated. Traditionally, most ADME studies have been carried out in vivo, usually in mice, rats, and dogs. However, increased knowledge of human drug metabolism, as well as the increased availability of human tissues, have led to a greater use of in vitro metabolism studies, using preparations from human tissues, in early drug development. The metabolic profile, as well as species differences in metabolism of the drug candidate can be obtained. Data obtained from these studies can help determine the human enzymes that are responsible for the metabolic clearance of the compound, and the choice of the most appropriate animal species to be used for in vivo evaluations. The metabolic profile could also be useful for characterizing a species-specific toxic and/or pharmacological effect of the compound. FDA guidelines for in vitro studies of drug metabolism and drug interactions have recently been published.

Biotransformation of most drugs occurs primarily in the liver, although some metabolism can also occur in the gut. In vitro methods that are used to study hepatic metabolism of drugs can be divided into whole-cell preparations, which include isolated perfused livers, liver slices, and hepatocytes, and broken-cell preparations, which include subcellular preparations and purified enzymes (61).

A significant part of the in vitro studies of human drug metabolism has been carried out using subcellular fractions. Subcellular fractions can be classified into three types: microsomes, which are vesicles formed from the endoplasmic reticulum during homogenization; the cytosol; and the S9 fraction, the fraction remaining after removal of nuclei and mitochondria from a liver homogenate. Therefore, the S9 fraction contains both the microsomes and the cytosol. These fractions contain enzymes that catalyze both Phase I and Phase II reactions. Phase I metabolism adds or exposes polar functional groups on a lipophillic substrate, whereas Phase II metabolism catalyzes the addition of a polar endogenous substrate to these functional groups, yielding a highly polar conjugate readily excretable from the body. The advantages of the subcellular preparations include ease of preparation and use, ease of cross-species comparisons, and good viability during long-term storage of the fractions. These fractions can be stored for at least 1 year without significant changes in the metabolic activity of the fractions. The subcellular fractions, as well as the individual purified enzymes discussed below, can be used to characterize the metabolic profile of a compound, to determine the enzymes responsible for the metabolic clearance of the compound, to investigate the formation of toxic metabolites, and to compare the profile of human metabolites with the profile generated by subcellular fractions obtained from other species. These systems can also provide early information on potential drug–drug interactions (61).

A large number of the drug metabolizing enzymes found in the subcellular fractions have been purified and characterized. Of the human enzymes involved in drug metabolism, the cytochromes P450, which constitute a superfamily of hemoproteins, have been the most widely studied. Over 200 P450 genes have been classified on the basis of structure into 36 gene families. Twelve of these gene families exist in all mammals examined to date, and three of these families, CYP1, CYP2, and CYP3, are thought to be responsible for the majority of hepatic xenobiotic metabolism. Under many conditions, a single P450 may be exclusively or primarily responsible for the detoxification or bioactivation of a particular compound (62). A major disadvantage of using purified enzymes is the amount of work required to prepare sufficient quantities of the enzymes needed to carry out studies. However, the availability of the cDNA for specific isozymes of human cytochromes P450 has made the production of large quantities of many of these enzymes possible.

One of the disadvantages of broken-cell preparations is that these preparations lack the functional integrity present in living organisms. In contrast, whole-cell preparations in general are more predictive of in vivo conditions since they have coupled Phase I and Phase II metabolism, competing enzyme pathways, normal cellular levels of cofactors, and an intact cellular membrane. Whole cell preparations include hepatocytes, liver slices, and intact isolated perfused livers.

Hepatocytes are whole-cell preparations lacking the intact architecture of liver slices or whole liver and are used either as suspension cultures or as monolayer cultures grown on a matrix of collagen or similar material. Hepatocytes in suspension lose viability after 4–6 hr in culture, whereas monolayer cultures are functional for a period of several days, although there is a loss of cytochromes P450 with time. A comparison of the metabolism of several model compounds by hepatocytes with that observed in vivo indicates that human hepatocytes are an excellent model of human drug metabolism (63).

Liver slices maintain the cellular architecture, structural heterogeneity, and intracellular communication between various cell types in liver and are not subject to potential damage of cellular membranes by collagenase, as is the case in the preparation of hepatocytes. The increased use of liver slices has been stimulated by the development of the Krumdieck tissue slicer, which allows the rapid preparation of uniform slices that are thin enough to allow adequate oxygenation of the whole slice during incubation while causing minimal damage to the hepato-cytes. Liver slices can be maintained in culture for periods up to 72 hr. Liver slices prepared in this manner have been shown to reflect accurately the metabolic capabilities of the liver in vivo (61,63).

The isolated perfused liver can be used to examine metabolism at the level of the whole organ. The organ remains viable for 4–6 hr, but viability declines rapidly after this time. Perfused livers can be used to measure uptake from the circulation as well as the release of metabolites into the circulation. However, the complexity of the system limits its utility for the routine study of drug metabo-lism.

A recent approach to the study of the role of the cytochromes P450 in drug metabolism and toxicology has involved the development of knockout mice which have altered or deficient drug metabolism (58). For example, a knockout mouse lacking CYP1A2 has been developed and has been used to show the utility of this approach for determining the role of specific enzymes in metabolic and pharmacokinetic processes.

IV. CONCLUSION

In this chapter, we have described approaches to the discovery and development of new chemical entities for the treatment of human diseases. Although all ap-proaches discussed above will not be used in the development of each compound, the basic pharmacological and toxicological processes and requirements that are necessary to advance a drug candidate to the IND stage, that is, selection of the lead molecule and demonstration of efficacy and safety, will be a part of the development of all potential drugs.

V. REFERENCES

1. Grever MR, Schepartz SA, Chabner BA. The National Cancer Institute: cancer drug discovery and development program. Semin Oncol 1992; 19(6):622–638.
2. Weinstein JN, Myers TG, O'Connor PM, et al. An information-intensive approach to the molecular pharmacology of cancer. Science 1997; 275:343-347.
3. Von Hoff DD. Human tumor cloning assays: applications in clinical oncology and new antineoplastic agent development. Cancer Metastasis Rev 1988; 7:357–371.
4. Algate DR. Application of the pharmacological screening process. Drug Metab Rev 1990; 22(6–8):809–820.
5. Maxwell RA. The state of the art of the science of drug discovery—an opinion. Drug Dev Res 1984; 4:375–389.
6. Kubinyi H. Strategies and recent technologies in drug discovery. Pharmazie 1995; 50:647–662.

7. Schacter LP, Anderson C, Canetta RM, et al. Drug discovery and development in the pharmaceutical industry. Semin Oncol 1992; 19(6):613–621.
8. Drug discovery. A casebook and analysis. In: Maxwell, ed, 1990.
9. Gallop MA, Barrett RW, Dower WJ, Fodor SPA, Gordon EM. Applications of combinatorial technologies to drug discovery. 1. Background and peptide combinatorial libraries. J Med Chem 1994; 37(9):1233–1251.
10. Doyle PM. Combinatorial chemistry in the discovery and development of drugs. J Chem Tech Biotechnol 1995; 64:317–324.
11. Burch RM, Kyle DJ. Mass receptor screening for new drugs. Pharm Res 1991; 8(2): 141–147.
12. Phillips DF. Making new drugs via combinatorial chemistry. JAMA 1996; 275(21): 1624–1626.
13. Burch RM. Mass ligand-binding screening strategies for identification of leads for new drug discovery. NIDA Res Monogr Ser 1993; 134:37–45.
14. Okun I, Veerapandian P. New methods to mimic nature in high-throughput screening. Nature Biotechnol 1997; 15:287–288.
15. Hodgson J. Pharmaceutical screening: from off-the-wall to off-the-shelf. The many routes to successful drug discovery. Bio/Tech 1993; 11:683–688.
16. Kirsch DR. Development of improved cell-based assays and screens in *Saccharomyces* through the combination of molecular and classical genetics. Biotechnology 1993; 4:543–552.
17. Borman S. Combinatorial chemistry. Researchers continue to refine techniques for identifying potential drugs in ''libraries'' of small organic molecules. Chem Eng News 1997; 75:43–62.
18. Hogan JC, Jr. Combinatorial chemistry in drug discovery. Nature Biotechnol 1997; 15:328–330.
19. Gold L. Oligonucleotides as research, diagnostic, and therapeutic agents. J Biol Chem 1995; 270(23):13581–13584.
20. Gold L, Alper J. Keeping pace with genomics through combinatorial chemistry. Nature Biotechnol 1997; 15:297.
21. Murray-Rust P. Bioinformatics and drug discovery. Biotechnology 1994; 5:648–653.
22. Boguski MS. Bioinformatics. Genetics Dev 1994; 4:383–388.
23. Mixtures PAHCoR. Comments on enantiomerism in the drug development process. Pharm Tech 1990; 46:161.
24. Veerapandian B. Three dimensional structure-aided drug design. In: Burger's Medicinal Chemistry and Drug Discovery. New York: Wiley, 1995:303–348.
25. Jones TR, Varney MD, Webber SE, et al. Structure-based design of lipophilic quinazoline inhibitors of thymidylate synthase. J Med Chem 1996; 39:904–917.
26. Appelt K. Crystal structures of HIV-1 protease-inhibitor complexes. Perspect Drug Discov Design 1993; 1:23–48.
27. Wlodawer A, Erickson J. Structure based inhibitors of HIV-1 protease. Annu Rev Biochem 1993; 62:543–585.
28. Hansch C, Fujita T. p-σ-π anaylsis. A method for the correlation of biological activity and chemical structure. J Am Chem Soc 1964; 86:1616–1628.

29. Free SM, Wilson JW. A mathematical contribution to structure-activity studies. J Med Chem 1964; 7(4):395–399.

30. Kubinyi H. The quantitative analysis of structure-activity relationships. In: Burger's Medicinal Chemistry and Drug Discovery. New York: Wiley 1995:497–571.

31. Kohler G, Milstein C. Continuous culture of fused cells secreting antibodies of pre-defined specificities. Nature 1975; 256:495–497.

32. Owens RJ, Young RJ. The genetic engineering of monoclonal antibodies. J Immunol Meth 1994; 168:149–165.

33. Faulds D, Sorkin EM. Abciximab (c7E3 Fab). A review of its pharmacology and therapeutic potential in ischaemic heart disease. Drugs 1994; 48(4):583–598.

34. Cancer. In: Principles and Practice of Oncology. Philadelphia: Lippincott-Raven, 1997.

35. Riethmüller G, Schneider-Gädicke E, Schlimok G, et al. Randomised trial of mono-clonal antibody for adjuvant therapy of resected Dukes' C colorectal carcinoma. Lancet 1994; 343:1177–1183.

36. Hanania EG, Kavanagh J, Hortobagyi G, Giles RE, Champlin R, Deisseroth AB. Recent advances in the application of gene therapy to human disease. Am J Med 1995; 99:537–552.

37. Crystal RG. Transfer of genes to humans: early lessons and obstacles to success. Science 1995; 270:404–410.

38. Ledley FD. Nonviral gene therapy: the promise of genes as pharmaceutical products. Hum Gene Ther 1995; 6:1129–1144.

39. Jolly D. Viral vector systems for gene therapy. Cancer Gene Ther 1994; 1(1):51–64.

40. Friedrich GA. Moving beyond the genome projects. Does the future of genomics-based drug discovery lie with the mouse? Nature Biotechnol 1996; 14:1234–1237.

41. Ferguson JA, Boles TC, Adams CP, Walt DR. A fiber-optic DNA biosensor microar-ray for the analysis of gene expression. Nature Biotechnol 1996; 14:1681–1684.

42. Lockhart DJ, Dong H, Byrne MC, et al. Expression monitoring by hybridization to high-density oligonucleotide arrays. Nature Biotechnol 1996; 14:1675–1680.

43. Blanchard AP, Hood L. Sequence to array: probing the genome's secrets. Nature Biotechnol 1996; 14:1649.

44. Drews J. Genomic sciences and the medicine of tomorrow. Nature Biotechnol 1996; 14:1516–1518.

45. Wilmanns C, Fan D, O'Brian CA, Bucana CD, Fidler IJ. Orthotopic and ectopic organ environments differentially influence the sensitivity of murine colon carci-noma cells to doxorubicin and 5-fluorouracil. Int J Cancer 1992; 52:98–104.

46. Fidler IJ, Wilmanns C, Staroselsky A, Radinsky R, Dong Z, Fan D. Modulation of tumor cell response to chemotherapy by the organ environment. Cancer Metastasis Rev 1994; 13:209–222.

47. Adams JM, Cory S. Transgenic models of tumor development. Science 1991; 254: 1161–1167.

48. Greenberg NM, DeMayo F, Finegold MJ, et al. Prostate cancer in a transgenic mouse. Proc Natl Acad Sci USA 1995; 92:3439–3443.

49. Shastry BS. Genetic knockouts in mice: an update. Experientia 1995; 51:1028–1039.

50. Kobayashi K, Oka K, Forte T, et al. Reversal of hypercholesterolemia in low density lipoprotein receptor knockout mice by adenovirus-mediated gene transfer of the very low density lipoprotein receptor. J Biol Chem 1996; 271(12):6852–6860.

51. Oshima M, Takahashi M, Oshima H, et al. Effects of docosahexaenoic acid (DHA) on intestinal polyp development in Apc^{delta716} knockout mice. Carcinogenesis 1995; 16(11):2605–2607.

52. Sikorski R, Peters R. Transgenics on the internet. Nature Biotechnol 1997; 15:289.

53. Wood D, Folk PI. Annual tests as predictors of human response. In: Handbook of Phase I/II Clinical Drug Trials. Boca Raton, New York, London, Tokyo: CRC Press 1997:35–49.

54. Ball SE, Scatina JA, Sisenwine SF, Fisher GL. The application of in vitro models of drug metabolism and toxicity in drug discovery and drug development. Drug Chem Toxicol 1995; 18(1):1–28.

55. Ashby J, Morrod RS. Detection of human carcinogens. Nature 1991; 352:185–186.

56. Rainer M. Toward using in vitro toxicology in the drug approval process. Bio/Tech 1990; 8:1248–1249.

57. Hidalgo IJ, Raub TJ, Borchardt RT. Characterization of the human colon carcinoma cell line (Caco2) as a model system for intestinal epithelial permeability. Gastroenterology 1989; 96:736–749.

58. Gan L-S, Eads C, Niederer T, et al. Use of Caco-2 cells as an in vitro intestinal absorption and metabolism model. Drug Dev Ind Pharm 1994; 20:615–631.

59. Guidelines for industry. Toxicokinetics: the assessment of systemic exposure in toxicity studies. Fed Reg 1995; 60:11264.

60. Mathieu M. New Drug Development: A Regulatory Overview, 1994. Waltham, MA: PAREXEL

61. Adams PE. In vitro methods to study hepatic drug metabolism. Emphasis 1995; 6: 1–6.

62. Halpert JR, Guengerich FP, Bend JR, Correia MA. Selective inhibitors of cytochromes P450. Toxicol App Pharmacol 1994; 125:163–175.

63. Wrighton SA, Vandenbranden M, Stevens JC, et al. In vitro methods for assessing human hepatic drug metabolism: their use in drug development. Drug Metab Rev 1993; 25(4):453–484.

3
The IND Process for New Drug Products

David M. Cocchetto
GlaxoSmithKline, Research Triangle Park, North Carolina

I. INTRODUCTION TO THE IND

A. What Is an IND?

An IND is an Investigational New Drug application, i.e., the documentation required for submission by the sponsor and clearance by the U.S. Food and Drug Administration (FDA) in order to use a drug product not previously authorized for marketing in the United States. The IND provisions apply to new drugs, new antibiotics, and new biologics. Critical review of the contents of the IND is the means by which the FDA protects the public health from new drugs with unproven safety and unproven efficacy.

B. When Is an IND required?

An IND is always required prior to initiation of a clinical study of an investigational new drug in the United States. In addition, an IND is required before initiation of a clinical study of a drug approved for some uses, but to be studied clinically for a new indication or at unapproved doses or if the new clinical study is intended to support promotion of the product. The following examples may be helpful.

> A sponsor wants to initiate animal toxicology studies of an investigational new drug in the United States. Is an IND required? *An IND is not required, because no studies in humans are proposed at this time.*
>
> A sponsor has a novel antihypertensive drug with supporting pharmacology, toxicology, and manufacturing information. *In order to initiate a*

single-dose pharmacokinetic study in humans in the United States, an IND must be submitted to the FDA.

A sponsor has a drug that is approved by the FDA for the treatment of hypertension. New clinical studies are planned to evaluate the drug in the treatment of congestive heart failure. *An IND is required, since the drug is investigational with respect to its unapproved use in patients with congestive heart failure.*

A sponsor has a drug that is approved by the FDA for the treatment of hypertension. The sponsor wants to initiate a new clinical study to compare the drug with a major competing antihypertensive product. Both drugs will be used at doses consistent with the FDA-approved labeling. *In this case, an IND is required if it is the sponsor's intent to use this study for promotion of its product.*

C.   What Is the Legal Basis for an IND?

The requirement for an Investigational New Drug application is defined in the law governing development of new drugs in the United States, i.e., the Federal Food, Drug and Cosmetic Act (FD&C Act). The FD&C Act became law in 1938, and it has had several major amendments since that time. Today, the fundamental requirements of the FD&C Act for new drugs are as follows:

Proof of safety
Substantial evidence of efficacy
Informative labeling for the product
Demonstration of manufacturing of the product to the desired strength, quality, purity, and identity

The FD&C Act requires that all drugs distributed in interstate commerce in the United States have proof of safety and substantial evidence of efficacy; an investigational drug (which by definition lacks such demonstration of safety and efficacy) may be administered to patients in the United States in order to gather evidence of safety and efficacy after such a drug obtains an exemption (i.e., an IND) for conduct of specific clinical studies for specific indications by specific clinical investigators in the presence of ongoing sponsor commitments to monitor these studies and provide certain information to the FDA.

The FD&C Act itself defines the requirement for an IND, but it does not provide more detailed information on the procedures and operational approaches to be used in drug development in order to satisfy these legal requirements. In order to provide operational details, subsequent to passage of the FD&C Act, the FDA developed the implementing regulations governing drug development. Most of these regulations are found in Title 21 of the Code of Federal Regulations.

The following list identifies the major regulations governing development of investigational drugs:

Part number in Title 21	Regulation
50	Informed Consent
56	Institutional Review Boards
201	Prescription Drug Labeling
202	Prescription Drug Advertising
211	Current GMPs
312	Investigational New Drug Application
314	New Drug Applications
320	Bioavailability and Bioequivalence Requirements

Beyond these regulations, which are enforceable as law, the FDA provides guidance documents on the drug development process. These guidance documents take the form of guidelines, "Points to Consider" documents, and "Information Sheets." Such guidances are informal communications from the FDA in that they reflect the FDA's best judgment at the time of their preparation, but neither the FDA nor sponsors are legally obligated to adhere to the provisions of guidances.

II. ESSENTIAL PRINCIPLES OF AN IND

The FDA uses an introductory part of its IND regulations (21 CFR 312.22) to present several important principles of the IND submission. These four principles should be carefully heeded since they provide insight into the key concepts used by the FDA in reviewing INDs and they can help the sponsor prepare IND documents that meet the FDA's expectations.

The first important principle is that *the IND must present adequate information to permit the FDA to evaluate the drug's suitability for use in the proposed clinical study.* An application that provides insufficient information to enable a specific and detailed review of all elements relevant to the proposed clinical study is unlikely to be allowed to proceed. Similarly, as clinical studies progress over the years under an IND, subsequent submissions to the IND must continue to present an adequate set of information to enable appropriate evaluation by the FDA of proposed clinical studies. For a clinical study in an IND to be acceptable to the FDA, it must meet the safety standard (i.e., human subjects will not be exposed to an unreasonable and significant risk); further, the FDA must be convinced that the study has an acceptable likelihood of providing data capable of meeting statutory standards.

The second important principle is that *the central focus of the initial IND should be the general investigational plan and the protocol for the first proposed human study*. These documents should inform the FDA of the history of discovery and nonclinical development of the drug, as well as the overall objectives of the first human study under the IND, in the context of the plan for other studies throughout the first year of this IND. A well-conceived, well-written general investigational plan places the development plan for the drug into perspective and can help the FDA anticipate the sponsor's needs for feedback and guidance. The specific aspects of the proposed protocol (i.e., dose, duration of administration, subject selection criteria) must be supported by appropriate nonclinical pharmacology and toxicology studies. If a new drug has had no prior human use outside the United States, and thus the initial study under the IND is the first study in humans, both the sponsor and the FDA understand that a highly detailed investigational plan must be contingent on the outcomes of the first clinical study, as well as other early studies. Sponsors are expected to exercise considerable discretion regarding the information submitted in each section of the IND, depending on the available information, type of drug, and the proposed human study. Therefore, a general investigational plan that outlines the important concepts of the proposed clinical development is usually acceptable.

The third important principle is that *the first proposed human study must be a logical extension of the supporting information in the IND; further, subsequent amendments to the IND that propose additional human studies must build logically on the previous submissions to the IND and be supported by additional relevant information*. For example, an initial IND for a novel antibacterial drug must include a proposed initial human study that builds logically on nonclinical pharmacology results (e.g., data from in vitro studies and in vivo animal studies showing antibacterial activity) and nonclinical toxicology results (e.g., the drug was tolerated in animal studies at exposures above that proposed for the first human use). Later in the IND process, a new clinical protocol (e.g., one that proposes to increase the duration of drug administration from 10 days to 30 days for selected patients) must build logically on appropriate supporting information reported to the IND. Such information would typically include the results of longer-duration nonclinical toxicology studies, as well as the safety results for subjects in prior clinical studies with shorter durations of treatment.

The fourth important principle is that the FDA's most important act in reviewing an IND is the ongoing need *to assure that human subjects who participate in the proposed study will not be exposed to unreasonable and significant risk*. Clearly, this focus of the review is consistent with the FDA's fundamental charge to protect the public health. Sponsors will be wise to provide information supporting safety that is as clear and as compelling as possible. In this regard, sponsors should bear in mind that it may be helpful to the FDA, in certain areas of therapeutics, for the sponsor to present background information on the safety of currently available therapies for the target disease. This approach can help establish the context for the FDA's assessment of the reasonableness of the safety aspects of the proposed human study in the IND.

III. CONTENTS OF AN INITIAL IND

The standard contents of an initial IND is described specifically in the regulations in Part 312. These contents are also listed in the FDA standard covering form for INDs, i.e., Form FDA 1571. Further explanatory guidance on the content and format of INDs can be found in regulatory documents (1,2).

The standard contents of an initial IND are listed in Table 1. The concept underlying this contents of an initial IND can be readily understood if you con-

Table 1 Standard Contents of an Initial IND

Item number	Contents of section
Item 1	Form FDA 1571
Item 2	Table of Contents
Item 3	Introductory Statement & General Investigational Plan
	a. Introductory Statement
	b. Summary of Previous Human Experience
	c. Withdrawal from Investigation or Marketing
	d. Overall Plan for Investigations
Item 4	Reserved
Item 5	Investigator's Brochure
Item 6	Protocol
Item 7	Chemistry, Manufacturing and Control Data
	a. Drug Substance
	b. Drug Product
	c. Description of Placebo
	d. Labeling
	e. Environmental Assessment
Item 8	Pharmacology and Toxicology Data
	a. Pharmacology
	b. Toxicology
Item 9	Previous Human Experience
Item 10	Additional Information
	a. Drug Dependence and Abuse Potential
	b. Radioactive Drugs
	c. Other Information

sider the contents within the six technical sections that comprise all regulatory submissions. The six technical sections of U.S. drug regulatory applications (i.e., Pharmacology & Toxicology, CMC, Clinical, Microbiology, Statistics, and Human Pharmacokinetics & Bioavailability) are illustrated in Fig. 1. In Fig. 2, the items in an initial IND are shown within the technical sections. This information and its associated documentation can be extensive. In the 1980s and 1990s, until 1996, initial INDs for new chemical entities presented this information in sufficiently complete detail to enable a comprehensive review, including review of raw data, not simply summaries of data. Typically, an initial IND would comprise 4000–6000 pages (e.g., 10 to 15 volumes of 400 pages per volume). For such initial INDs, the nonclinical pharmacology and toxicology information typically comprised the largest portion of the IND.

Regulatory reform efforts in the 1990s led to the FDA's issuance of its guidance (in November 1995) regarding streamlining the contents of an initial IND to specifically support an initial Phase I study (2). FDA's guidance states that "if the guidance specified in this document is followed, IND submissions for Phase 1 studies should usually not be larger than 2 to 3, three inch, three-ring binders" (i.e., approximately 1200–1800 pages). Obviously, successful implementation of this guidance could lead to substantial reduction in documenta-

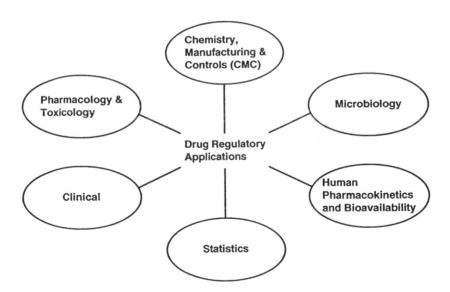

Figure 1   Six technical disciplines that comprise all drug regulatory applications in the United States.

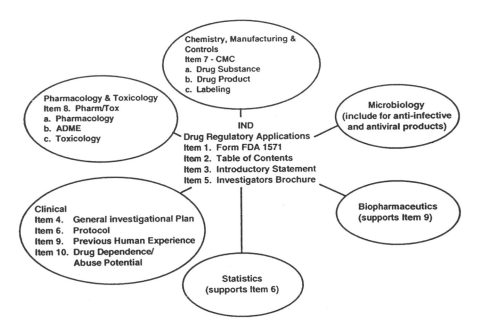

Figure 2 Diagrammatic representation of each item in an initial IND.

tion needed for an initial IND. Given the youth of this new guidance, its implementation bears close observation.

IV. REQUIREMENTS FOR NONCLINICAL TOXICOLOGY STUDIES TO SUPPORT HUMAN USE OF AN INVESTIGATIONAL NEW DRUG

A critical component of an initial IND is the results of nonclinical toxicology studies that support human use of the investigational drug. Fundamentally, nonclinical toxicology studies are conducted to explore and characterize the spectrum of the drug's toxicity in vitro and in animals. Some of these nonclinical studies (i.e., preclinical studies) must be completed before the drug may be administered for the first time to humans. Such preclinical studies provide the sponsor with some expectation of which organ systems are likely to exhibit toxicity-related findings in humans, as well as an expectation of the magnitude of drug exposure at which such toxicities may occur. Therefore, an adequate characterization of the drug's toxicity is an essential precursor to initiation of human studies of the drug. After initiation of the first study in humans, additional nonclinical studies must be conducted concurrently with human studies. It is critical to establish close coordination between nonclinical and clinical testing, since nonclinical testing must progress to longer durations of exposure and characterization of the drug in special populations (e.g., juvenile animals) ahead of proposed clinical studies using these longer durations of treatment or special patient populations. Successful coordination enables the relevant aspect of the clinical program to begin without toxicology-related delays. Each new proposed human study must build logically on the results of appropriate toxicology studies which are reported to the IND (as Information Amendments) prior to submission to the FDA of the new human protocol.

Typically, each new drug undergoes a series of toxicology studies in animals, beginning with single-dose studies (i.e., acute toxicity studies) and progressing through subchronic and chronic toxicity studies. Characterization of the toxic effects of a drug in animals with repeated drug administration over time provides some insight into the drug's likely effects in humans, given that many drug-induced effects are related to the dose, frequency of administration, duration of administration, and various pharmacokinetic measures of drug exposure. It is important to consider a typical series of toxicity studies that would be conducted before the first human use of a new drug in the United States. Although the information that follows is representative of a typical series of studies, each new drug must have customized aspects to its nonclinical toxicology program, depending on the unique chemical, pharmacological, and toxicological properties of the drug, as well as the specific proposed therapeutic use of the drug in humans. Several authoritative reviews and regulatory guidelines are available to describe the requirements for nonclinical toxicology studies in the United States (3–9). These requirements have not changed radically since publication of the Goldenthal guidelines in 1968 (3).

Assume, for example, that a new drug is being developed for oral administration for treatment of a human disease. Table 2 lists a typical series of toxicology studies that should be completed and reported in the initial IND to support initiation of human studies. Usually, each acute and repeat-dose toxicity study assesses at least three different doses of the drug in order to characterize the dose–response relationship of toxic effects on various organ systems in both male and female animals. If toxicologically adequate, this series of studies would support repeat-dose administration of the drug to human subjects for up to 4 weeks, i.e., the longest duration of repeat-dose administration in animals. The rationale for this series of studies bears explanation.

> Acute and repeat-dose toxicity studies provide a screen for initial detection and characterization of the spectrum of the drug's toxicity on all major organ systems. Note that the classical single-dose LD_{50} study (i.e., deter-

Table 2 Example of Nonclinical Toxicology Studies Needed Before Initiation of Studies in Humans of a New, Orally Administered Drug

Type of study	Species or test	Route of administration
Acute toxicity studies	Rat	Oral
	Rat	Parenteral (IV or IP)
	Mouse	Oral
	Mouse	Parenteral (IV or IP)
Repeat dose-studies	Rodent, 2 weeks dosing	Oral
	Nonrodent, 2 weeks dosing	Oral
	Rodent, 4 weeks dosing	Oral
	Nonrodent, 4 weeks dosing	Oral
Toxicokinetic (ADME) studies (as components of acute and repeat-dose studies)	Rodent and nonrodent	Oral and parenteral
Antigenicity testings	Guinea pig or rabbit	Dermal application
Mutagenicity testing	Assay for genetic mutations in bacteria (e.g., Ames test)	
	Assay to detect clastogens (e.g., rodent bone marrow micronucleus test or human peripheral lymphocyte test or mouse lymphoma assay)	

mination of a dose that is lethal to 50% of animals) is not required or routinely recommended by the FDA (10).

Toxicokinetic components of these acute and repeat-dose studies enable correlation of findings with measures of drug exposure across different species.

Mutagenicity studies provide initial evidence that the drug is not a mutagen, as reflected by detection of point mutations, frame shifts, or aberrations in individual chromosomes. Lack of mutagenicity is important since chemical mutagens are more likely than nonmutagens to pose a higher risk of heritable damage via germ cell mutations, as well as being more likely to be carcinogenic in humans.

Antigenicity testing is required for drugs that can contact skin. Such testing provides a means of screening for a drug's sensitization ability.

Again, this series of toxicology studies should be sufficient to support human studies with up to four weeks of dosing.

For some drugs, the sponsor may want to assure that the status of toxicology studies does not limit the rate of progress of Phase I and II studies in humans. In such cases, the sponsor may be wise to complete 3-month repeat-dose studies in rodents and nonrodents, as well as major parts of the reproductive toxicology studies. Specifically, the sponsor may complete Segment I (study of fertility and reproductive performance) in a rodent species (usually rat) and Segment II (study of organogenesis) in male and female rodents and nonrodents (usually rabbit). Submission of this larger set of results to the IND usually supports clinical trials well into Phase II with repeat-dose administration to male and female patients for up to 3 months. However, as originally described in the Goldenthal guidelines in 1968, some situations still merit completion of Segment I in female rodents, Segment II (rodent and nonrodent), and preliminary evidence of clinical safety and efficacy in male humans in order to justify inclusion of female humans of child-bearing potential in Phase II and III clinical trials. Note that it is usually acceptable to complete the Segment III study (study of perinatal and lactation periods) in a rodent species later during the IND period.

A second example may also be helpful. In some cases, the goal of the sponsor is to introduce a lead member of a novel series of new chemical entities into human investigations as rapidly as possible. An initial IND for an orally administration drug, for example, could be submitted with results of single-dose acute toxicity studies in rat and mouse, 7-day repeat-dose toxicity studies in rodent and nonrodent (e.g., dog), and 2-week repeat-dose toxicity studies in rodent and nonrodent. These toxicity studies will usually be sufficient to support initiation of a single-dose, dose-ranging study of the safety and pharmacokinetic properties of an orally administered drug as the first study in humans. This IND could subsequently be amended to supply the FDA with the results of the 4-week repeat-dose toxicity studies in rodent and nonrodent (e.g., rat and dog), as well as results of human studies (for single doses and multiple doses for up to 3 days), as a precursor to initiating human Phase I or II studies that require drug administration for up to 4 weeks.

Initiation of clinical investigations in special patient populations may require supporting nonclinical studies. To enable inclusion of pediatric patients in U.S. clinical trials, juvenile toxicity studies should be completed in rats, with drug administration beginning in animals at the fourth day of age and proceeding through 21 days of age. Typically, three different doses of drug and a control are assessed. In some cases, juvenile toxicity studies may also be done in a nonrodent species (e.g., dog) when pediatric use of the drug is a major anticipated clinical use or when the class of drug is known to be associated with pharmacological effects on development. Of course, in practice, many sponsors and some divisions of the FDA do not consider it prudent to initiate clinical studies in pediatric patients until they have collected an appropriate amount of laboratory and clinical safety data, as well as pharmacokinetic data, in adults. Further, some sponsors obtain clinical experience in descending order by age, i.e., first obtaining clinical experience in adults, then proceeding to study adolescents, then studying older children, then younger children, and finally infants.

In summary, for the United States, the following toxicology studies are generally needed to support various clinical trials:

Proposed duration of drug administration (oral or parenteral) in humans	Minimum duration of treatment in toxicology studies (R = rodent and NR = nonrodent)	
	Phases I and II	Phase III
1 day	2 weeks R and NR	
3 days	2 weeks R and NR	2 weeks R and NR
7 days	4 weeks R and NR	3 months R and NR
4 weeks	4 weeks R and NR	3 months R and NR
3 months	3 months R and NR	6 months R and NR
≥6 months		6 month rodent and 12 month nonrodent

Each toxicology study should be done with drug administration via the intended clinical route. Each study should elicit sufficient toxicity findings to enable characterization of the toxicity profile of the drug, within the constraints of the studies completed to date. For drugs with limited bioavailability by the intended clinical route of administration, adequate characterization of the toxicity profile may be facilitated by conduct of some repeat-dose toxicology studies using parenteral administration of the drug. Typically, the duration of human use in Phases I and II may be as long as the duration of animal studies. However, in Phase III, longer-term animal studies must be complete, since the duration of human use cannot (in general) exceed one-half the duration of treatment in animal toxicology studies.

V. THIRTY DAY WAIT FOR INITIAL IND

The FDA must have time to review an initial IND before the investigational drug is shipped and the first clinical investigation is initiated. This review time is essential to protect the public health because the FDA must assure that, based on the evidence presented in the initial IND, it is reasonable to proceed with the first proposed clinical investigation. The more specific nature of the FDA's review is described in a separate section below. The 30-day review clock begins on the day of the FDA's receipt of the initial IND, not on the day the sponsor mails the application. Thirty days after the FDA receives the IND, unless the FDA has notified the sponsor that the proposed clinical investigation is subject to a clinical hold, the IND becomes effective and the first proposed clinical investigation may be initiated. The sponsor may not send or deliver the investigational drug to any investigator named in the IND until the IND has become effective (unless the FDA has authorized otherwise).

The reader should note that the FDA does not "approve" INDs; rather, the FDA allows acceptable INDs to come into effect so that human investigations can proceed. The regulations do not require an active step with verbal or written notification by the FDA to the sponsor so that the sponsor is notified that the IND is in effect. By default, the IND goes into effect 30 days after the FDA receives it, assuming that no clinical hold has been imposed. Many sponsors, as well as divisions of the FDA, are uncomfortable with this passive aspect of the regulations. These sponsors and divisions typically rely on teleconferences to learn verbally whether the FDA will allow the IND to come into effect.

VI. FDA REVIEW OF AN INITIAL IND

A. FDA Divisions that Receive INDs for Drugs

Initial INDs for investigational drugs are sent by the sponsor to the appropriate reviewing division of the FDA's Center for Drug Evaluation and Research (CDER). Each of the 15 reviewing divisions is responsible for sustaining medical/scientific expertise and regulatory responsibility for drugs within a specific therapeutic area. For example, The Division of Neuropharmacological Drug Products reviews drug products that exert their effects through actions on the central or peripheral nervous systems, such as anxiolytics, antidepressants, and anticonvulsant drugs. The Division of Antiviral Drug Products reviews, for example, antiretroviral drugs, as well as drugs active against the herpes simplex virus. These 15 reviewing divisions are organized into five Offices of Drug Evaluation (ODE), each of which reports to the Office of Review Management within the CDER. The organizational structure of the CDER, as well as the names of the current Directors of each ODE, can be readily viewed on the FDA's web site (http://www.fda.gov/cder/).

Each reviewing division maintains a cadre of reviewers in three of the six technical disciplines found in drug regulatory applications, i.e., physician/medical reviewers, pharmacologists/toxicologists, and microbiologists (e.g., in the case of the Divisions of Anti-Infective Drug Products and the Division of Antiviral Drug Products). Reviewers in the other three technical disciplines are administratively located outside the reviewing division, but are assigned to the reviewing division through a matrix organization. That is, the Chemists are in the Office of New Drug Chemistry, the Statisticians are in the Office of Biostatistics, and Pharmacokineticists/Biopharmaceutics Reviewers are in the Divisions of Pharmaceutical Evaluation within the Office of Clinical Pharmacology and Biopharmaceutics. In some cases (such as the Division of Antiviral Drug Products), these matrix chemistry, statistical, and biopharmaceutics reviewers are co-located in office space within the reviewing division to which they are assigned.

INDs and New Drug Applications (NDAs) are assigned by therapeutic category to the relevant FDA reviewing division. Within that division, a review team is assembled to work in a multidisciplinary collaborative effort to review the IND or NDA. The review team consists of a regulatory/scientific reviewer from each of the six technical disciplines plus a review coordinator (entitled Consumer Safety Officer or Project Manager or Regulatory Health Coordinator). The members of the review team are illustrated in Fig. 3. Each of these members will evaluate the acceptability of the application, first from the perspective of their own technical discipline and then from an integrated perspective in concert with the reviewers across all six disciplines. In view of this review system at the FDA, it is wise for the sponsor of the application to perform a similar multidisciplinary review and defense of the application in the course of preparing and submitting the application.

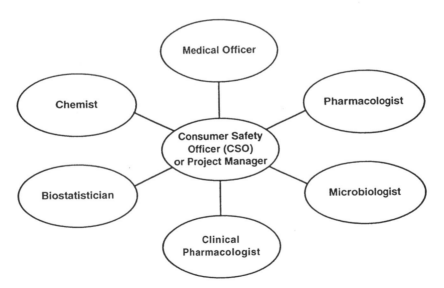

Figure 3 Members of the FDA's review team for a drug regulatory application.

B. Nature of FDA Review of an Initial IND

FDA reviewers ultimately assess an initial IND against a set of specific criteria. These criteria are as follows:

> The IND contains sufficient information to allow reviewers to assess risk to humans who will enter the proposed study.
> Humans will not be exposed to unreasonable or significant risk of illness or injury from the drug.
> The proposed clinical investigator is qualified by training and experience to conduct the proposed study.
> The Clinical Investigators Brochure is not misleading, erroneous, or materially incomplete.

Upon completion of their review, each primary and supervisory reviewer at the FDA must sign an internal review cover sheet to signify that it is reasonable and appropriate to proceed with the proposed clinical investigation.

VII. FDA USE OF CLINICAL HOLD

FDA reviewing divisions have at their disposal a specific regulatory mechanism to delay initiation of a clinical study which they find objectionable or to suspend conduct of an ongoing clinical study which has become objectionable. This regulatory mechanism, called a "clinical hold," is "an order issued by the FDA to the sponsor to delay a proposed clinical investigation or to suspend an ongoing investigation" (21 CFR 312.42). The clinical hold order may apply to one study governed by an IND, more than one study governed by an IND, or all studies governed by an IND. The consequences of a clinical hold are significant, and thus INDs must be constructed in such a way as to provide sufficient information to avoid clinical holds. If a proposed clinical protocol is placed on clinical hold, no human subject may receive the investigational drug under that protocol. If an ongoing clinical protocol is placed on clinical hold, no new human subject may be recruited into the protocol and no new human subject may receive the investigational drug; the disposition of subjects already enrolled in the protocol must be agreed between the sponsor and FDA.

The grounds for imposition of a clinical hold are specific and detailed. For ease of reference, these regulatory grounds are presented in detail in Table 3. In essence, a clinical hold may be imposed if there is a significant safety hazard to humans receiving the drug, if the investigational plan or protocol is so deficient that it cannot meet the stated objectives, if the clinical investigator is not qualified to conduct the investigation, or if the contents of the Clinical Investigators Brochure is fundamentally flawed.

Table 3 Grounds for Imposition of a Clinical Hold on a Clinical Protocol Conducted Under an IND

Situation	Grounds for clinical hold
Clinical hold of a Phase I clinical protocol	1. Humans subject are or would be exposed to an unreasonable and significant risk of illness or injury. 2. The clinical investigators named in the IND are not qualified by reason of their scientific training and experience to conduct the investigation described in the IND. 3. The Investigator Brochure is misleading, erroneous, or materially incomplete. 4. The IND does not contain sufficient information required under 21 CFR 312.23 (format and content of the IND) to assess the risks to subjects of the proposed studies.
Clinical hold of a Phase II or III clinical protocol	Reasons 1–4 above also apply in this case, plus one additional criterion: 5. The plan or protocol for the investigation is clearly deficient in design to meet its stated objectives.
Clinical hold of any clinical protocol that is not designed to be adequate and well controlled	Reasons 1–5 above also apply in this case, plus one or more of the following 7 additional criteria: 6. There is reasonable evidence the investigation that is not designed to be adequate and well controlled is impeding enrollment in, or otherwise interfering with the conduct or completion of, a study that is designed to be an adequate and well-controlled investigation of the same or another investigational drug. 7. Insufficient quantities of the investigational drug exist to adequately conduct both the investigation that is not designed to be adequate and well controlled and the investigations that are designed to be adequate and well controlled. 8. The drug has been studied in one or more adequate and well-controlled investigations that strongly suggest lack of effectiveness. 9. Another drug under investigation or approved for the same indication and available to the same indication and available to the same patient population has demonstrated a better potential benefit/risk balance. 10. The drug has received marketing approval for the same indication in the same patient population. 11. The sponsor of the study that is designed to be an adequate and well-controlled investigation is not actively pursuing marketing approval of the investigational drug with due diligence. 12. The Commissioner determines that it would not be in the public interest for the study to be conducted or continued.

VIII. SUBSEQUENT SUBMISSIONS TO AN IND

After submission of an initial IND and its acceptance by the FDA, the sponsor's effort to develop the drug continues, leading to collection of new information and the need to submit this information to the FDA. The FDA must be kept informed of the evolving, increasing scientific knowledge of the drug. The objectives of subsequent submissions to the IND are to maintain the IND in ongoing good regulatory standing, as well as to assure that new information is submitted to the FDA before action is initiated by the company. For example, implementation of a new facility for manufacturing drug product should be adequately documented and submitted to the FDA before initiation of use of resulting drug product in human studies governed by the IND.

The types of submissions to an established IND are as follows:

	Reference in Title 21
Protocol Amendments (new protocols, protocol amendments, new investigators, and changes in investigators)	21 CFR 312.30
Information Amendments	21 CFR 312.31
Response to FDA Request for Information	
IND Safety Reports	21 CFR 312.32
IND Annual Reports	21 CFR 312.33
Response to Clinical Hold	21 CFR 312.42 (e and f)
General Correspondence (e.g., request for a meeting)	

These submissions are required by the IND regulations in order to assure that the sponsor provides the FDA, on an ongoing basis with diligence, with new information as it becomes available on the investigational drug. The FDA's criteria for review of these subsequent submissions are essentially the same criteria as applied to the initial IND, i.e.:

> Submissions continue to build logically on the base of scientific information about the drug.
> Submissions support the conclusion that humans will not be exposed to unreasonable or significant risk.
> The evolving clinical plan or new protocol must be adequate in design to meet its stated objectives.

IX. SUMMARY

The IND process for novel investigational drugs gives the sponsor the opportunity to prepare a logical and integrated collection of scientific information to support the first clinical investigation under the IND. After submission and acceptance of the initial IND, the IND process gives the sponsor the opportunity to build logically and efficiently on the knowledge base about the drug so that subsequent clinical investigations will continue to be justified on the basis of this growing knowledge base. As the investigational process continues, the sponsor must continue to coordinate parallel, integrated development in each of the technical disciplines of drug development (i.e., clinical; statistical; chemistry, manufacturing, and controls; nonclinical pharmacology and toxicology; human pharmacokinetics and bioavailability; and microbiology). Such integrated growth of knowledge in each of these technical disciplines is a logical means to lead to construction of an approvable New Drug Application.

REFERENCES

1. Final rule. New drug, antibiotic, and biologic drug product regulations ("IND rewrite"). Fed Reg 1987; 52(53):8798–8857.
2. Food and Drug Administration. Guidance for industry: content and format of investigational new drug applications (INDs) for Phase 1 studies of drugs, including well-characterized, therapeutic, biotechnology-derived products. Washington, DC: Food and Drug Administration, U.S. Department of Health, Education, and Welfare, November 1995.
3. Goldenthal EI. Current views on safety evaluation of drugs. FDA Papers 1968 (May):13–19.
4. General Considerations for the Clinical Evaluation of Drugs. Washington, DC: Food and Drug Administration, U.S. Department of Health, Education and Welfare, September 1977.
5. General Considerations for the Clinical Evaluation of Drugs in Infants and Children. Washington, DC: Food and Drug Administration, U.S. Department of Health, Education and Welfare, September 1977.
6. Traina VM. The role of toxicology in drug research and development. Med Res Rev 1983; 3:43–72.
7. Hoyle PC, Cooper EC. Nonclinical toxicity studies of antiviral drugs indicated for the treatment of non-life-threatening diseases: evaluation of drug toxicity prior to Phase I clinical studies. Regulatory Toxicol Pharmacol 1990; 11:81–89.
8. Scales MDC, Mahoney K. Animal toxicology studies on new medicines and their relationship to clinical exposure: a review of international recommendations. Adverse Drug React Toxicol Rev 1991; 10:155–168.
9. Cartwright AC, Matthews BR, eds. International Pharmaceutical Product Registration: Aspects of Quality, Safety and Efficacy. London: Ellis Horwood, 1994:411–552.
10. LD50 test policy: notice. Fed Reg 1988; 53:39650–39651.

4

Performance and Interpretation of Laboratory Tests

W. Leigh Thompson*
Eli Lilly and Company, Indianapolis, Indiana

Rocco L. Brunelle
Eli Lilly and Company, Indianapolis, Indiana

Michael G. Wilson
Michael G. Wilson and Company, Inc., New Palestine, Indiana

Symptoms, signs, and laboratory tests are the inputs to health decisions about prognosis, diagnosis, and treatment. The quality with which they are elicited and interpreted limits the quality of health decisions.

Symptoms are God's reminders to visit your physician or modify your behavior. Symptoms are elicited from patients or their companions, and a skilled practitioner knows not only what questions to ask, but in what order, with what flavoring, and with careful observation of the nonverbal and verbal responses.

Signs are detected by the health practitioner using her or his five primary senses: seeing a rash, hearing a murmur, feeling the pulse, smelling the fetor hepaticus of liver failure, and tasting the sweet urine of a patient with diabetes mellitus. The best practitioners have a sixth sense, poorly defined, that the patient is sick or dying, that the patient is recovering, or that the patient is faking. When a nurse with this sixth sense tells a physician that the patient is going sour, a bright physician hastens to patientside.

God provided us with a few sensors for a narrow bandwidth of energy spectra more suitable for living than diagnosing. Our elegant eye–brain visual system, which can detect the subtle yellowing of jaundice under the tongue, has been supplemented with shorter-wavelength detectors of Röntgen rays, magnetic resonance imaging (MRI) detectors of electron spin in radio frequency fields,

---

* Retired

and longer-wavelength infrared detectors of thermography and the echoes of ultrasound. The skin's limitation to direct vision has been supplemented with fiber optic extenders into our innermost secrets.

Our 20- to 20,000-Hz ears, which can hear a subtle murmur in a neonate, have been supplemented by ultrasonic visualizers of fetal heartbeats.

Our temperature receptors, which feel fever, are supplemented by precise trends in core and surface temperatures.

Our touch receptors, which detect an erratic pulse, have been supplemented by noninvasive monitors of blood circulation and gas transport.

Our olfactory and gustatory chemoreceptors, which modulate our diet and detect diabetes mellitus from urine taste, have been supplemented by a host of microchemical reactions that can measure many chemicals, even a single gene, in biological samples taken from the body, sampled via intrusive needles, or soon through noninvasive glucose sensors worn like a watch.

Formerly it took decades to hone the skills of the expert clinician, who, like Sherlock Holmes, could amaze with her online integration of subtle symptoms and expertly elicit signs to elaborate an elegant differential diagnosis, progress through a sophisticated decision tree, and focus on the proper decisions about prognosis and disease management.

Today a clerk can report that the computer signaled that the patient's blood serum bilirubin concentration reported value is, in someone's estimate, abnormal. The training, experience, expertise, and patientside time of the clinician that was formerly revered has been complemented by highly reimbursed laboratory tests that properly supplement but sometimes supplant that clinician's intellect.

Perhaps because these tests can be counted and accounted with imagined precision, they have become the reimbursement scaffolding that seems to replace both physicians and patients in formulating diagnoses (e.g., hyponatremia) or treatment (e.g., a limit of 4 days inpatient care with no more than two sodium measurements per day). Older clinicians will remember when health decisions were made by those who touched, saw, heard, smelled, and tasted the patient directly, not vicariously or vacuously.

In 1769, James Watt patented the steam engine that began the industrial revolution. Objects that had been handmade with parts finely honed to fit together perfectly were now stamped out of machines that made interchangeable parts. Workers too became interchangeable as their tasks were simplified so that they did not need to speak a common language, require training, or learn to understand more than the simple repetitive task they did amidst time–motion and other efficiency studies.

Medicine withstood the industrial revolution for two centuries, continuing as a cottage industry *feeforsaurus*. Today, laboratory tests are just part of the managed-care race to the industrial revolution of medicine, where customers (patients) have interchangeable parts and workers (physicians and nurses) are dumbed down to simple tasks described by numerical codes. Imagine Sir William Osler performing a 17.3 (office visit routine) or Halsted describing his mastectomy procedure as a 376 and racing to discharge every such patient in 3 days.

Let us consider how to interpret laboratory tests, individually and multidimensionally, and how the astute clinician braids them with symptoms and signs into an elegant relevance diagram (the linear transform of an exponential decision tree) to enhance the quality of health decisions, refine prognostic divinations, and formulate a health plan with the patient.

Sample identification: Everyone considers the linkage of the patient sample with the identification of the patient, the date and time of sampling, the bodily source of the sample, the processing and transport of that sample, the date and time of analysis, and the technique used in analysis. Fewer consider the position of the patient, prior food or exercise and meals, the duration of tourniquet ischemia, circadian or menstrual cycles, prior medications, or subtle lysis of or leakage from blood cells and platelets. Repeating a sample with an unusual test result, perhaps with a few confirmatory tests and observations, can help validate the legitimacy and consistency of the original observation or spark an inquiry into errors and neglected factors. Miracles do occur, but less frequently than laboratory error (1,2).

Test performance: Imagine that you just discovered your ability to quantify the concentration of myocardial actin elements (MACE) in blood serum with a noninvasive ray gun and you wish to adjust the red and green lights on the ray gun so that red will indicate myocardial ischemia and green will indicate no ischemia. Your first concern may be sensitivity. Should your settings be such that only very severe ischemia is indicated, or do you wish to include mild ischemia as well? Using a ''gold standard,'' such as following closely the course of typical patients with all the standard tests, you discover a range of settings from high levels that only turn red for the most severe ischemia to low levels that turn red for many patients who do not have ischemia. Sensitivity (true positive rate) is the fraction of patients with a condition (such as ischemia) who have a positive test (the red light turns on). In terms of true (T) and false (F) positive (P) and negative (N) test results, sensitivity is $TP/(TP + FN)$. You might find a red light setting that made your test pathognomonic with no false positives—if the red light is on, the patient is certain to have ischemia by gold standard tests (3,4).

Specificity (true negative rate) is your other concern. Specificity is the fraction of patients without the condition who have a negative test: $TN/(TN + FP)$. If patients with a red light are immediately injected with an expensive and dangerous drain opener or have a rotorooter procedure, you may wish to minimize false positive tests.

A graphical representation of sensitivity and specificity on a single test that is commonly used is taken from radio receiver operating characteristic curves (ROC) in which noise (1 − specificity) is on the abscissa and signal (sensitivity) on the ordinate (5). The upper left (0,1) is perfect sensitivity and specificity—all positive tests indicate the condition and all patients with the condition have a positive test. If the test has no ability to discriminate between patients with and without the condition, the characteristics of the test are a straight line from lower left (0,0) to upper right (1,1). Most tests, characteristics describe an upwardly convex curve above the diagonal and a point may be selected (defining the TP, TN, FP, and FN proportions) for desired performance.

For your MACE assay you would test many patients with very diverse characteristics and health conditions with your ray gun and with all the conventional gold standard tests to construct the ROC curve of your device. Then you would consider which operating point on the ROC curve to select for switching from a green to red light.

If a false negative sends the patient home to die of myocardial infarction, you might want a very sensitive test. But if false positives lead to expensive, dangerous treatments, you might want a more selective point. There is no perfect answer to adjusting the cost–quality function of a test, but the test cannot be considered in isolation from the patients to whom it is applied and the decisions that will be conditioned by the test result.

Pretest probability of the condition being diagnosed should be considered as well. Suppose you find your MACE ray gun to have an excellent ROC with a point that has sensitivity and specificity of 0.98. Suppose you used it to screen the first 1000 patients entering your emergency department. If this population has a prevalence of myocardial ischemia of 0.1%, then your test is 98% certain of detecting the one patient with myocardial ischemia, but your red light would also brighten for 20 other patients who do not have this condition. Would your test seem better if it were applied only to patients with chest pain, or to patients with chest pain plus an abnormal electrocardiogram?

Information theory and Bayes' law best describe the value of one or a group of laboratory tests. If the probability of the patient having the disease or condition before testing (pretest probability) is 0 or 1, the test adds no value to the classification of that patient and thereby imparts no useful information for the purpose of classification. In information theory, the test has 0 bits of information.

If the test alone provides perfect information to classify the patient, it contains 1 bit of information. The extent by which the test reduces uncertainty about the classification can be expressed as a fraction of one bit of information. Shannon and Weaver (6) developed this information theory as an expression of the information and noise in an audio signal transmitted via telephone.

The information content of a test in an individual patient can be calculated from the probability of the patient having disease before the test [$p(D+)$], the true positive rate or the probability of a positive test given that the patient has disease [$p(T+|D+)$], and the false positive rate [$p(T+|D-)$]. Informational content is 0 when $p(D+)$ is 0 or 1 and reaches a peak at some intermediate p(D+).

George Diamond et al. (7) derived the equations for calculation of information content of diagnostic tests and showed how the average information content and its variance can be calculated over a population of patients.

Diamond et al. applied information theory to the ST segment depression on an exercise test in a population of patients who later had coronary artery disease determined by angiography (their gold standard). In an ordinal (categorical)-scale analysis they segregated responses by ST depression: 0.5 or more, 1.0 or more, etc. The information content of this test was greatest near a pretest probability of 50%, determined from symptoms, where there was maximum uncertainty about classification of the patient before applying the test. Even so, considering all patients given the test, the average information content was only 0.11 bit. Had the test been perfect for this population of patients, the average information content would have been 0.72 bit.

They also performed a compartmental analysis in which each ST segment was analyzed on a continuous scale rather than solely in classes such as 0.5 or greater. Such continuous-scale analysis increased informational content by 41%. For example, in a patient with a pretest probability of 0.5, a positive ST segment depression of 1.0 mm or more increased the probability of coronary artery disease to 0.81 overall, but if the depression were negative (less than 1.0 mm), the posttest probability was reduced to 0.29. See how this can easily demonstrate the test value to a patient and be used to calculate the cost-effectiveness of this test.

Categorical analysis using the actual ST depression further sharpened the informational content. A positive ST depression led to a posttest probability of 0.68 for 1.0-mm depression to 0.98 for 2.5-mm depression. Similarly a negative ST depression led to posttest probabilities of 0.19 for 0-mm depression to 0.48 for 0.5-mm depression.

The importance of pretest probability cannot be overemphasized. In this study, Diamond et al. (7) found that the ECG stress test contained 0.05 bit of information when applied to asymptomatic patients (with a pretest probability of 4.5%), as compared with 0.28 bit when applied to patients with atypical angina (pretest probability 49.9%). One might conclude that in routine testing of asymptomatic patients in a clinical trial, the informational content of all those tests would be at a minimum and their cost–benefit therefore problematical.

Sometimes diagnostic tests are described by likelihood ratio. This is the ratio of true positive rate to false positive rate. It neglects prevalence of disease and is not weighted for the frequency of occurrence of the observation. In some cases it correlates negatively with information content and therefore is a misleading tool (7). Combining the results of multiple tests to provide a discriminant function may enhance sensitivity and specificity. A combination of serum concentrations of bilirubin, gamma glutamyltransferase, alkaline phosphatase, alanine aminotransferase, and aspartate aminotransferase will sharpen the discrimination of patients with clinically significant liver dysfunction from those without. With modern numerical methods, many functions can be explored for different patient classes. One function might minimize false positives and negatives when applied to Caucasian men who are more than 50 years old and who claim not to smoke or drink ethanol. Another function might be found to be better for other patient groups.

Thus tests should not be considered in isolation. Patient characteristics may change your operating point that switches from expected to notable, prevalence must be considered, and combinations of tests may be more informative than individual tests.

Now let us focus on the use of laboratory tests in clinical trials in which outcomes of patients are related to different classifications (e.g., diagnoses or strata) or different interventions (e.g., placebo and experimental therapies). We would employ laboratory tests (8), as well as signs and symptoms, in six ways:

1. To select patients for inclusion in a trial
2. To exclude from the trial patients who might be unsuitable
3. To prehoc stratify patients into groups expected to have differences in outcomes
4. To protect patients during the trial if signals indicated the need for a change in treatment
5. To detect unexpected consequences of treatment
6. To assess outcomes themselves

Inclusion criteria should be considered carefully in any trial. The definition of those included may be narrowed to minimize variability, but this also restricts generalization of the results. If you study drug kinetics in young, healthy, Caucasian, nonobese men who do not smoke, drink, exercise, or abuse drugs while they are eating a defined regular diet and have only normal routine blood and urine chemistry laboratory test results, will these observations help you select doses to use in a population of patients who actually use your new drug? If you are testing a drug for treatment of anemia, should all patients have a blood hemoglobin concentration less than 10 g/L, or should menstruating women have blood hemoglobin concentrations less than 9 g/L, or should all patients have blood hemoglobin concentrations less than those expected in 99% of healthy patients of similar age, gender, race, smoking, and ethanol drinking habits?

Exclusion of patients who will die, disappear, or be removed from a trial before its conclusion will minimize concerns about analyzing results in such patients together with those that complete the trial. Thus patients with test results suggesting drug or ethanol abuse, pregnancy, metastatic cancer, or other rapidly lethal conditions might be excluded.

Likewise, patients with chronic diseases that fluctuate in intensity may be excluded if exacerbations of the concomitant disease may be confused with effects of the illness being studied or its treatment. Thus, patients with chronic active hepatitis might be excluded, lest exacerbation of this illness be confused with liver toxicity of a treatment.

However, one may not wish to exclude healthy elderly, young, or obese subjects or those with stable diseases unlikely to confound your observations, to ensure that your results can be generalized to most of the population of patients to apply your recommended prognoses or treatments.

Prehoc stratification is a powerful tool that should be considered in any trial. Random allocation attempts to distribute patients evenly among groups so they are otherwise comparable in all characteristics except those you use to define the groups (e.g., active drug or placebo).

If you can predict characteristics that you expect to correlate with the outcome of interest, then proactively, prospectively ensure that patients with these characteristics are distributed evenly among the groups. Thus in treating an illness you might prehoc stratify on the severity or duration of the illness at intake and, if age or gender or both might affect outcome, you could also stratify on those characteristics.

During a period of observation of any patients, some will develop illness that requires special attention. Patient safety can be improved if, in addition to symptoms about which you have instructed the patient, signs are assessed at periodic physical examinations, and laboratory tests are employed at appropriate intervals.

Active treatments and placebos will cause adverse events that are undesired and often unexpected. Are such events causally related to treatment or assignment of patients to groups, or are they unrelated to your protocol and manifestations of concomitant drugs, behaviors, and illnesses? Such events should be well characterized by careful assessment of signs, symptoms, and laboratory test results over their duration so that similar events can be clustered and alternative causation explored.

Sometimes laboratory test results may themselves define the outcomes of interest. Treatment of diabetes mellitus might be defined by the concentration of glycosylated hemoglobin or treatment of moderately severe depression might be defined by the score of the Hamilton Depression Scale.

In any of these uses, one must assess which test results are usually expected and which are notable. Epidemiologically one might assess a symptom, sign, or test result in a well-characterized population of subjects and describe the distribution of results.

Scales: For a dichotomous scale variable there may be a binomial result—present or absent. Thus, all the population might be found to have a detectable heartbeat. A classification scale would assign subjects to discrete sets such as blonde, brunette, or red-haired. For an ordinal-scale variable you might assign continuous or discontinuous numerical values in which the ratios of values are not meaningful: $+$, $++$, $+++$. A ratio scale has a defined zero and ratios among values are meaningful. A patient who loses from 160 to 140 pounds has the same proportional weight loss as one who goes from 120 to 105 pounds.

How precise must be your measurement? Would you count the pulse until you could assert a heart rate of 72.6 min^{-1}? In this case, you palpate many heart beats not to achieve precision in defining the rate but to detect the infrequent abnormal beat. If you feel only 100 heartbeats, you have a 95% probability of detecting at least one abnormal beat if abnormal beats make up 3% or more of all heartbeats.

If you measured heart rates in many patients, how would you describe the distribution of heart rates in your population? Perhaps there would be many between 65 and 75 min^{-1}. There might be a few less than 35 min^{-1} and a few greater than 130 min^{-1}. For many biological variables the distribution approximates a mathematical function described by Gauss and often called the normal distribution.

Close examination of most variables will show that this approximation is a poor fit in the tails of the distribution, partly because living beings are more unusual than the Gaussian function would predict and partly because samples may include members from other populations.

If one is interested only in the central tendency of the distribution, the mean, median, or mode, then the tails are relatively less important.

In medicine and in clinical trials, however, it is the unusual observation that is of greatest interest. We are less concerned about patients with relatively low levels of liver test results, but we are intensely interested in those with unusually high levels. Unfortunately, our statistics generally address the center of distributions and we are unaccustomed to tests that define whether just the tails fit a Gaussian curve or how to test just the tails. In a clinical trial of a new diuretic you might ask whether the mean serum urate concentration is different among the treatment groups, but a more important observation might be of patients with high urate concentrations.

Because we often lack sufficient observations to test whether the tails fit a mathematical function precisely, it is best to use nonparametric tests.

Modern numerical methods using computers provide sophisticated distribution-free analyses of the tails of distributions and help us define notable observations as distinguished from expected observations.

Most laboratories will provide a reference range for their tests (9,10). Many assume that this range will include 95% of healthy subjects. But how is health defined? Often these are observations of a few young, Caucasian, nonobese males who do not smoke, drink ethanol, or abuse drugs. Unusual values from this sample may be censored just because they are several standard deviations from the mean and make the curve messy. In one case we found the reference range to be constructed from eight employees, but the results from one were censored.

Errors in defining reference ranges or alert values can greatly complicate a large clinical trial. The average New Drug Application to the Food and Drug

Administration contains about 573,000 laboratory test results—the sponsor might be evaluating thousands of results each day.

For a more useful reference range in clinical-trial patients, we examined routine laboratory test results of 5560 consecutive patients, withdrawn from prior therapies, who were attempting to qualify for trials of hypertension, cardiac dysrhythmia, or peptic ulcer (1).

Reference ranges of the major central laboratory that performed all the assays were said to exclude 2.5% of healthy subjects in each tail. But in this sample, only 4 of 36 analyte distributions defined 1.25% to 3.75% of the values as falling beyond the reference ranges.

In examining a large number of published reference ranges for routine analytes, we could not find any that reliably predicted the outliers for our populations of patients.* Therefore, we defined clinical-trial candidate reference ranges using 20,102 patients similar to those described above (2). This population resembled closely the general U.S. population, as 54.9% were female (U.S., 52.8%), 78.2% were Caucasian (U.S., 84.1%), 59.8% were less than 50 years old (U.S., 67.4%), 64.5% said they were nonsmokers (U.S., 70.2%), and 51.5% said they did not imbibe (U.S., 59.2%). These values were collected from two large well-known central laboratories by Patrick J. Simpson and Randy L. Walker of Eli Lilly and Company (1,2). The first and 99th percentile values for each of 36 analytes are shown in Appendix A at the end of this text.

Then we tested to see if any patient characteristics influenced the distribution of analyte results. It is known, for example, that hemoglobin concentrations are smaller in women, low neutrophil counts are more common in blacks, and men have higher concentrations of creatinine, urate, gamma-glutamyltransferase, and urea. Rocco L. Brunelle, Michael G. Wilson, and Gregory G. Enas of Eli Lilly and Company (1,2) performed Brown-Mood tests to see if patient characteristics influenced the proportion of patients segregated into the tails of the analyte values. For 39 blood and urine analytes, significant ($p < .05$) differences were found in 50% of the tails (<1% and >99%) of distributions according to gender (male or female), 46% according to race (Caucasian or other), 47% according to age (<50, >49 years), 39% by smoking (current by history, yes or no), and 36% by ethanol consumption (recent by history, yes or no). In many cases, the differences were quite large (12).

For example, the upper 99th percentile for gamma-glutamyltransferase is 94 U/L in Caucasian men over 49 years of age who smoke but deny drinking

---

* Subsequent to our initial publications, approved guidelines for the definition and determination of reference ranges were published by the National Committee for Clinical Laboratory Standards in 1995 (11). That work of the EPTRV proved to be a most useful basis for the development of the NCCLS guidelines. Basically, the a-posteriori method as described by the NCCLS protocol guideline was the methodology employed to construct our ranges.

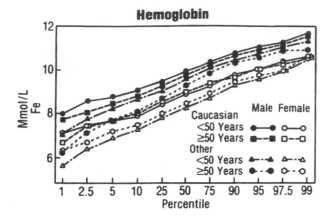

Figure 1 Blood hemoglobin concentrations in 20,102 subjects applying for clinical trials on a probability plot in which a Gaussian distribution is linear. Eight demographic groups are shown.

ethanol and 460 U/L in similar patients who are non-Caucasian and admit to imbibing ethanol. Similar creatinine kinase activities upper tails vary from 218 U/L in young Caucasian women who smoke but do not drink to 2770 U/L in young non-Caucasian men who smoke and drink.

Consider the distribution of blood hemoglobin concentrations. This illustration shows a Gaussian probability distribution on the abscissa. On this scale, a

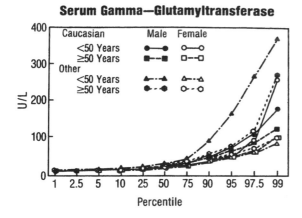

Figure 2 Blood serum gamma—glutamyltransferase activities in subjects applying for clinical trial. Gaussian distributions would be linear. Note that few of these values are within textbook reference ranges for this analyte.

Gaussian distribution would be a straight line. Note that hemoglobin values are relatively Gaussian throughout. Also note that values tend to be greater in males and non-Caucasian subjects. Because the sample was drawn from hundreds of investigators throughout the United States, these hemoglobin measurements reflect some subjects living at relatively high altitudes and some who were not excluded by a history or signs and symptoms of anemia or polycythemia from participating in this initial blood sampling to qualify for a clinical trial. Clearly these patients are not a healthy population, but they may be representative of ambulatory subjects who are not seriously ill and who are volunteering for participation in a clinical trial.

Contrast this with the distribution of activities of serum gamma-glutamyl-transferase. Obviously, the higher values are not described well by Gaussian statistics. Probably some of these patients have values influenced by imbibing ethanol. Serum creatinine kinase distributions are similar.

Neutrophil concentrations are not Gaussian. Note the S curves on this probability distribution. Also observe that non-Caucasians (mostly blacks in this population) have distinctly lower neutrophil counts at the lower tail.

The effects of age on the serum creatinine concentrations is apparent especially in non-Caucasians.

Thus, it is prudent to use reference ranges from a population of patients that resemble your individual patient. To this end, we (2) constructed 32 reference ranges for dichotomized values of gender, race, age, smoking, and drinking ethanol as described above. These are used routinely by many laboratories and regula-

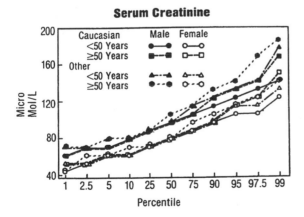

Figure 3 Serum creatinine concentration in 20,102 consecutive patients applying for participation in clinical trials. No patient values were censored. Older patients have higher values of creatinine.

Neutrophils

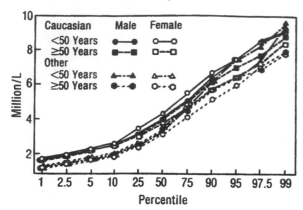

Figure 4 Blood neutrophil counts in an uncensored population of patients applying for clinical trials. Non-Caucasians, mostly Blacks, have lower neutrophil counts which may be confused with neutropenia.

tors in defining notable versus expected analyte values. The first and 99th percentile values for the 32 demographic groups are reprinted in Appendixes B to E. Almost all of these tests were performed in adults. The difficulty of establishing pediatric reference ranges has been emphasized (13,14).

Are 1% tails suitable? Remember, you are trying to identify notable results. In this reference population we can predict what proportion of patients will have notable results using the 1% and 99% tails. If the analyte results are not correlated, we would identify $1 - (.98)^{36} = 52\%$ of patients as having one or more notable values. If we repeated the observations at five intervals, and the results were not correlated, we would identify 97% of patients as having one or more notable values.

Are the first and 99th percentiles appropriate for panic values that lead to immediate notification of the investigator and sponsor? Probably not. Kost (15) surveyed U.S. medical centers to establish a consensus of critical values for urgent clinician notification.

Reference ranges describe one measurement in a defined population. But what of intraindividual variation between repeated measurements? To estimate this, we sampled 3556 patients from the population above who had duplicate samples drawn at intervals of 1–2 weeks (1). The largest 1% of decrements and increments between paired samples were called delta limits. These were not found to be related to the patient characteristics. The delta limits (2) are reprinted in the appendixes. You may find them a useful standard against which to compare intraindividual variation in your clinical trial patients.

At the start of a trial, one might exclude patients with underlying liver dysfunction by excluding any with five liver test values exceeding the 99th percentile for that patient's demographic group. You would expect a positive correlation among these analytes and therefore you would exclude less than 5% of your population. If you were willing to exclude up to 10% of your applicants, you might also exclude those with creatinine kinase and creatinine values that exceed the 99th percentile and those with neutrophil, platelet, or erythrocyte values that fall below the first percentile.

During the course of your patients' participation in the protocol, routine laboratory values that fall outside the reference values for the demographic group or changes in analyte values since baseline that fall outside the delta limits can be flagged for special observation. If significantly more patients in one treatment group have notable values for an analyte, that suggests a causal relationship should be explored.

We prefer to monitor continuously the proportion of test results after baseline that fall outside the appropriate reference range or delta limit for each treatment group. We also group all five liver tests and examine only the high values, all five kidney tests, etc., and monitor the proportion of patient liver tests after baseline notable by reference range or delta limit for each study group. Thus a patient with very abnormal liver test values would have 10 values entered, but a patient with one isolated high test value would have only one or two entries. If there is a significant difference among groups, this deserves further analysis.

Another test among groups is to rank for each analyte the most extreme values observed after baseline and the most extreme change from baseline. Thus the largest serum bilirubin concentration, either as a concentration or transformed into a percentile for that patient's demographic group, would be assigned a rank of 1. Then sum these ranks across all five liver tests. The patient who had the worse liver tests and changes in tests might have a summed rank as small as 10. Test the distribution among groups of these summed ranks for the top 5% of patients. If the summed ranks in the group given a new drug are significantly smaller (more extreme) than those in the group given placebo, then a causal relationship should be explored.

What is three times the upper limit of normal? Is this thrice the upper limit of a reference range? This point is just an arbitrary large value. No patient would survive a serum sodium twice the upper limit of normal, but a creatinine kinase or gamma-glutamyltransferase thrice normal is common. A limit might be more useful as the point that would be exceeded by only one in one thousand "usual" subjects.

REFERENCES

1. Thompson WL, Brunelle RL, Enas GG, Simpson PJ. Routine laboratory tests in clinical trials: interpretation of results. J Clin Res Drug Devel 1987; 1:95–119.

2. Thompson WL, Brunelle RL, Enas GG, Simpson PJ, Walker RL. Routine Laboratory Tests in Clinical Trials. Indianapolis, IN: Eli Lilly, 1990:1–63.
3. Thompson WL. Decision Quality for Health Professionals, Patients, and Managed Care. Indianapolis, IN: Eli Lilly, 1993:1–144.
4. Barnett RN. Medical significance of laboratory results. Am J Clin Pathol 1968; 50: 671–676.
5. Metz CE, Goodenough DJ, Rossman K. Evaluation of receiver operating characteristic curve data in terms of information theory, with applications in radiology. Radiology 1973; 109:297–306.
6. Shannon EC, Weaver W. The Mathematical Theory of Communication. Chicago: University of Illinois Press, 1949.
7. Diamond GA, Hirsch M, Forrester JS, Staniloff HM, Vas R, Halpern SW, Swan HJC. Application of information theory to clinical diagnostic testing. The electrocardiographic stress test. Circulation 1981; 63:915–921.
8. Wallach JB. Interpretation of Diagnostic Tests. 7th ed. Philadelphia: Lippincott Williams & Wilkins, 2000.
9. Solberg HE, PetitClerc C, Dybkoer R. Approved recommendation (1986) on the theory of reference values (parts I–VI). J Clin Chem Clin Biochem 1987; 25:337–342, 639–644, 645–656, 657–662, and 1988; 26:593–598.
10. Galen RS, Gambino SR. Beyond Normality: The Predictive Value and Efficiency of Medical Diagnoses. New York: Wiley, 1975.
11. Sasse EA, Aziz KJ, Harris EK, Krishnamurthy S, Lee HT, Ruland A, Seamonds B. How to Define and Determine Reference Intervals in the Clinical Laboratory; Approved Guideline. Villanova, PA: National Committee for Clinical Laboratory Standards, pub. C28-A, 1995.
12. Wilson MG. Lilly Reference Ranges. In: Chow S-C, ed. Encyclopedia of Biopharmaceutical Statistics. New York: Marcel Dekker, 2000.
13. Burritt MF, Slockbower JM, Forsman RW, Offord KP, Bergstralh EJ, Smithson WA. Pediatric reference intervals for 19 biologic variables in healthy children. Mayo Clin Proc 1990; 65:329–336.
14. Whitley RJ. Reference values in pediatric medicine (editorial). Mayo Clin Proc 1990; 65:431–435.
15. Kost GJ. Critical limits for urgent clinician notification at U.S. medical centers. JAMA 1990; 263:704–707.

5
Issues in Endpoint Selection

Karen D. Weiss
Center for Biologics Evaluation and Research, United States Food and Drug Administration, Rockville, Maryland

Jay Philip Siegel
Center for Biologics Evaluation and Research, United States Food and Drug Administration, Rockville, Maryland

I. INTRODUCTION

The goal of any clinical trial is to yield valuable and reliable scientific information that can ultimately guide medical practice. To that end, appropriate attention to study design, including the selection of reasonable and relevant trial endpoints, is essential for success. Trial endpoints are events or measurements that reflect the effects of an intervention on the study participants. Most trials are designed to collect data on many different endpoints, the nature and number of which will depend on the condition or disease of the individuals who are in the study, the anticipated pharmacological and toxic effects of the intervention, and the objective of the clinical investigation. In the initial studies, where safety and dosing information is of prime interest, study endpoints usually are measurements of pharmacokinetics and safety. In later clinical development, there is growing emphasis on evaluation of activity and, ultimately, efficacy. Efficacy is generally evaluated by using adequate and well-controlled clinical trials designed to show that the intervention meaningfully affects the trial's efficacy endpoints.

Efficacy endpoints either directly characterize the clinical benefits of the intervention or are surrogates believed to predict clinical benefit. The choice of efficacy endpoints involves selection of an outcome measure, determination of when and how to measure it, and determination of how to analyze the results. These choices have profound effects on the success of a trial.

II. DESIRABLE CHARACTERISTICS OF ENDPOINTS

Several characteristics should be considered when selecting an endpoint. An endpoint should be *feasible* to measure, meaning that it should be possible to obtain the endpoint measure in all or nearly all subjects. Factors such as the following may result in endpoint data being missing from a substantial number of patients:

> Patients may refuse to consent to the endpoint measuring procedure.
> Patients may die or withdraw before endpoint measurement.
> Patients may miss the critical visit for endpoint measurement.
> Technical problems may invalidate some data.

Missing data may substantially reduce the ability to draw valid inferences from a trial; appropriate selection of an endpoint can reduce the amount of missing data and its effect on the study.

An endpoint should be *sensitive* to the desired effects of the interventions under study. Selection of an endpoint sensitive to the hypothesized differences in treatment effects between the experimental and control arms will increase the likelihood of demonstrating a difference (i.e., power) or decrease the size of study required to demonstrate a difference.

An endpoint should be *clinically meaningful*. In general, an endpoint should be a direct measure of an important benefit to patients, such as longer survival, less pain, or improved physical functioning. Endpoints based on scoring systems should be validated to ensure they reflect true clinical benefit. Endpoints that do not directly measure benefit (e.g., laboratory tests, x-rays) are of value as primary efficacy measures only when they correlate with and predict clinical benefit.

It is desirable that an endpoint be one whose meaning can be *readily communicated* to those who will receive the results of the trial. Communication of the results of a trial and the nature and magnitude of a drug effect, whether in a manuscript, a presentation, or a package label, is easier if endpoints have a readily understood clinical meaning (e.g., percentage survival at 1 year), than if alternative endpoints are used (e.g., an unfamiliar scoring system). Selection of endpoints that are readily communicated potentially can enhance the impact of a trial on medical practice.

It is desirable that an endpoint be *objective*, particularly in trials in which subjects or investigators may be unblinded or in which the study treatment has unblinding effects. Many factors may introduce bias into the assessment of an endpoint that is subjectively assessed by patients or assessors; objective endpoints reduce bias.

III. MEASUREMENTS AND EVENTS

Some endpoints assess events, while others provide a measurement of an outcome. Events occur at a specific point in time and their assessment is binary, i.e., either the event has occurred or it has not. Examples of events are death, stroke, cure of infection, progression to AIDS, myocardial infarction, or a flare of asthma. In contrast, measurements have several or many potential values that may change over time. Examples of measurements include blood pressure, strength, weight, CD4+ cell count, tumor size, quality of life scored on a standard scale, and visual acuity. Several factors may affect the decision to use a measurement-based or an event-based endpoint. Measurements can detect a broad range of change in the outcome measure in each patient; therefore, measurement-based endpoints will often be more sensitive and yield greater power than event-based endpoints. Measurements, however, may detect very small changes, and therefore may raise more questions about clinical meaningfulness.

IV. CUTPOINTS

In clinical trials, measurements are sometimes turned into binary, eventlike endpoints through the establishment of one or more cutpoints. For example, rather than assessing the change in measurements of CD4+ cell count, weight, or visual acuity, one can assess the prevalence of a drop in CD4+ cell count below 200 cells/μL, a loss of at least 5 kg body weight, or improvement of vision by two lines on an eye chart. Such approaches generally sacrifice sensitivity because changes that do not involve crossing the cutpoint are ignored in the analysis.

Despite such loss of sensitivity, cutpoints are often used in an attempt to ensure that only clinically meaningful changes affect the endpoint. In determining what size of change to consider meaningful when creating a cutpoint, two separate considerations are relevant. First, because of the variability inherent in all measurements, one may wish to choose a size of change that has a high probability of reflecting real change rather than measurement variation. Second, one may wish to choose a size of change that indicates clear and meaningful clinical benefit.

With regard to the first consideration, that is, distinguishing real changes from measurement variation, it is important to note that a sufficiently large clinical trial may be able to detect real differences between treatment groups of a magnitude within the range of error or variation for individual measurements. For example, suppose that in a clinical trial of an antiretroviral agent for HIV infection, the plasma viral load, on average, remained unchanged in the control group and showed a twofold decrease in the treatment group. If a twofold change is within the measurement error of day-to-day variation of the measurement, one may not be able to determine for an individual patient in the treatment group whether the twofold decrease in level of viremia was a real drug effect. However, in a sufficiently large trial, statistical analysis may lead to the conclusion that the observed twofold difference between treatment groups was highly unlikely to arise by chance because of measurement error or day-to-day variation. One could therefore conclude that a true drug effect was demonstrated. Because statistical assessments may thus help distinguish small but real changes from measurement variation, it is generally not necessary to use cutpoints for this purpose.

As noted above, cutpoints and minimum change size may be used not only to ensure that observed changes do not arise from measurement error or random variation, but also to ensure that such changes are sufficiently large to indicate clear and meaningful clinical differences. One should note that although changes exceeding a specified size or crossing a specified value may be more meaningful than smaller changes, smaller but real changes often also provide some level of benefit. Where small changes imply small benefit, one should consider choosing the more sensitive endpoint (i.e., the endpoint that incorporates all changes) as the primary endpoint, reserving a cutpoint for use in secondary and exploratory analyses. When cutpoints are used in the primary analysis, supportive analyses that include analyses without cutpoints and analyses using other cutpoints will generally be of value.

V. LANDMARK AND SURVIVAL ANALYSES

A landmark analysis of an event endpoint assesses the proportion of patients in whom an event has occurred by a specific point in time. It does not take into account how soon before that time point the event occurred. This type of analysis is most appropriate when the time during the trial at which an endpoint occurs is of far less clinical significance than whether or not the endpoint occurs at all. Typically, this situation arises in relatively short trials in which the risk of an endpoint event potentially affected by the study intervention is largely limited to a short period after enrollment. Trials of treatments for acute sepsis syndrome and acute myocardial infarction often use landmark mortality at 28 or 30 days as a primary endpoint, thus essentially considering all deaths before this time point as equally bad outcomes.

A time-to-event analysis (frequently called a survival analysis, even when the endpoint does not involve mortality) takes into account the timing of an endpoint event (1). The outcome of a patient who experiences an adverse outcome event (e.g., death, tumor progression) early is considered (i.e., is ranked as) worse than that of a patient who experiences the event later.

An example of a trial with a time-to-event endpoint is the study of Avonex® (interferon beta-1a) in primary relapsing, remitting multiple sclerosis. The primary endpoint was the time to progression in disability (2). In this study, all subjects had some degree of disability at the onset, and all were expected to progress in disability eventually. Delay in the progression of disability was clinically meaningful and desirable.

Usually, time-to-event analyses are displayed graphically by using Kaplan-Meier survival methods, and nonparametric rank tests are used to test for differences between groups (3). These methods facilitate meaningful graphic presentation and analysis of survival data when the length of follow-up on patients enrolled early in the trial is substantially longer than the follow-up on patients enrolled more recently.

Although use of cutpoints may make a measurement-based endpoint more like an event, use of time-to-event analyses may make an event-based endpoint more like a measurement. For interventions that only delay events or that both delay and prevent events, a time-to-event analysis is likely to be more sensitive to differences in effect than a landmark analysis. However, particularly in short-term studies such as those described above, a time-to-event analysis may detect differences of little clinical meaning. Theoretically, for example, a new treatment that reduces mortality in an acute disease might appear inferior to the control group if the deaths in the treatment group occurred a few days earlier than the deaths in the control group.

When a landmark analysis is chosen for the primary endpoint, it is important that the time point selected for the analysis be late enough so that it captures most of the events potentially affected by the intervention(s), but not so late that many endpoint events (e.g., deaths) are captured that are likely unrelated to the disease or treatment under study. If the time point is too early, not only might sensitivity be lost, but also the validity and reproducibility of the endpoint findings may be impaired by the fact that minor variations in the time of occurrence of important, treatment-related events could result in the event not being counted at all.

Although a single analysis of the primary endpoint is desirable (see below), it is often advisable to plan prospectively and perform landmark analyses as well as time-to-event analyses at several time points. The results will usually correlate strongly; if they do not, the outcome data should be explored for unexpected relationships to time.

VI. RECURRENT EVENTS

For diseases manifested by recurring events, such as asthma with periodic attacks or multiple sclerosis with periodic relapses, and for treatments intended to reduce the frequency of such events, assessment of the frequency of recurrence of the primary endpoint event over the study period may be more useful than a time-to-event or landmark analysis. Not uncommonly, this is accomplished by counting the total number of events in each treatment group and dividing by the number of subjects or subject-years. However, the validity of this method rests on assumptions that often are incorrect, for example, the assumption that patients who have experienced a first event on study are no more or less likely to experience further events than are patients who have not experienced one. A few individuals in one treatment arm who experience multiple events could lead to erroneous conclusions about treatment effect. To avoid this phenomenon, it is usually more appropriate to analyze recurrent-event data by using ranks, that is, to rank outcomes from least desirable (i.e., most events) to most desirable (i.e., no events) and to evaluate groups by comparing ranks.

VII. MULTIPLICITY

Use of a single primary efficacy endpoint is generally desirable in Phase III trials. With increasing numbers of endpoints comes increasing concern regarding Type 1 error, that is, erroneously declaring that an endpoint was affected by the intervention. Type 1 error is particularly of concern in Phase III efficacy trial(s) in which the outcomes are intended to form the basis for establishing the product's efficacy and safety. A study with one primary endpoint is more likely to generate a straightforward analysis and therefore minimize ambiguity in interpreting the results. This type of study also often allows the trial to be more focused, simplifies the trial design and improves the power of the study.

In cases in which it is not known which efficacy outcome is most likely to reflect the drug effect or which efficacy effect is most clinically relevant for a new therapy in a specific disease setting, it is often useful to evaluate multiple efficacy endpoints in a Phase II trial. Although such a study may not give definitive results about the product's effect on each endpoint, the results may be used to identify the endpoint(s) most appropriate for Phase III testing.

If, in planning a Phase III trial, more than one clinical outcome is thought to be critical to the primary evaluation, several approaches are available to limit Type 1 error. Some approaches retain multiple primary endpoints with correct application of statistical tests that adjust for multiplicity and preserve overall Type 1 error rates (4–6). As a result of these adjustments, the effect on any one of the endpoints must be more definitive (i.e., larger in magnitude and associated with a lower nominal p value) to ensure statistical significance. Thus, when compared with selection of a single endpoint, these approaches to correcting for multiplicity generally reduce the power to observe a drug effect on each of the individual endpoints. Alternative approaches involve assessing multiple outcome variables as part of a single primary endpoint through use of a composite endpoint or a scoring scale, as described below.

VIII. COMPOSITE ENDPOINTS

A composite of several types of events may serve as a single endpoint in a clinical trial. For example, in persons who test HIV-positive, a commonly used endpoint has been progression to AIDS, defined as the occurrence of any one of several AIDS-defining illnesses (7). By including several types of events, a composite endpoint increases the likelihood that a subject will experience an endpoint event and avoids the problem of multiplicity. Thus, the power of the study is increased, and fewer study subjects are needed to show an effect of a given magnitude.

Results on composite endpoints are most readily interpretable when all components of the composite have similar levels of clinical impact and when any differences in effects between study treatments occur in the same direction for all components. If these conditions are not met, a small effect on a high-clinical-impact component of the composite, such as mortality, may be out-weighed in the analysis by a larger but less important effect on a relatively minor component of the composite, such as morbidity. Nonetheless, it is often not possible to satisfy these two conditions. Although the conditions are desirable, they are not requirements. Many composites include mortality or another event of singularly important clinical consequence together with less important events. Divergent effects on components may occur.

Weighting or ranking of components of the composite may be employed to compensate for the disparate clinical effect of the components, though neither weighting nor ranking is entirely satisfactory. Weighting outcomes involves subjectively assigning individual values according to each outcome's relative clinical effect. Ideally, the weighting method should be validated before use in an efficacy trial. Rank-ordering outcomes still requires some subjectivity, but often general consensus can be reached on a limited number of ranks (e.g., mortality, then survival with morbidity, then survival with no morbidity). Such ranking diminishes the likelihood that an effect on a less important outcome will outweigh an opposite effect on a more important outcome. However, ranking components only partially accounts for differences in impact; such ranking does not take into account differences in the degree of superiority of some ranks over other ranks or differences in the impact of outcomes within a rank.

Regardless of whether the components are weighted or ranked, an analysis should be undertaken showing how each component is affected by the intervention. This allows better understanding of the treatment effects, including an assessment of whether a benefit in one component has occurred at the expense of another component.

Another potential concern regarding the use of a composite endpoint is that the ability to communicate results may be impaired. It is relatively easy to communicate a finding of a statistically significant decrease in the incidence of a specific event, by giving the estimated effect size and confidence interval. In contrast, when a treatment causes a statistically significant decrease in the incidence of a composite of events, particularly with no clearly significant effect on the individual elements of the composite, it is harder to communicate the nature and extent of clinical benefits demonstrated.

In some settings, use of a composite endpoint offers the potential to diminish problems with missing data. In serious diseases, the ability of a therapy to affect the occurrence of a particular undesired event (e.g., end-stage renal failure, stroke, amputation), may be complicated substantially by the occurrence of a significant number of deaths before the endpoint is reached. By combining death with the undesired event in a composite endpoint, the patients who die would be counted as dying because of treatment failure, and a valid measure of clinical benefit may be able to be developed with fewer missing data. The EPIC trial comparing ReoPro® (abciximab), which is a platelet glycoprotein IIb/IIIa inhibitor, and placebo in prevention of ischemic complications in patients undergoing a percutaneous intervention successfully used a composite endpoint. The components were death, myocardial infarction, or an unplanned urgent revascularization procedure for recurrent cardiac ischemia. Mortality was very low in the trial and not different between treatment and control arms, but treatment-associated reduction in the incidence of the other components of the composite led to a positive result (8,9).

IX. SCALES AND INDICES

One type of outcome measure that frequently involves a composite of several events or measures is the use of a scale or index. Scales and indices used in clinical trials are generally disease-specific, such as the ACR20 for rheumatoid arthritis, the Expanded Disability Status Scale (EDSS) for multiple sclerosis, the National Institute of Health Stroke Scale (NIHSS), and the Crohn's Disease Activity Index (CDAI) (10–13). Most scales or indices comprise individual measures of physical or psychosocial function pertinent to the particular disease. Typically, a scoring system is developed that assigns points for each level of functioning achieved, usually on each of several outcome measures. The points are summed to derive a single numerical score. Thus, many scales and indices are weighted composites and carry the same potential cautions and advantages discussed above. Some scales have been subjected to rigorous validation in earlier studies, offering an advantage over some other composite endpoints. However, even if validated, a scale not in widespread clinical use may not communicate as readily the nature and degree of drug effect as would a single event or simpler composite.

As with other composite endpoints, when scales are used, it is often helpful to look at the effects of an intervention on the subparts of the scale or index to ascertain differential effects. Many scales and indices are a mixture of objective as well as subjective assessments. When the treatment has unblinding side effects, it is particularly reassuring if the more objective elements are affected in the same general manner as the more subjective components.

As described above for other measurement endpoints, scores on scales or indices may be analyzed as binary, eventlike endpoints by using cutpoints. This practice may help ensure that the findings are clinically meaningful, but may decrease the information, power, and sensitivity of the measurement. In the setting of acute stroke, trials are often conducted by using a dichotomized stroke scale in which complete or near-complete recovery is a success, and all other scores that indicate lesser degrees of recovery, including death, are failures.

A scale or index should be assessed to determine the extent to which patient scores are reproducible among different raters (interrater reliability). The usefulness of any scale or index to describe a given condition should be made in the context of the following features of validity.

> Criterion validity—How well does the test measure up to a generally accepted measure of patient outcome?
> Construct validity—How well does the test measure what it is supposed to measure?
> Content validity—How appropriate are the choice and weighting of each component of the scale/index/questionnaire?
> Face validity—Are the individual components assembled in an overall measure that makes sense?
> Discriminant validity—Can the test discern the smallest change that would appear clinically significant (14)?

Quality of life (QOL) assessments have gained considerable attention as endpoints in clinical trials, particularly for chronic disorders. QOL indices are usually based on questionnaires that patients or their caregivers answer over the course of the trial. Typically, assessments are made in each of several QOL domains that cover different aspects of physical and mental well-being. Because QOL may be influenced by many factors in addition to treatment and because assessments are subjective in nature, randomization and masking greatly facilitate making valid inferences about any results observed in a trial. The factors affecting QOL vary among diseases and treatments; therefore, disease-specific QOL questionnaires should be developed and validated for the particular disease being studied and, similarly, for any treatment adverse effects that may significantly affect QOL (15). The QOL scale should be sufficiently sensitive to the course of disease and the therapy to detect meaningful changes. The length and amount of detail in the QOL questionnaires should not be so great that compliance becomes an onerous task, for if this happens, the likelihood that the QOL questionnaires will be completed may decrease. Special care should be taken in the acquisition, analysis, and reporting of QOL data (15,16); a detailed discussion of these issues is beyond the scope of this chapter.

X. SURROGATE ENDPOINTS

Ideally, the primary efficacy endpoint(s) should be a direct measure of clinical benefit. Such endpoints are clinically meaningful, facilitate communication of observed benefits, and generally allow quantification of benefit that can be weighed against toxicity to assess net clinical value. However, direct measurement of clinical benefit may require large, lengthy trials or may otherwise be impractical or impossible to accomplish. Therefore, in many trials, efficacy of a therapy is measured indirectly by using surrogate endpoints. Surrogate endpoints are laboratory or other measurements that do not directly indicate clinical benefit but that are expected to correlate with or predict clinical benefit. The principal concern with the reliance on a surrogate endpoint to establish efficacy is that the surrogate endpoint is not clinically meaningful in its own right and that the ability of the surrogate to predict clinical benefit may be overestimated.

Use of a surrogate endpoint is often considered when direct measures of clinical benefit arise (are available) only after a lengthy period of observation. For example, the principal clinical sequelae of chronic hepatitis C are the development of end-stage liver failure, hepatocellular carcinoma, or death. These outcomes typically occur many years to decades after diagnosis, therefore using them as endpoints to assess new treatments for chronic hepatitis C would require very lengthy trials. In the trials of interferons for treatment of chronic hepatitis C infection, decreases in levels of circulating liver enzymes, improvements in liver histopathology, and, more recently, loss of detectable virus in the plasma have been used as surrogate endpoints because these types of improvements are thought to indicate a decreased likelihood of serious, long-term clinical sequelae. Similarly, in trials of antiviral agents for the treatment of patients with early HIV infection, effects on CD4+ lymphocyte counts and on plasma viral levels can be measured well before any effect might be observed on clinically significant events such as AIDS-related opportunistic infections, and they are thought to predict such effects for some types of interventions.

Another reason for using surrogate endpoints is that they may be more sensitive to drug effects. Often measures such as blood pressure, tumor size, or CD4+ cell count, are used as surrogates for clinical events such as stroke, death, or progression to AIDS. As noted above, measurement endpoints are generally more sensitive to drug effects than are event endpoints and thus allow greater power.

A third reason for using surrogate endpoints is that they are often more objective measures than are the true clinical endpoints. For example, measurements on x-rays of arthritic joints may be more objective than assessments of inflammation or pain, and changes on magnetic resonance imaging (MRI) scan in a patient with multiple sclerosis may be less subjective than reports of disability. Use of objective endpoints can offer substantial benefits in protection against bias, particularly in unblinded trials and trials partially unblinded by drug effects.

Despite the attractive features of surrogate endpoints listed above, considerable caution should be observed in using a surrogate as the primary endpoint in an efficacy trial. Surrogates may prove to be less reliable predictors of benefit than one had hoped. Although more detailed discussion of this issue can be found elsewhere (17,18), two common pitfalls will be highlighted here. First, a marker should not be assumed to be a good surrogate simply because it correlates with prognosis of the disease, absent treatment. For example, the presence of pulmonary metastases is undoubtedly a poor prognostic sign in patients with a primary adenocarcinoma; however, the excision of the metastases, although improving the "surrogate," may not alter prognosis at all and is highly unlikely to restore to the patient a prognosis comparable to that of a patient who had not developed a metastasis. Second, a surrogate marker should not be assumed to be valid simply because it has been validated as a surrogate for efficacy in trials of other treatments for the same disease acting by a different mechanism. For example, increases in circulating CD4+ lymphocyte counts have predicted clinical benefit for some antivirals used to treat patients with HIV, but similar increases in response to an infusion of CD4+ lymphocytes are of unknown value.

In her review article in *Science*, Nowak states "the vast majority of clinical trialists contacted by *Science* agree on one thing: the most potentially damaging flaw in clinical trials today is the inappropriate substitution of 'surrogate' markers for well-defined clinical endpoints . . ." (19). The Cardiac Arrhythmia Suppression Trial (CAST) is a classic example in which a drug effect on a surrogate marker that correlates strongly with prognosis did not predict an effect on the clinical outcome (20). Individuals who have experienced an acute myocardial infarction (AMI) are at increased risk for ventricular arrhythmias and sudden death. Based on observation, ventricular arrhythmias were considered to be an effective surrogate endpoint to predict sudden death. Encainide and flecainide were in common off-label use to suppress asymptomatic arrhythmias after AMI because of the belief that suppression of these ectopic beats would improve survival. In CAST, patients in whom the drugs had been shown to suppress high-risk arrhythmias were randomized to receive drug or placebo. The trial was halted after an interim analysis indicated that the treatment was associated with an *increase* in sudden death and total mortality, despite the reduction in arrhythmias (21).

Use of a surrogate as the primary efficacy outcome in a Phase III trial is least likely to be misleading when the surrogate has been validated for the drug (or class of drugs) and the disease. Validation of the surrogate is accomplished by assessment of both the clinical and the surrogate endpoint in the same trials to establish that most or all of the clinical effects of the drug on the clinical endpoint can be predicted by effects on the surrogate (22). Rigorous validation of a surrogate requires much clinical outcome data, and such data are not commonly available, particularly before a drug is proven effective. Generally, one can only make an educated guess at the likelihood that the surrogate will correctly predict benefit, based on epidemiological, pathophysiological, or clinical trial data linking the surrogate with the clinical outcome. In 1992, the Food and Drug Administration issued regulations that permitted market approval of drugs or biologics for serious or life-threatening diseases based on clinical data demonstrating an effect on an endpoint deemed reasonably likely to predict clinical benefit. This type of product approval is generally contingent on the postmarketing acquisition of additional trial data that confirms the clinical benefits of the drug (23). Importantly, although surrogates may allow determination of efficacy in a shorter or smaller trial, sometimes the critical factor dictating the number of patients and the duration of treatment is not the determination of efficacy but rather the need for safety data. When a large or long trial is necessary to generate controlled safety data, the benefits of a surrogate efficacy endpoint may be substantially diminished.

A significant problem often arises in assessment of net clinical benefit when surrogate efficacy endpoints are used to assess agents with significant toxicity. Even when a surrogate endpoint is determined to be reasonably likely to predict clinical benefit, it is rarely possible to make a precise estimate of the amount of clinical benefit predicted by a given change in the surrogate. Therefore, assessment of net clinical benefit requires weighing uncertain benefit of unknown magnitude against significant toxicity.

After an acute myocardial infarction, thrombolytic agents increase coronary artery patency (surrogate) and improve mortality (clinical endpoint), but they may also cause a hemorrhagic stroke. One might well determine that a 1% decrease in mortality makes an acceptable associated 1% increase in stroke rate. However, even if one assumed that improved patency is likely to predict improved survival, because the quantitative relationship between patency and survival is unknown, one could not determine how acceptable improved patency made a 1% increase in stroke rate.

Despite their problems, surrogates have important roles in clinical development. They can be of substantial value as secondary or supportive endpoints in

Phase III trials, providing further information about the nature of a drug's effects. Surrogates are particularly likely to be useful as efficacy endpoints earlier in clinical development (e.g., in Phase II). Although uncertainty about the validity of the surrogate may necessitate use of a clinical benefit endpoint in an ultimate efficacy trial, reliance on clinical benefit endpoints in all trials of a drug could be extremely costly and time-consuming and may prevent development. Trials with surrogate markers may be used effectively to determine if an agent is sufficiently promising to warrant investment of the time, effort, and money to conduct a trial measuring clinical benefit and may also be used to determine the optimal dose, regimen, target population, or concomitant medications for such a trial (24). Decisions based on such trials may be suboptimal if the surrogate is not valid. However, because a clinical benefit trial will ultimately be performed in Phase III, use of a surrogate in earlier trials will not lead to an incorrect final determination that an ineffective treatment is effective.

XI. SUMMARY

The choice and the analysis of endpoints is a critical issue in design of a clinical trial. Desirable characteristics of an endpoint include feasibility of measurement, sensitivity to drug effects, meaningfulness, objectivity of measurement, and usefulness in communicating results. These characteristics will depend, in part, on the type of endpoint chosen (e.g., events, measures, composites, scores, surrogates). Careful consideration of the characteristics of potential endpoints will generally facilitate the development and selection of an appropriate endpoint.

REFERENCES

1. Friedman LM, Furberg CD, DeMets DL. Fundamentals of Clinical Trials. 3d ed. St Louis: Mosby, 1996:223–245.
2. Jacobs LD, Cookfair DL, Rudick RA, et al. Intramuscular interferon beta-1a for disease progression in relapsing multiple sclerosis. MSCRG. Ann Neurol 1996; 39: 285–294.
3. Collett D. Modelling Survival Data in Medical Research. London: Chapman & Hall, 1994:15–51.
4. Westfall PH, Tobias RD, Rom D, et al. Multiple comparisons and multiple tests. SAS Institute, 1999:1–11.
5. Proschan MA, Waclawiw MA. Practical guidelines for multiplicity adjustment in clinical trials. Control Clin Trials 2000; 21:527–539.
6. Gong J, Pinhero JC, DeMets DL. Estimating significance level and power comparisons for testing multiple endpoints in clinical trials. Control Clin Trials 2000; 21: 313–329.

7. 1993 revised classification system for HIV infection and expanded surveillance case definition for AIDS among adolescents and adults. MMWR Morb Mortal Wkly Rep 1992 (Dec 18); 41(RR-17):1–19.

8. Use of monoclonal antibody directed against the platelet glycoprotein IIb/IIIa receptor in high-risk coronary angioplasty. The EPIC investigation. N Engl M Med 1994; 330:956–961.

9. Stolman DS, Siegel JP, Walton MK, et al. Design issues in clinical trials of thrombolytics and antithrombotic agents. In: Sasahara AA, Loscalzo J, eds. New Therapeutic Agents in Thrombosis and Thrombolysis. New York: Marcel Dekker, 1997:49–75.

10. Felson DT, Anderson JJ, Boers M, et al. American College of Rheumatology. Preliminary definition of improvement in rheumatoid arthritis. Arthritis Rheum 1995; 38:727–735.

11. Kurtzke JF. Rating neurologic impairment in multiple sclerosis: an expanded disability status scale (EDSS). Neurology 1983; 33:1444–1452.

12. Clark WM, Hourihane JM. Clinical stroke scales. In: Herndon RM, ed. Handbook of Neurologic Rating Scales. New York: Demos Vermande, 1997:161–186.

13. Best WR, Becktel JM, Singleton JW, Kern F Jr. Development of a Crohn's disease activity index. National Cooperative Crohn's Disease Study. Gastroenterology 1976; 70:439–444.

14. Fayers PM, Machin D. Quality of Life: Assessment, Analysis, and Interpretation. West Sussex, U.K.: Wiley, 2000:3–27, 45–71.

15. Naughton MJ, Shumaker SA. Guest contributors assessment of health-related quality of life. In: Friedman LM, Furberg CD, DeMets DL, eds. Fundamentals of Clinical Trials. 3d ed. St. Louis: Mosby, 1996:185–203.

16. Testa MA, Simonson DC. Assessment of quality-of-life outcomes. N Engl J Med 1996; 334:835–840.

17. Fleming TR, Prentice RL, Pepe MS, Glidden D. Surrogate and auxiliary endpoints in clinical trials, with potential applications in cancer and AIDS research. Stat Med 1994; 13:955–968.

18. Wittes JW, Lakatos E, Probstfield J. Surrogate endpoints in clinical trials: cardiovascular diseases. Stat Med 1989; 8:415–425.

19. Nowak R. Problems in clinical trials go far beyond misconduct. A close look at clinical trials. Science 1994; 264:1538–1541.

20. Echt DS, Liebson PR, Mitchell LB, et al. Mortality and morbidity in patients receiving encainide, flecainide, or placebo. The Cardiac Arrhythmia Suppression Trial. N Engl J Med 1991; 324:781–788.

21. Rapaport E. Limitations of clinical trials. In: Pitt B, Julian D, Pocock S, eds. Clinical Trials in Cardiology. London: Saunders, 1997:43–71.

22. De Gruttola V, Fleming TR, Lin DY, Coombs R. Perspective: validating surrogate markers—are we being naïve? J Infect Dis 1997; 175:237–246.

23. 57 Fed Reg 58942, December 11, 1992 (codified at 21 CFR 314 and 601, Appendix 4).

24. Fleming TR. Surrogate markers in AIDS and cancer trials. Stat Med 1994; 13:1423–1435.

6

Dix, Cent, Mille: Proof of Principle with $10 Million, 100 Patients, and 1000 Days

W. Leigh Thompson*
Eli Lilly and Company, Indianapolis, Indiana

I. INTRODUCTION

The product decision to invest enormous sums in pivotal studies of safety and efficacy of a new treatment should be made when the probability of success has grown to 90% from the 10% on choosing a new molecule. This point can be reached in less than 1000 days after 100 patients for $10 million. For optimal speed, minimal waste resources, enhanced ethics, and maximal information from each subject, the chemistry, toxicology, and clinical studies should not be done *en bloc* in series, but rather elegantly braided together in a stronger, shorter continuum of data capture, analysis, and utilization to plan the next dose. A clear focus on the goal—a better-quality investment decision—will aim this braid straight to that target with no unraveling of unnecessary studies, with conservation of living subjects, and with maximum decision-critical information per minute. Only three things are needed to achieve this new paradigm of efficiency: clear thinking, an elegant informatics system for all data and users, and a plan based on the relevance diagram of the product decision.

II. GOAL

The goal of early therapeutics development research is to reach a critical decision on continuing investment into pivotal large studies—the *product decision*. This

---

* Retired
Note: See Appendices on pp. 439–449 for Routine Clinical Analyte Test Results.

decision point should be after most predictable failures when the probability of successful marketing is high. About 90% of new molecules chosen for development fail before marketing or are soon withdrawn from market. After the first dose in a human the failure rate is 78%. To reduce the failure rate to 10%, how many chemical tests, toxicology protocols, and patient studies must be performed?

Data from the Center for the Study on Drug Development, the Centre for Medicines Research, industry benchmarking surveys, and Eli Lilly and Company suggest that late failures of truly innovative and medically important therapies occur with:

> Unpredictable toxicity in animals, such as carcinogenicity despite negative tests for genotoxicity
>
> Unpredictable infrequent severe clinical reactions, such as aplastic anemia or agranulocytosis, with no animal or clinical premonitory signs
>
> Unexpected early marketing of equivalent, better or cheaper competitive treatments
>
> Avoidable errors in the planing of manufacture, marketing, pricing, reimbursement, or pharmacoeconomic proofs of cost-effectiveness

If all the avoidable and predictable failures are eliminated, the probability of global marketing should be nearly 90% for most drugs after careful comprehensive studies of about 100 patients who have the target illness and are given appropriate doses of the new molecule for periods of up to 3 months. Enough should then be known to write a comprehensive product label and to complete sufficient studies of the markets, disease epidemiology, and competition to allow a very well-informed, high-quality *product decision*.

For many decades we have followed a rubber-stamp paradigm of completing in a lockstep series:

> Chemistry studies: analytical standards, analytical assays for feed and biological samples, bulk synthesis routes, formulations, formulation stability, metabolism, impurity identification, kinetics, metabolite identification and synthesis
>
> Animal studies: efficacy in too many animal models; in-vitro and ex-vivo toxicology; in-vivo acute, subacute, and chronic toxicology; metabolism and kinetics in many species
>
> Phase I clinical studies: often in healthy homogeneous volunteers examining kinetics and symptoms, signs, and laboratory tests suggesting adverse events
>
> Phase II efficacy and safety studies: in relatively healthy homogeneous patients with a single target disease and no concomitant confounding factors

Such studies are often done in series, with toxicology demanding completion of the chemistry before they will set doses, clinicians demanding final reports of the toxicologists, and each group of *prima donnas* focusing only on their own navels. This wastes chemists, animals, and patients as well as time, money, and expertise.

If studies are restricted to homogeneous subjects, it may provide no basis for predicting product performance in a heterogeneous marketplace, and it is exactly this error that has caused many of the postmarketing product withdrawals.

Everyone should realize the goal is not submitting a New Drug Application (NDA), gaining market approval, obtaining an appropriate price, or initial launch—it is *sustained dominance of the global market.*

III. BRAID ELEGANCE

Contrast the plodding *en block* linear ooze described above with smoothly integrated, seamless streams of data from chemistry, toxicology, and clinical studies deftly interwoven into a comprehensive *knowledge braid* that reaches a high probability of future success with the least time, money, effort, and expertise. To accomplish this elegant braiding requires only a global focus on two critical elements—the *ethics* of human exposure to innovative molecules and a *single purpose* of predicting success and failure with the least effort. Nothing should be done that is not entirely ethical, but also, nothing should be done that is not essential to reach a product decision at which you have a 90% probability of regulatory, reimbursement, and pricing approvals in the desired markets. This is no time for hidden agendas, meanders unraveling the braid, or "feel good" studies.

Why should we change the successful paradigms of the past? They served us well in an era of high profitability, low competition, leisurely research and marketing, and risk-averse avoidance of change. We might not have liked the lengthening times and escalating costs, but we could then afford them and the devil of change was ominous. Today, faster, more efficient decisions are imperative. A new molecule in 2001 requires $1 billion investment to pay for the failures and for global support of the launch. The Centre for Medicines Research estimates that about 40 new molecules are launched worldwide annually at a current investment of $50 billion. If research investments are 16% of sales, the average molecule must achieve $6 billion in sales over its lifetime. If 1 million patients use the treatment each year for 10 years of exclusivity, each must pay $600 (wholesale) to achieve this reimbursement of the investment. Currently one must invest for 15 years to reach launch in the United States and about 12.8 years worldwide. About 11% of new drugs that begin development, with teams focused on them, will be launched. Perhaps one in four that is launched will earn a true profit beyond the fully allocated investments. Surely new drugs are the most prolonged, most risky of investments.

IV. LINEARITY VERSUS HYPERLINKING

Before Gutenberg abolished illiteracy with cheap linear codes for thoughts, people could recite oral histories in different verse orders or study stained glass windows and statues in any order. After Gutenberg we learned the first page before the second, courses proceeded from front cover to back, and you didn't spoil the mystery by peeking at the last page.

Henry Ford developed the mindless linear assembly line. The chassis was built first, then the axles were applied before the wheels went on. Workers from different countries, speaking different languages, could be minimally trained to perform a single mindless function, such as adding the left rear wheel. No communication was needed, and all the cars were identical, black, with interchangeable parts—not the perfectly fitted, hand-crafted parts of a skilled artisan, but inexpensively standardized modules linearly assembled.

Linearity was embellished during World War II by multiple assembly lines making an airplane or submarine with product streams, each from its own assembly line, arriving in proper order. Today we have refined this to just-in-time resourcing, but the linear thinking hasn't changed—in fact, it has spawned the mathematical/management discipline of linear programming.

A. Hyperlinking Media

Your eye–brain isn't linear. It soaks up all the data available, processes it in priority order, and acts upon it before you consciously think *chasm, tiger,* or *stop sign.* Speech leaps from one thought to the next. Transcripts of my lectures are ungrammatical nonsense as I leap among media and thoughts.

Hyperlinked multimedia may restore in one generation the sentient capacities of *homo sapiens*, and make her more worthy of her species appellation. How do these new tools simulate our natural eye–brain? The MIT Computer Sciences Laboratory "smart room" sucks up images from CNN, print from *The Wall Street Journal*, references from NLM, audioclips from your message machine, and your own musings. It then braids these data for you by concept, learned from observation of how you use the materials, the order you prefer to use it, and how long you spend with each subject. It then presents to you new material in your priority order—leaping from image to text to sounds almost as effortlessly as your eye–brain to create a knowledge braid optimal for your interests. As these tools become more user-seductive and we learn to communicate through virtual reality and real-time language translators that seamlessly assume our individual knowledge levels, we will become less and less conscious of them as tools, as today we are not conscious of the technology of TV, just its content.

Children who learn from hyperlinked multimedia encyclopedias seem to retain their creativity. They explore rich solution spaces with intuitive quests for solutions that work, rather than being immobilized by fear of failure and mired in linear analysis of what might be perfect. They just *do it*. Soon the World Wide Web will vanquish the linear chains of Gutenberg and liberate our right brains.

B. Hyperlinking Research

In rethinking decision research we need to be facile in braiding chemistry, toxicology, and clinical studies into a tight synergistic web of data, all of which are quickly validated, organized, analyzed, and displayed before the next step.

When climbing a mountain you seamlessly integrate data from positional sensors, tension sensors in muscles, vision, wind sensors, etc., before each step. Similarly, we need to acquire all the essential data, just in time, valid, analyzed, displayed, and integrated into our decision for our next step. And each step, even if it seemingly veers off to a ridge, should be the optimal path to the goal—the *best possible product decision.*

What chemistry tasks are essential for your next toxicology study? What toxicology tasks are essential for your next clinical study? Must the formulation used in the first human be that which you will market worldwide? Of course not. Consider what must be, what is essential, what is *sine qua non* for each step of toxicology and clinical studies. Make each task modular and complete the modules just in time—*no module before its time* means no wasted resources.

V. REDESIGN OF CLINICAL RESEARCH

If your goal is predicting market acceptance of your product from a few human studies, should you study healthy, young, nonobese, Caucasian, nonsmoking males taking no drugs or ethanol, eating a prescribed diet, and having no sex or exercise while incarcerated in a closed ward for weeks? By definition these are the subjects *least* likely to be taking your drug when you market it. What will they tell you? They will have very little variability in the kinetics of your drug. The halftimes will be almost identical and the confidence limits about the plasma concentration–time curves will be very narrow. The graphs in the publication will be beautiful.

Unfortunately, these data will not predict the responses to the drug of children, fat old French women, Native Americans athletes, patients with multiorgan failure taking many other medicines, and patients with aberrant drug metabolizing enzymes.

Diversity is key. You cannot predict the average weight of fruit at a green-grocer by measuring precisely with a micrometer the diameter of grapes. Although diameter is a good surrogate of weight, grapes are not representative of all fruit. Your sample should include apples, watermelon, kiwis, limes, etc.

Study diverse patients early. Include only patients with your target disease, but ensure that they vary in age, gender, race, size, obesity, diets, habits, activities, smoking, ethanol use, concomitant ills, and use of concomitant prescription, over-the-counter, illicit, and health products. Consider a multidimensional grid representing values of each of these patient variables and disperse your patients widely in this space of patient characteristics.

When Lilly examined the effects of some of these variables on routine laboratory tests, we found that many of these factors caused large differences in the test results. So we created 32 reference probability distributions for each laboratory test to be able to interpret the results seen in trials of patients differing in age, gender, race, smoking, and use of ethanol. Lilly employs a single clinical protocol in two dozen countries simultaneously to achieve the diversity needed for proper prediction of market responses.

What of pivotal trials? Must they also be diverse? Use the data from the decision-phase research to design these trials. You might restrict the young or the very old, but you should plan on reflecting that lack of knowledge in your label. At least you will have meaningful data, from all sources, on which to base the design of those pivotal trials.

Must these first decision clinical trials be pivotal proofs of safety and efficacy? Of course not. They are exploratory to fill in your vision of the vast space of patient responses to different doses. Later you can design elegant, precise dose–response pivotal trials with all the good clinical practices to prove your point to regulators, payors, practitioners, and patients.

VI. THE FIRST HUMAN

Should the first human be healthy? Why? Won't you learn more from patients? If the target disease makes the patient so fragile that he is at special risk for an unexpected serious adverse reaction, begin with a healthy volunteer but move quickly to patients. Phase I trials can include both volunteers and patients braided together.

There are not many such diseases. Life-threatening hepatitis B severely compromises patients. Fialuridine, a nucleoside that seemed very promising in a National Institutes of Health (NIH) trial in hepatitis B, killed five patients despite liver transplants through very delayed unexpected toxicity. This toxicity was not observed in extensive animal and prior clinical studies in several patient populations. Perhaps the toxicity is only manifest in humans with fatally progressive chronic hepatitis B. Healthy volunteers might have contributed nothing or even false encouragement to these trials. If the deaths had been in healthy volunteers instead of patients, would that be more ethical?

Patients may respond favorably to a new treatment. They may manifest improvement in at least surrogate endpoints and thereby contribute more information for their risk of participation. As a reward, they can be promised that they will be allowed to participate in later pivotal efficacy trials and they may be promised compassionate use of the drug until a regulatory decision is made about its marketing, pricing, and reimbursement.

A. Labeled First Dose

Gather the most information from each patient. In the first patient, besides tolerance of a small dose, determine the metabolic routes and kinetics of the drug by using a labeled dose. Use a stable label such as deuterium and mass spectrometry to trace the metabolites or use a radioactive tracer.

Before I have taken small doses of radioactive test drugs, I have asked about the distribution and persistence of the label in two appropriate species after single doses. If the label does not accumulate in any special organ, such as eyes or testes, and if it is eliminated promptly, then I would not be concerned about any damage from the label.

If the drug is excreted in urine of several species, then my kidneys will probably eliminate it. If the drug is metabolized by a pathway defined in animals, and if I am known to have similar pathways, then the drug should not persist unduly.

This concept could be tested further by measuring the metabolism of the drug in ex-vivo preparations of human liver microsomes, or even individual human drug-metabolizing enzyme isoforms. Having identified the specific isoform that metabolizes the drug ex-vivo, I could be tested with a safe common drug to ensure that I have a normal level of activity of that specific isoform via which to eliminate the test dose promptly. My own blood could be tested ex-vivo to examine the binding of test drug and label to cells and proteins and to see if any ex-vivo transformation of the substance occurs.

B. First Dose

Examining the distribution of test substance among my blood cells, proteins, and water, one can calculate what dose, if fully absorbed and distributed only in my blood, would achieve a plasma water concentration one-half to one-third that which produced any detectable change in any other species. Perhaps that is an appropriate first dose. For many molecules, the first humans can be dosed for 1 day based on acute toxicology in two species. That day of dosing can begin with an intravenous-labeled dose, and 23 hours later, depending on the results, a larger oral dose.

Analyzing my exhaled air, saliva, urine, feces, sweat, stomach juices, blood cells, blood plasma proteins, and plasma water over time should provide an accurate picture of how I have absorbed, distributed, metabolized, and excreted the small dose of labeled drug.

How should that first dose be administered? Should it be in a beautiful capsule filled with excipients and analyzed for purity and stability? Of course not. It should be freeze-dried, dissolved at bedside, and consumed in an appropriate beverage or instilled in the stomach through a small feeding tube inserted into the stomach (bypassing the taste buds).

C. Intravenous Dosing

Even more appropriate, in my opinion, would be to give the first doses by intravenous infusion. One can start with a very very small dose and gradually increase the infusion rate over several hours, perhaps sampling plasma concentrations as a guide. One can mimic any pattern of absorption from other administration sites using a programmed pump and intravenous infusions. One can also give unlabeled material by mouth and labeled material intravenously to measure absolute bioavailability and define gastrointestinal absorption and presystemic elimination.

VII. THE NEXT HUMANS

All the important data from the first patient should be available in 48 h. Consider the toxicokinetic data in several species. At what blood concentrations have the animals begun to manifest effects? What were the concentrations in the first human? Considering the acute toxicity in animals, should you next give a dose to the second human that will achieve one-third or two-thirds the minimal effective plasma water concentration in animals? Give the second patient labeled material and complete the studies in 48 hours. From the first patient you have begun to recognize which samples are the most important to analyze immediately. As you approach the minimally effective dose, institute efficacy and surrogate efficacy assessments.

A. Blinding

If you wish to believe data, especially subjective data about adverse events, blind the patient and investigators and determine why the sponsor should not also be blinded. Placebos are inexpensive, although they may be toxic. They have saved many drugs when an influenza epidemic swept through the laboratory and altered liver tests and created many adverse events. Placebo use does add data, but without placebos you will have difficulty interpreting data. Did those patients really have drug-induced bizarre dreams, trouble thinking, and penile erections? Avoid exsanguinating a patient with unnecessary samples after a placebo dose, but do blind everyone appropriately. Blind the switch from placebo to active drug—often subjects anticipate adverse events at this moment.

B. Dose Escalation

For each new patient, use all the data at hand from chemistry, toxicology, and prior patients to choose the dosage regimen. Control each patient through rapid analysis of plasma drug concentrations. If a patient has unexpected slow elimination, perhaps a multiple dose should be reduced. If a patient has unexpected low plasma concentrations, quickly study the patient and determine why. If the patient has an adverse event, does it correlate with plasma concentrations? Will sensitive psychomotor tests predict subtle brain effects that indicate drug passage through the blood–brain barrier?

This Bayesian approach of using all data was employed in the transition from traditional LD_{50} testing to more modern methods. In olden LD_{50} testing, large batches of animals were each given one dose and observed for death. Perhaps seven doses would be tested at once, with 10 animals of each gender per dose. Perhaps the survivors were 20/20, 19/20, 17/20, 13/20, 8/20, 3/20, 0/20. One could calculate that the LD_{50} was between the fourth and fifth dose and you could estimate the most likely value and its confidence limits. But this would use 140 animals.

Instead, dose the first animal with your best estimate of the LD_{50}. If that animal lives, dose the next animal with a larger dose. If that animal dies, dose the next with a smaller dose. Continue a march through a few animals, converging rapidly on the domain of the LD_{50}. If you model this you will find there to be great efficiencies in using all data in planning the next dose. If you were paid to minimize the number of rodents employed in such testing, I am sure you would use an efficient Bayesian dosing regimen.

C. Dose–Response Versus Dose Ranging

Never do dose ranging. Dose ranging allows the investigator to escalate the dose within a patient, or from patient to patient, using only a vague protocol. Historically, this technique leads quickly to maximum tolerated doses, often overshooting the minimal effective dose by 10-fold or more. When Federico Dies, MD PhD, at Lilly studied penbutolol, a beta-blocker, he found that the efficacy was fully manifest at one-tenth the dose at which it was marketed by another firm in

Europe. Bob Temple, MD, of the FDA can rattle off the names of more than a dozen similar overdosage errors made through dose ranging.

Instead, do parallel, predefined dose–response studies in which the dosage of each patient is carefully planned based on the plasma concentrations and responses of prior patients. If doses cause adverse events, the algorithm should diminish future doses. If doses are ineffective, the algorithm should augment future doses. This algorithm can be decided in advance and implemented blindly, with periodic reassessments.

The dose–response escalating algorithm for the first patients is a variant of the *adaptive allocation* algorithm I prefer for pivotal trials. This is a prospective, triple-blinded (the sponsor is also blinded), randomized dose–response design in which the first patient has equal probability of assignment to placebo, small, medium, or large dose, or active comparator. A control variable is chosen to express the patient's response to therapy. This variable may be just the global opinion of the patient or investigator. It must correlate positively with the primary efficacy variable, but it can be any surrogate.

Suppose the patient assesses the treatment on the Goldilocks scale: *too little, too much, just right*. If the first patient's assessment is too much, the probability of assignment to that specific therapy or any larger doses of it is reduced. If the assessment is too little, the probability of assignment to that therapy or any smaller doses of it is reduced. If the assessment is just right, the probability of assignment to that treatment is increased slightly.

As the study proceeds, more and more patients are allocated (blindly and randomly) to doses and products that are effective and not toxic, and fewer and fewer patients are assigned to doses that are less effective or less safe. The exact behavior of the algorithm can be modeled easily for different dose–response curves for the population being tested.

Adaptive allocation helps regulators who insist on placebos see that placebos will be used, in at least a few patients, throughout the study. For regulators who abhor placebos, they can see how placebo allocations will diminish if placebos don't work. A larger proportion of patients are on *helpful* doses, thereby enhancing the ethics of the investigation and the power of the study to provide helpful information in the marketplace.

D. Toxicology

What toxicology do you need for the first tiny labeled dose in a human? I would ask about the kinetics, tissue distributions, behavioral signs, laboratory tests, and autopsy results in two appropriate species given very large single doses. Depending on these findings, I might also ask about the effects of multiple doses given over 2 weeks, but in many cases I would be interested only in the single large doses.

Are fertility studies needed if the first patients are sterilized or otherwise infertile? Think of the savings if you have not perfected a lovely formulation, completed stability studies, or have started chronic toxicology if a few doses in humans shows the drug to be unsuitable. *Just in time* and *only what is relevant* for the decision are the tests to apply.

E. Chemistry

What chemical tests are needed? I would want to have reasonably well characterized material used in the toxicology studies and in me to ensure that no new toxic contaminant has appeared in my dose, but if we are doing only single-dose or short-term studies in animals there will be little need for stability studies, testing animal feeds containing the test drug, etc. Using labeled material early can be a major help before sophisticated assays are perfected.

If metabolism in the first human is unexpected, and significant metabolites are seen that have not been observed in animals, one might wish to return to other animal species and strains to find one in which the human metabolites can be evaluated. Perhaps this metabolite will cause dose-limiting toxicity. Perhaps knowing the toxicity of this metabolite in animals will make one wish to abort the project or alter plans about the tolerated dose.

F. Effects

As the plasma concentration is increased, with larger doses one may begin to see effects in the patients. Hopefully there is an acute surrogate that will predict efficacy. Relate these effects to plasma concentration profiles. Soon you will be ready for multiple doses.

The first multiple-dose patient might be given just a few doses. Shouldn't this be one of the single-dose patients in whom you can predict precisely the plasma concentration profiles after multiple doses from studying the single dose? Later patients might be treated for as long as test animals have indicated repetitive dosing to be safe.

In every patient, dosing should be based on *all* the knowledge gained from all prior animal and clinical studies, from everything known about that patient, and from the best prediction of what plasma concentrations will be achieved after the dose.

G. Protocols

Using all information before each dose is safer and more ethical, but it makes it impossible to write a rigid protocol in advance. In some cases doses will escalate rapidly as plasma concentrations in humans are less than expected. In other cases doses will advance slowly. Sometimes multiple doses may begin with the third or fourth patient. Sometimes they will begin after 10 or more patients have been given single doses.

H.   Fail Fast/Smart

Failure lurks with every dose. Suppose the first dose is eliminated at startling speed by a unique human enzyme. Suppose the first dose is not absorbed from the gut. Suppose the first dose has nearly complete presystemic elimination in the liver. These may abort the project after one or a very few patients. We should always prepare for failure and plan our studies to minimize the number of patient exposures and overall patient risk as well as time and effort to failure. Tom Watson of IBM always admonished his scientists to *fail fast*. I would say *fail smart*. Science respects failures that inform and denigrates stupid successes.

I.   Kinetics Versus Dynamics

In these early studies you are separately determining the relation of plasma concentrations to dose and biological effects to plasma concentration. Both kinetics and dynamics show variation with patient age, gender, race, diet, disease, habits, etc. Diversity is key to predicting responses in your marketplace to your product. Select diverse patients and study them intensively to learn the predictors of responses.

J.   Rechallenge

The single-dose patients are excellent choices for the first multiple-dose trials. Single-dose patients also can be rechallenged for specific studies of kinetic variables. Study the same patient given a test dose together with drugs that will alter plasma protein association or urine pH. To define oral absorption, give a second test dose together with divalent cation-containing antacids or after a proton pump inhibitor or during diarrhea, which can be induced with oral hypertonic mannitol or sorbitol. Give a test dose together with activated charcoal to see if this is effective therapy if a child overdoses on a dose taken home. Give a dose into the duodenum, jejunum, ileum, cecum, or rectum, or sample the *succus entericus* to see if drug appears in the bile or intestinal secretions.

These are the patients in whom a second dose can define absorption from nasal installation, a skin patch, sublingual administration, rectal suppositories, enemas, enteric coated capsules timed to disintegrate in the cecum, or regular enteric coating. If the material is not irritating, and you have tolerated one dose, why would you want special toxicity studies for these unusual routes of administration? I wouldn't.

Measure subtle psychomotor effects of the test drug alone and when given together with concomitant drugs such as ethanol and sedatives. Will driving behavior deteriorate further? Should future clinical trial patients be warned?

K. Ethics vs. Regulations

Must these studies be done under strict U.S. FDA Good Laboratory Practices, Good Manufacturing Practices, Good Clerical Practices rules? No. They must be ethical. You must carefully think through the risks, benefits, and ethics. You should engage an appropriate ethical review committee in your culture to ensure that the studies will be viewed as ethical when described in your news media. You should ensure that the investigators and the local ethical review committee(s) are cautious, conservative, ethical, and attuned to the risks and benefits of the volunteering patients. Ensure that the investigators and their ethical review committees monitor the patients and the study thoroughly and ensure that they receive prompt reports of any safety concern. Consent must be truly informed and the patients must be protected and followed meticulously. Do no studies in the homeless vagrants who populate so many Phase I farms—maybe that is where the word "farmacology" began.

Must these studies be suitable for submission to the U.S. FDA as pivotal trials? Of course not. These decision-phase studies must permit you to design and effect the most elegant and efficient pivotal proofs of safety and efficacy with proper doses, patients, and test procedures. But these early decision-phase patients themselves are only to provide you with the best-quality product decision about further investments and to prepare for those pivotal trials. Obviously, all data will be considered by all regulators. With proper design and interim analyses, however, many decision-phase protocols can be extended and expanded through product decision to serve as one or both pivotal studies.

L. Braiding

Some of the long stream of chemical testing must be done before the first toxicology study. Some will be needed for the first human. If the project has not failed, other chemistry studies will be needed before multiple doses or before using solid dosage forms or inhalation techniques. Unexpected human metabolites or new contaminants will necessitate further chemistry studies. Certainly much will be required before the pivotal trials. But if 9 of 10 projects fail, think how many chemistry studies can be saved by doing them just in time, as they are needed.

Some toxicology will be needed before the first human dose. The findings in that first patient will guide additional toxicology. New rodent strains or other species might be needed to simulate the kinetics and metabolites in humans. If a key metabolite is observed only in humans and ferrets, perhaps ferrets would be a good model to test.

VIII. ANIMAL TESTING

We need more diversity in test animals. We have stuck to a few strains of mice and rats because they are predictable and cheap, but are they as helpful as they might be? Wouldn't one animal metabolizing a new drug exactly the way it is metabolized in humans be far more useful than thousands of animals that don't metabolize it? Why don't we use rodents expressing selected human drug metabolizing enzymes? Would you be interested in cancer promotion in transgenic animals with knocked-out tumor suppressor genes or promoted oncogenes? If plasma protein association is a dominant feature, why don't we have animals expressing human plasma albumin? Would it be more informative to do our studies on variegated herds of mice and rats from many different strains, of different ages, levels of obesity, etc? If you knew that certain of these diverse creatures had unusual responses, wouldn't that be interesting? Is it better to be ignorant of these observations? Do we pursue ostrich research in the same sand box over and over?

IX. INFORMATICS

A single user-seductive informatics system is fundamental to the elegant braiding of data from chemistry, toxicology, and clinical studies into a coherent stream of information predicating good decisions. Data should be captured directly from all sources with as little human intervention as possible. Human hands and brains err. Instead, have the implanted chips in animals signal their movements, eating, and weight as they pass over scales. Why pay psychiatrists to ask patients how they sleep, eat, and make love? Ask the patients directly, using questionnaires, touchtone telephones, pen-pads, computer games, desktop and portable computers, and interactive TV.

Validate the data quickly with human and machine audits. If the weight of the patient is recorded as 30 pounds less than on the last visit, ring a bell and ask what limb has been amputated. Organize the data into a single relational database that can be easily queried by the unsophisticated, or prepare and test standard queries in advance. Especially effective are predefined extractors that download data into familiar simple spreadsheet programs that can be easily integrated with graphics and text for high-level desktop publishing of reports.

Include in the informatics system electronic mail, bulletin boards, online databases such as Medline, and the ability to facilitate high-level meetings. A one-round Delphi questionnaire before the meeting is helpful in eliminating time wasted discussing subjects on which everyone agrees. The Delphi results can order the agenda according to the disparity of opinions. Real-time voting during meetings, whether same-place or videoteleconferencing, will guide discussion, show disagreements, and speed closure of each topic as constant re-voting displays convergence during discussions.

Many meetings can be held in *choice time, choice place* rather than in same time, same place. Some can contribute during flights to other business locations. Others will review the data at night. Why restrict insight and innovation to 9 to 5 in one time zone?

A. Decision Trees

Decision research should follow a decision tree through a series of decisions. Most decisions can be mapped in advance. Many variables that will help you make the decisions can be mapped. Each of these can be estimated, with the information you have at the beginning, and then the estimates can be refined as you proceed through the decision tree. Some variables will be defined precisely and become deterministic. In many cases you will be surprised to find that only a few observations of the variable will refine your estimates enough to make further refinement irrelevant for the following decisions. This is one of the most important features of decision analysis in research—you can measure precisely the value of information and pay for information only if it will influence a subsequent decision.

At the beginning of decision research, write the product label. This exercise will expose a number of decisions that must be made and the knowledge that will help you make better-quality decisions. From this, design the decision tree of your decision-phase research. Estimate all the variables from the information you have. Then see how the variables will alter subsequent decisions. For the most critical variables, see if they can be studied first. Don't follow a rubber stamp, but design the studies dynamically, the order in which they will be completed, as well as the extent of data to be collected. If the next datum will not influence a decision, save it until an affirmative product decision is made. *No datum before its time—all data just in time.*

B. Relevance Diagrams

Ron Howard, ScD, invented the relevance diagram as a linear transform of the exponential decision tree. On one page you can represent 10–20 decisions and 50 or more nodes representing variables. The relationships are shown by arrows that indicate which variables are relevant (influenced by) other variables. If you were to estimate the halftime of a new drug in the first human, you might predicate your estimate on the halftime in animals, the age of the patient, the liver and kidney function of the patient, etc.

A well-constructed relevance diagram is the map to research. The decisions are highlighted. Before each decision there are variables you should estimate and variables you should measure directly. You can test the value of additional information at any node. Some variables will surprise you with the importance of precise information, but the studies can be designed specifically to acquire that information with only the precision that will improve the quality of the decision.

The science of decision analysis, and especially its relevance diagram, is perhaps the modern elegant hyperlinked multimedia embellishment of the World War II operations research, linear programming, PERT charts, and flow diagrams. It focuses attention on the critical decisions, defines the timing and precision of tests, and provides a framework for discussion. It minimizes waste of intellect and energy, speeds the flight of this braid to its decision goal, and keeps everyone on track and focused.

X. RESULTS

A. Savings

Designing elegantly braided decision research from a relevance diagram should save half or two-thirds of traditional time, effort, and expertise. A few drugs might not reach 90% probability of success at product decision if they have very delayed effects. You may have to make the product decision based on surrogates such as plasma cholesterol concentration or markers of bone metabolism without knowing for sure that the drug prevents heart attacks or vertebral fractures until you have treated thousands of patients for years. But your investment decision will be based on decision-phase studies of surrogates designed in elegant braided fashion.

B. Value

What value is created in discovery, in decision-phase research, or in registration research leading to launch? If the probability of launch is only 0.1, then your expected value is 10% of the product's value at launch. When you reach first human dose, and an industry-average 0.22 probability of regulatory approval, your expected value has increased 120% from the 0.1 probability point. At product decision, if your probability of successful launch is 0.9, you have increased your expected value 900% from the start of decision research. These expected values might be the maximum you should expect a partner to pay for your project. If the partner is risk-averse, he will pay even less until you have eliminated much of the risk. At what point should a small inventor firm try to sell its product?

C. Value/Assets

Examine the assets employed to move the project from milestone to milestone. From molecule selection (start) to completion of single-dose animal studies including toxicokinetics should cost $1–3 million but might increase the probability of success from 0.1 to 0.15. From there to the first human might cost $1–3 million but increase the probability to 0.22. From there to the 20th human might cost $1–3 million, but increase the probability to 0.4. From there to the 100th patient at appropriate doses might cost $2–6 million, but increase the probability to 0.9. If the certain-to-launch present certain equivalent value is $300 million, examine a risk-neutral track of value generated per assets employed:

0.05 ($300M)/$2M = 7.5
0.07 ($300M)/$2M = 10.5
0.18 ($300M)/$2M = 27
0.5 ($300M)/$4M = 37.5
Overall: 0.8($300M)/$10M = 24

More expected value per asset employed is generated as research proceeds toward the product decision. After the product decision, however, there may be the need to spend $100M to eliminate that last 0.1 of uncertainty and harvest the value in the marketplace. This expense can be predicted accurately and there is little associated risk after the product decision.

If the firm undertaking the pivotal studies is successful and spends $100M to reap the equivalent of $300M, that would seem to be a good investment. How much should be shared with the originator who has spent perhaps $30M on discovery and $10M on development? Perhaps $100M to the originator will provide a 250% profit and leave a 200% profit to the new owner.

D. Failure

Unfortunately, the above summary neglects failure. If nine discovery projects fail for this one to succeed, and if each costs $30M, who will have paid the $270M? In decision-phase research the developer will be careful to evaluate the project at each milestone and use an options model to decide whether to make the next investment. Thus failure in development will usually cost less than $10M of development investments, but may cost all of the $30M of discovery investments unless a second molecule, with greater probability of success, can emerge from the same discovery efforts.

E. Synergies

A small firm may have its future fixed to one product or a cluster of related products and either thrives or dies on its success. A large firm diffuses the risk and funds failures from successes. As long as a small firm can raise funds, it will continue decision-phase research to reap the greatest value when it strikes a deal with a partner to harvest the value. Unfortunately, when the product begins to pale, fund raising becomes more difficult.

Another reason for synergy among large and small firms is that only the large firms can afford asset-intensive combinatorial and computational chemistry, high-throughput robotic screens, process and pilot plant chemistry, and manufacturing excellence. However, the frontier of biology moves quickly and at low cost into genes and gene products. Small companies linked with academia can exploit inexpensive biological tools to move rapidly through these emerging technologies to select biological targets suitable for screening with chemical libraries.

Surely this can be the magic of large company chemistry and small company biology, if these collaborations can be braided elegantly into thoughtfully planned and efficiently executed projects. Such collaborations in discovery can be fashioned to use the more risk-neutral and risk-diffusing large enterprise to help buoy the smaller, more fragile enterprises.

XI. CONCLUSION

Why haven't we always done research this way? We treat patients one at a time, using all available knowledge. The early statisticians and trial design specialists were explorers who valiantly sifted through data to generate hypotheses and test them. They used all the data they could find. Then frequentist statistical thinking began to dominate. It arose from agriculture research in which large fields could be planted in various ways, manured, and, much later, the crops harvested and assessed. The frequentist would then make inferences about the population from which the samples were drawn and about future samples that could be drawn from the same population. These slow, plodding, smelly trials may be suitable for crop cycles, but patients are at your door needing care. You can't send them away until the study is harvested. You must treat them using all your knowledge now.

The second problem with traditional frequentist statistics is that it focuses on the central tendency—the mean. For approval, the U.S. FDA demands two studies that have shown the means of two samples, for example, your test drug versus placebo—to vary enough that the alpha error is .05 or less. But we don't treat patients in herds. Unfortunately, the U.S. FDA thinks of patients in just that way. What is the proper dose of digoxin if you treat 100 patients each with the same dose? The answer might be 0.5 mg per day orally, but some with hyperthyroidism and atrial fibrillation will be undertreated and others with hypomagnesemia or hypokalemia or renal failure will be overdosed.

This is what is so malignant about the U.S. FDA restricting access to drugs until their frequentist statistical studies of herds has resulted in data that pleases them, rather than focusing on the patients in need now. It also leads the U.S.

FDA to believe that their crisply defined sets of diseases are correct, when every practitioner knows that patients come in very fuzzy sets of joint pain, not classical Still's Disease, or cancer, not the stage IIIB lymphopenic tumors that made up the herd that won drug approval. No wonder so many cancer patients are treated *off-label*—their practitioners are classical Bayesians who use all information to select the best treatment regimen and view patients as individuals, not members of herds.

Today, with hyperlinked data and high-dimensional multivariate analyses, patients can be studied as though they were individuals with some common features. By studying such patients thoroughly, we can learn the predictive characteristics that will allow us to choose the best therapy. We may not always be correct, but we can always make the best decision based on all the available information. That is why it is so critical that the U.S. FDA stop its embargoes on data that do not fit its definition of approved, crisp diagnostic sets in its approved labels. Under any circumstances such censorship is insulting to health practitioners charged with the best care of their patients. When the patient is suffering and dying, such censorship is immoral, unethical, and reprehensible.

Why use half a brain if you have both halves? We are the victims of the left-brain, frequentist, post-hoc thinking. After the study is over, we analyze it to death and we become the world's best Monday morning quarterbacks (perhaps Tuesday morning, after the Monday night game). But we've lost the resilience of our ancestors who learned to cope, predict the best they could, innovate, try, and make it work. Of course, those primitive Bayesians must have known how to bet when in the past they sailed thousands of miles in Polynesia with the stars and a few sticks or today open a hot belly and master whatever they find.

Tomorrow our newborns will be problem solvers in virtual reality, surfing libraries, sampling historical CD-ROMs, invoking sophisticated analysis programs, and consulting online oracles all for that third-grade term paper. They will visit museums where there are pens, dictionaries, newspapers, and linearly scheduled TV programs, and they will wonder how the Nowanderthals ever survived without real-time translators, voice input, and attention-focusing knowbots. Too futuristic for you? Remember how shocked you were at *2001: A Space Odyssey*, when it appeared, and how contemporary it seems today.

We can leap forward toward tomorrow, enhancing the ethics of our research by reducing needless patient exposures and reducing the time and cost of therapeutics development, through elegant braiding of chemistry, toxicology, and clinical studies supported by comprehensive informatics and a relevance diagram map. There will still be risk and failure and expense, but more patients will live through earlier access to innovative treatments, and more patients will be able to afford them.

7

Clinical Drug Trials in Pediatrics:

Dilemmas of Clinical Drug Trials in Pediatric Populations

Allen Cato
Cato Research Ltd., Durham, North Carolina

Myron B. Peterson
Cato Research Ltd., Washington, D.C.

I. INTRODUCTION

Because of unique physiological, ethical, legal, and economic factors, drug development in the pediatric population (patients aged 16 years or younger) is a complex process. Approximately 80% of the prescription drugs approved by the U.S. Food and Drug Administration (FDA) and marketed in the United States are not approved for use in children or are restricted to older age groups because of limited clinical trials. Thus, children have been denied the benefit of many advances in therapeutics and remain, as Dr. Harry Shirkey (1) described them some 33 years ago, therapeutic orphans.

The failure to conduct pediatric drug trials for the proper labeling and formulation of drugs is directly related to the following six factors:

1. Study expense is too large for a small potential market.
2. Small patient numbers limit the feasibility of statistical analysis.
3. Ethical issues are more complex in children.
4. Approval process may be prolonged because of patient recruitment issues.
5. Pediatric clinical investigators are few in number.

6.   Once approved and marketed for adults, drugs will be used off-label
     for children, so why conduct pediatric trials?

Other mitigating factors, such as questions of delayed toxicity, mutagenesis, and pharmacokinetic variability, are also germane to the pediatric age group.
These factors, however, do not normally impose a barrier to drug development
in children, although specific cases may prevent the initiation of clinical trials
with certain drugs.

Despite these issues, pediatric clinical trials and testing can be properly conducted if careful steps are taken to ensure the safety of the subject and of the drug.
Recent regulatory efforts to require pediatric studies to be a part of the labeling
process for all drugs, with some exceptions, are certain to increase the numbers
of pediatric clinical trials in the near future. This focus on the need to improve
drug development in children came to the fore when Dr. David Kessler, a pediatri-
cian, was commissioner of the FDA. His recognition of the drawbacks of off-label
prescribing practices in pediatrics was largely responsible for the stepped-up efforts
by regulatory authorities to intervene in this process in recent years.

The decision to conduct a pediatric drug study and the relative timing of
such a study, is based on the following underlying factors:

1.   Severity of the disease
2.   Availability of alternative therapy
3.   Safety/efficacy versus toxicity ratio
4.   Distribution of the disease in pediatric populations
5.   Duration of the disease
6.   Practicality of conducting the study
7.   Regulatory influence

This chapter discusses each of these seven decision points and provides specific
examples that demonstrate the application of these principles. Special emphasis
is placed on regulatory changes of the past decade.

II. FACTORS AFFECTING THE STUDY OF A DRUG IN THE PEDIATRIC POPULATION

A. Severity of the Disease

The basis for determining the necessity and urgency of conducting clinical trials
in the pediatric population is related directly to the severity of the disease process.
For this discussion, we will classify disease process "severe with high mortality"
(e.g., HIV), "clinically significant, but not usually fatal" (e.g., hepatitis), or "minor" (e.g., acne). The greater the severity of the disease, the greater is the obligation to conduct trials in younger patients.

B.   Availability of Alternative Therapy

The need to identify a new drug in the pediatric population depends on whether suitable alternatives exist. There may be no available therapy to treat a disease, the therapy available may result in significant treatment failures, or it may be associated with unacceptable side effects. Often overlooked is the fact that an otherwise acceptable therapy may be unavailable in a dosage formulation suitable for infants and children. Appropriate dosage sizes, lack of liquid formulations, and strange tastes decrease compliance with treatment modalities, directly or indirectly. In many instances, parents must divide an adult tablet to obtain the appropriate dose prescribed for their child. This practice often results in imprecise dosing, with a poor therapeutic response. At times, drugs are prepared in liquid forms by pharmacies in a well-intentioned attempt to aid parents. This effort, however, gives rise to formulations that have not been tested for expiration, stability, or efficacy. In effect, the lack of adequate drug formulations renders a therapy unavailable for children.

C.   Safety and Efficacy Versus Toxicity Ratio

The balance among safety, efficacy, and toxicity is a major concern in the decision to engage a pediatric subject in drug research. From birth through adolescence, a child is constantly changing, both physiologically and metabolically. These dynamic changes contribute to the increased susceptibility of these individuals to certain types of undesirable effects from drugs. Consider the following examples.

Delayed toxicity.   Certain completely unanticipated types of toxicity have been shown to develop long after exposure to the offending agent. Examples include retrolental fibroplasia (a scarring of the retina that occurs in children months to years after exposure to oxygen in the neonatal period), and uterine cancer (has been linked to the offspring of mothers exposed to diethylstilbestrol while pregnant (2–4).

Mutagenesis.   During the early developmental years, individuals are especially vulnerable to genetic alterations from drug effects.

Drug interactions.   Unique and important drug interactions occur in the pediatric population. For example, infants have special needs for certain dietary components, such as vitamins, amino acids, and calcium, to maintain normal growth and development. The efficacy of these dietary elements may be enhanced or diminished by drugs. Calcium (found in milk), for example, significantly interferes with the absorption of some antibiotics, limiting their therapeutic effectiveness. In addition, antibiotics can alter the intestinal flora, potentially resulting in diminished absorption of certain vitamins. Although the same may be true in adults, one normally does not attach the same importance to these ancillary interactions because the effects on cognitive and physical development in adults are not an issue.

Pharmacokinetics. The absorption, distribution, metabolism, and excretion of drugs in children can be dramatically different than in adults (5), substantially restricting the ability to extrapolate data from adults to children. The pharmacokinetic behavior of chloramphenicol, for example, is markedly different in neonates because hepatic glucuronidation is not well developed in infants. When this antibiotic was first administered (off-label) to neonates, excessive concentrations of chloramphenicol occurred and were associated with abdominal distention, hypotension, hypoxia, and poor perfusion. The gray appearance secondary to poor perfusion gave rise to the term ''gray baby syndrome'' used to describe this condition. Consequently, chloramphenicol is now contraindicated in the neonatal population.

Bioavailability. For all the reasons previously discussed, infants and children usually require drug formulations unique to their age group to assure adequate delivery of a drug.

D. Distribution of the Disease in Pediatric Populations

The distribution of a disease in the pediatric population determines not only whether the drug will be studied, but also how such studies will be timed in the continuum of drug development. If the disease is rare with no alternative therapy, or if it occurs primarily in children, deviations are permitted from the usual safety and efficacy requirements. In such cases, a Phase I study may be initiated directly in children, permitting pediatric pharmacological evaluations to begin in the absence of comparable data from adults. After minimal pharmacokinetic studies have been completed, it may be reasonable for pilot efficacy studies to proceed in children, and greater flexibility may be extended to investigators with regard to efficacy requirements. Additional leeway is often granted concerning the frequency and amount of doses that may be used without extensive preclinical studies.

If a disease occurs in both adults and children, the initial single-dose and short-term multiple-dose studies are usually initiated in adults (frequently in normal volunteers) to define a dosage range suitable for human pharmacological and toxicological effects. If and when pediatric investigation ensues, the initial studies are usually conducted in pediatric pharmacology research units (PPRUs), which have with adequate facilities and personnel to carefully monitor and execute the pharmacokinetic bioavailability and clinical studies. These units are funded by the National Institute of Child Health and Human Development and constitute a formal network that was established to provide access to large numbers of infants and children with a correspondingly large number of diseases. These research units are also geographically distinct, thus distributing both the risk and the benefit of clinical investigation across the entire pediatric population.

Subsequent pediatric investigation is conducted in small numbers of children and usually consists of studies using single-dose schedules or short-term multiple doses with an escalating dose schedule. Pilot studies assessing efficacy are initiated only after studies establishing evidence of pharmacological activity and toxic dosage ranges are completed in the adult population, unless an indication is limited to children.

E. Duration of the Disease

The duration of the disease to be investigated with a new compound affects the timing of the investigation. The normal investigative period involved in attaining FDA approval consists of four phases of study (Phases I through IV clinical trials). If a disease is acute and short-lived, pediatric patients are usually studied during Phases I and II. When the disease is chronic, however, pediatric trials are usually not initiated until Phase III or Phase IV. Some drugs, such as psychoactive compounds, must be administered to children over many months or years. In such cases, special preclinical tests should be completed before the initiation of pediatric trials. Such studies would include animal studies testing for the effect of the compound on growth, development, pubescence, and reproduction—the effects of long-term administration. Typically, these studies are not completed until Phase III. Studies in pediatric patients should be scheduled so that the effects of the test drug can be assessed during various stages of development, especially during periods of rapid growth and development.

F. Practicality of Conducting the Study

A factor often overlooked when addressing the lack of pediatric drug trials for new drug development is the practicality of conducting the study. The number of investigators trained in pediatric pharmacology is quite limited. In addition, the number of pediatric patients available to participate in a study may be insufficient, either because the disease is much less common in the pediatric population, or because the pediatric population is scattered, rendering the study impractical. Although the latter problem has been partially addressed by the advent of the PPRUs network, it still can pose a significant barrier to clinical trials in certain types of patients.

The measurements necessary to obtain a definable endpoint may be unobtainable in neonates and infants. Pulmonary function tests, for example, are not easily performed in subjects under the age of 6 years. This clearly can affect asthma studies and may cause the investigator to use alternative endpoints, such as asthma questionnaires that provide less objective data. Validated, subjective test procedures, such as measurements on a visual analog scale, are obviously impossible when a patient has not yet learned to speak. Hence, methodology, or lack thereof, may be crucial. Furthermore, it was only a short time ago that the clinical laboratory was adapted adequately to use the smaller volume of biological fluids available in pediatric patients to measure drug bioavailability, chemistries, electrolytes, and other parameters needed to evaluate drug safety and efficacy. Even now, many tests do not lend themselves to use in the pediatric population because of blood volume considerations in small children.

Finally, trials conducted early in the development of a drug often involve either hospitalized patients or patients who can be grouped together and kept under close supervision. This poses limitations when studying children, where the importance of being permitted to remain in the secure and comforting environs of home is tantamount. Thus, pediatric clinical trials must be designed to limit patient inconveniences such as discomfort, travel distance, and time. Outpatient trials, which may be more convenient, usually come later in the course of drug development.

G. Regulatory and Legal Issues

When initiating pediatric studies, many important, sometimes political, regulatory and legal issues must be considered. Regulations affecting pediatric drug trials differ widely from country to country. Even in the United States within the FDA, opinions often vary, although in many cases this variation results from the many clinical and practical issues discussed above.

In the United States, many regulatory issues are governed by Institutional Review Boards (IRBs), which play a major role in deciding the timing, conduct, and design of pediatric investigational trials. The IRB (or a proxy IRB) must review every pediatric drug protocol submitted to the institution. The composition of the board is specified by law and must include individuals such as priests, homemakers, and other nonmedical personnel. Given such a mix of participants, it is hardly surprising that opinions vary widely from institution to institution regarding pediatric trials. This situation is further complicated by the fact that not every IRB has members with experience or training in the conduct of clinical trials involving children.

One specific important regulatory and legal concern is the difficult issue of consent versus assent. Some people argue that it is impossible for a child of any age to give true informed consent. It is certainly impossible for an infant even to assent to a clinical trial, much less give informed consent. Clearly, the parent or guardian must give consent for the child, but removing consent from the individual most affected by the trial further complicates the approval process.

Also complicating this process is the rise in the numbers of single parents and the often-contentious custody issues surrounding these situations.

Finally, judicial findings play a major role in the decision to study a drug in a pediatric population, as exemplified by the story of Bendectin™. Bendectin was the only FDA-approved drug ever indicated for use during pregnancy for nausea and vomiting. First marketed in 1956, it was subsequently used by 33 million pregnant women. Inevitably, liability suits were brought against the manufacturer, Merrell-Dow, by the parents of deformed babies whose mothers had ingested Bendectin during pregnancy. The scientific facts were impressive. Numerous teratology studies in multiple animal species had failed to show any association of Bendectin with teratological risk. Perhaps most impressive were the results of several large epidemiological studies in humans, which assessed subjects exposed to Bendectin and failed to suggest any teratological potential. The sad fact is that many congenital abnormalities occur in babies; there is a baseline incidence of these defects regardless of maternal ingestion of any medication.

Despite these facts, Merrell-Dow was found liable in a legal case brought by parents of a child born with limb-reduction deformities after in-utero exposure to Bendectin. A flood of lawsuits followed this verdict, as one would expect. The company's insurance premiums tripled in 3 years, reaching $1 million per month, with sales of Bendectin exceeding $15 million per year. With 325 suits pending, Merrill-Dow ceased production of Bendectin in 1983. Thus, a judicial, rather than scientific, decision leading to the subsequent withdrawal of Bendectin left the medical community with a significant therapeutic void, because severe cases of nausea and vomiting during pregnancy may lead to serious maternal nutritional deficiencies linked to damaging effects in the fetus.

III. EXAMPLES OF DRUG DEVELOPMENT

To illustrate how the factors outlined in the Introduction may be used in practical applications (i.e., before submitting a New Drug Application to the FDA), consider the following two examples.

A. Example 1: Tracrium™

Tracrium (atracurium besylate), is a nondepolarizing neuromuscular blocking agent with an intermediate duration of action (45 min).

1. *Severity of the disease*. This compound was intended for use during surgery, and hence would be considered a clinically significant agent.
2. *Availability of alternative therapy*. No other agents of intermediate

duration were available; the commonly used neuromuscular blocking agents available for children at that time were either very short or very long in duration of action. Furthermore, all previously available neuromuscular blocking agents caused significant cardiovascular side effects (e.g., bradycardia, hypertension, tachycardia, malignant hyperthermia) in a portion of the pediatric population.

3. *Safety/efficacy versus toxicity ratio.* Because Tracrium was only to be administered as a single dose, there was no reason to expect any delayed toxicity. Moreover, because its effects were of intermediate duration, its actions were expected to approximate the duration of surgery in many pediatric cases. Furthermore, at the time of administration, minimal cardiovascular effects at therapeutic doses had been observed in 500 adult patients during Phase II trials, and no significant abnormal laboratory or electrocardiogram data had been found.

4. *Distribution of the disease in pediatric populations.* Surgery occurs uniformly often in the pediatric population.

5. *Regulatory influence.* Because of the safety/efficacy ratio previously demonstrated in adults, it was easy to enlist the approval of the IRBs. Additionally, parents and children were cooperative and freely gave consent to participate. One center required at least verbal assent for children age 7 and older, and another required only parental consent.

6. *Duration of the disease.* Surgery is acute.

7. *Practicality of conducting the study.* Surgery is a frequent occurrence in the pediatric population. In addition, all patients were necessarily hospitalized and under the direct care of an anesthesiologist with ready systems for life support. Good follow-up also was available. One complicating factor was that preoperative and postoperative chemistries are not routine for uncomplicated pediatric surgery cases, and thus this information had to be included in the informed consent. These two otherwise unnecessary venipunctures did have the potential for negatively influencing patient entry. Therefore, to optimize the entry rate and obtain safety data, a quota system was devised wherein the protocol required the collection of laboratory safety data from at least 30% of patients studied. When the study was conducted, investigators were actually able to obtain data from 47% of the patients between 2 and 10 years of age; however, no laboratory data was collected in the patients between 1 month and 2 years of age.

When the New Drug Application (NDA) for Tracrium was approved by the FDA, adequate dosing instructions for pediatric patients were included in the approved package insert.

B. Example 2: Flolan™

Flolan (prostacyclin/epoprostenol sodium) is an example of a drug that was studied in the pediatric setting very early in the course of its development. Flolan is a naturally occurring substance, synthesized primarily by vascular endothelial cells. It is the strongest vasodilator and antiplatelet aggregation agent known. Given its pharmacological profile, the drug was studied very early in its development in relation to a disease called persistent fetal circulation of pulmonary hypertension of the newborn.

1. *Severity of the disease.* Persistent fetal circulation is an extremely severe disease, with a mortality rate of >90% in those newborns who fail to respond to conventional treatment.
2. *Availability of alternative therapy.* The only treatment available was hyperventilation and 100% oxygen. This combination was considered to be a relatively low-risk therapy, but the failure rate was unacceptably high, at approximately 40% treatment failure.
3. *Safety/efficacy versus toxicity ratio.* Owing to the extreme pharmacological potency of the drug, hypotension, flushing, nausea and vomiting, and headaches were known to occur. Offsetting these limitations was its short pharmacological half-life, which is 3 min in adults and is similar in children.
4. *Distribution of the disease in pediatric populations.* Persistent fetal circulation occurs only in neonates, at or shortly after birth.
5. *Regulatory influence.* Given the severity of the disease and the unfavorable outcome for those patients who fail to respond to conventional therapy, the FDA, IRB, and parental consent were all favorable.
6. *Duration of the disease.* The course of the disease is acute, with recovery or death within days.
7. *Practicality of conducting the study.* Considerable negatives weighed against the decision to proceed with the study: the frequency of the disease was rare, with only one or two resistant cases per year in large medical centers; neonatologists are not usually trained in drug development; and cardiac catheterization was required (a procedure that might not otherwise be needed) to make the measurements necessary for entrance into the study and to measure efficacy. On the positive side, however, the patients were always hospitalized.

The decision was made to proceed with the Flolan study. Only the worst cases were enrolled. Unfortunately, after accumulating approximately 12 patients, the study was suspended because of lack of sufficient data demonstrating efficacy. One very interesting and surprising bit of data emerged: neonates could tolerate 5 to 10 times the dosages of Flolan that would make adults quite ill.

This drug was subsequently used to treat primary pulmonary hypertension, a disease of unknown etiology that occurs in both children and adults. The first treatment of primary pulmonary hypertension with Flolan was given to an 8-year-old child in 1980 (6). The first adult study for the same indication was performed later, in 1982 (7). This indication was pursued and Flolan was finally approved for primary pulmonary hypertension in New York Heart Association Class III and Class IV patients. No approval has ever been granted for use in pediatric patients.

These two examples demonstrate the decision-making process that goes into a drug development plan. In one case, the decision was successful. In the case of Flolan, the study was not successful, and the trial was suspended with the possibility that another study might be attempted after more was known about the drug. It is curious indeed that this occurred for a related, although not identical, indication in adults. Children with the same disease were never studied; thus this potent agent is now used off-label in the pediatric population because no alternative treatment exists for the disease.

IV. RECENT DEVELOPMENTS IN PEDIATRIC REGULATIONS

The fact that, for years, very few drugs were labeled safe and effective for pediatric use led the FDA to issue labeling requirements in 1979 (8) to address this problem. These regulations required that specific pediatric indications be described in the Indications and Usage section and the recommended pediatric doses in the Dosage and Administration section of the drug label. Recommendations for pediatric use had to be based on substantial evidence derived from adequate and well-controlled trials in the pediatric population, unless the requirement was waived. If safety and efficacy could not be proved, or if the drug posed specific hazards to children, specific comments were to be included in the Pediatric Use section of the label.

Although the intent of these new regulations was to promote pediatric labeling, it had the opposite effect because it called for enhanced data collection in children, which was often difficult or impractical to gather. During a 5-year period (1984–1989), the American Academy of Pediatrics found that about 80% of all drugs approved had no pediatric use information.

Because of concerns related to inappropriate use or nonuse of these drugs, the FDA wrote a new pediatric rule in 1994 (9). This rule was an attempt to both clarify the FDA position vis-à-vis the 1979 requirements, and at the same time simplify the requirements for industry to provide adequate pediatric information. The requirement that pediatric labeling must be based on adequate and well-controlled trials in children was amended to allow submissions of other data when these trials were not or could not be performed. This essentially permitted the extrapolation of adult data to pediatric populations, although additional pediatric safety and pharmacokinetic information had to be submitted upon request. This rule also increased the responsibility of the sponsor to justify those instances when pediatric labeling should not occur. Finally, the fact that inactive ingredients can pose hazards to children was also recognized. Still very little progress was made after the 1994 rule. In 1996, only 15 of 40 new molecular entities (NMEs) thought to have pediatric applications included any pediatric labeling. By 1997, only 9 of 27 potentially useful NMEs included pediatric use information.

When it became clear that voluntary compliance would not achieve the stated goal of increased pediatric labeling, the FDA issued a new rule in 1998 (10). This rule mandates pediatric studies for all NMEs, new active ingredients, new indications, new dosage forms, new dosing regimens, and new routes of administration. Waivers may be given and deferral of information may be granted at times. Furthermore, if a sponsor is not compliant, legal proceedings may be initiated.

Drugs that have already been marketed may also be affected if at least one of the following is true:

1. Substantial pediatric use occurs for the marketed indications, and lack of labeling may pose significant risk.
2. Increased therapeutic benefit can be achieved over existing therapy in pediatric patients, and lack of labeling may pose significant risk in this population.

At present, substantial use is defined as 50,000 children with a specific disease or condition. In a pediatric subpopulation (e.g., neonates), 15,000 patients must have a specific disease or condition. Meaningful therapeutic benefit means significant improvement in prevention, diagnosis, or treatment of disease compared with marketed products that are labeled for pediatric use. Increased patient compliance, decrease or elimination of drug reactions, and efficacy and safety in a new subpopulation also constitute significant improvement.

The 1998 rule also requires the constitution of a panel of pediatric experts to advise the FDA on matters concerning the conduct of pediatric clinical trials, including ethics, trial design, and questions pertaining to substantial use and significant therapeutic benefit.

Waivers are granted when it is clear that no pediatric benefit exists—that is, that the number of cases is small and the therapeutic benefit is minimal or nonexistent. Examples of diseases that meet these criteria are breast cancer, Alzheimer's disease, osteoarthritis, and lung cancer, all of which result in automatic waivers. Waivers may be requested if too few patients exist with a pediatric disease, or if those who are affected are geographically dispersed and hence too difficult to study. If evidence suggests that a drug would be ineffective or unsafe in children, a waiver may also be granted.

A deferral of pediatric information until after approval may be granted if safety and efficacy data need to be on hand before conducting pediatric trials, or if conducting the pediatric studies would result in a delay in the development process, thus limiting the availability of the therapeutic agent to adults. If a new drug is not likely to offer benefits over and above those drugs already approved for children, pediatric data submission may also be deferred. In such instances, until pediatric studies are conducted, the approved label must advise against use in children and, if appropriate, suggest other drugs in the same class that have been labeled for pediatric use.

To further increase compliance with pediatric labeling, Congress has provided economic incentives in the form of a 6-month extension of exclusivity within the Food and Drug Administration Modernization Act of 1997 for products (antibiotics and most biologics are excluded) that have exclusivity or patent rights. Exclusivity extensions are granted via three steps: (a) the sponsor receives a written request from the FDA; (b) the sponsor reports the results of the requested studies; and (c) the FDA determines whether the report meets the terms of the written request.

Written requests from the FDA are sent in response to a proposal from a sponsor, manufacturer, or an interested party on behalf of either the sponsor or the manufacturer. The proposal is submitted under an appropriate Investigational New Drug (IND) Application or NDA, and can include references, planned studies, analyses, description of suitability for children, and so forth. Analysis of the literature alone is not acceptable. If the proposal is adequate, the FDA sends a formal written request to the applicant that details exactly what needs to be done and a time frame that must be followed. Upon receipt of the report, the FDA makes a determination based on a review division's findings, which are endorsed by a pediatric panel. Granting of exclusivity is not connected to approval; the pivotal factor is whether the applicant complied with the terms of the written request. As of April 1, 2001, 218 proposed pediatric study requests had been received, and 188 written requests had been issued. In addition, as of February 26, 2001, 38 total exclusivity determinations had been made, of which, 27 were approved. As of March 1, 2001, 16 changes to pediatric exclusivity labeling had been made.

Congress has recently requested that the FDA publish an annual list of drugs that may produce benefits in children. These are termed "essential drugs" for children and are targeted as a developmental priority for children. As far back as 1979, the American Academy of Pediatrics' Committee on Drugs made a list of hundreds of drugs in 33 therapeutic groups thought to be useful for children, but not labeled as such. This list was created under contract with the FDA. However, no effort was made to rank these drugs, and the FDA never took official action concerning this list. In 1984, a second list of 103 drugs was made, under contract, and sent to the FDA. Again, no attempt was made to rank the drugs. Subsequently, the FDA did request a list of 10 important drugs used parenterally in neonates, which finally resulted in some progress: pediatric information was eventually added to five of these drugs.

The recent request from Congress includes every drug approved for any indication found in children. Also included is a priority section consisting of drugs that are already approved for an adult indication, which have the same potential pediatric indication and, if approved for children, would result in a significant benefit over products already marketed. Any such drug must meet the additional criterion of being prescribed at least 50,000 times yearly, and it must be needed for additional therapeutic or diagnostic use.

At present, this list is used for internal FDA review purposes, but it will likely find wider application in the future. Industry investment in pediatric drugs is disproportionately concentrated in antimicrobials, probably because of market potential. Other important drugs such as sedatives or hypnotics, inotropes, and antiarrhythmics are not labeled for pediatric use or are not available in appropriate formulations for children. For example, Adenocard™ IV (adenosine), a drug widely used in children to convert supraventricular tachycardia to sinus rhythm, has never been studied in a controlled trial in the pediatric population. Proper application of a carefully designed priority list will be one way of helping to correct this imbalance.

V. CONCLUSIONS

Although pediatric clinical trials are difficult to conduct, well-designed studies can and should be conducted for drugs that will be, or may be, used in children. The FDA is developing guidelines for pediatric clinical trials that address trial design, the use of placebos, and the role of data and safety monitoring boards in modulating these studies. Off-label use of drugs for children is a practice that should be discouraged, because it is essentially the use of a drug that has not been approved by the FDA. An adult indication does not directly translate to a pediatric indication, and it is not acceptable for a physician to assume the risk of using a drug off-label merely because it has not been tested in children.

The new regulations described above represent an important step toward correcting the inequities that exist between adults and children in contemporary drug development.

REFERENCES

1. Shirkey H. Therapeutic orphans. J Pediatr 1968; 72:119–120.
2. Olitsky SE, Nelson LB. Disorders of the retina and vitreous. In: Behrman RE, Klieg-man RM, Jenson HB, eds. Nelson Textbook of Pediatrics. Philadelphia: Saunders, 2000:1925–1931.
3. Herbst AL, Cole P, Colton T, Robboy SJ, Scully RE. Age-incidence and risk of diethylstilbestrol-related clear cell adenocarcinoma of the vagina and cervix. Am J Obstet Gynecol 1977; 128:43–50.
4. Mattingly RF, Stafi A. Cancer risk in diethylstilbestrol-exposed offspring. Am J Obstet Gynecol 1976; 126:543–548.
5. McManus MC, Peterson MB. Developmental pharmacology. In: Todres ID, Fugate JH, eds. Critical Care of Infants and Children. New York: Little, Brown, 1996:570–581.
6. Watkins WD, Peterson MB, Crone RK, Shannon DC, Levine L. Prostacyclin and prostaglandin E1 for severe idiopathic pulmonary artery hypertension. Lancet 1980; 1(8177):1083.
7. Rubin LJ, Groves BM, Reeves JT, Frosolono M, Handel F, Cato AE. Prostacyclin induced acute pulmonary vasodilation in primary pulmonary hypertension. Circulation 1982; 66:334–338.
8. 44 Fed Reg 37434, June 26, 1979.
9. 59 Fed Reg 64240, December 13, 1994.
10. 63 Fed Reg 66631 (Part 231), December 2, 1998.

8
Electronic Capture of Clinical Trial Information

Daniel C. Cato
Cato Research Ltd., Durham, North Carolina

David B. Thomas
Roche Molecular Systems, Inc., Pleasanton, California

I. INTRODUCTION

The drug development process has matured into a system used primarily for capturing information on paper. Although this process is entrenched in industry procedures and is well understood, documented, and accepted, it is also recognized as somewhat inefficient and costly. To date, the greatest progress in moving clinical trial information by electronic modes has been in the transfer of patient testing results from centralized laboratories to trial sponsors' databases. This technical innovation was made by the central laboratories that had the electronic technologies available through their own laboratory information systems and saw an opportunity to attract business from clinical trial sponsors by offering efficient transfer of testing information to the sponsor.

For more than 20 years, various proposals have been made for expanding electronic data capture to encompass an increased portion of trial information. The motivation behind these proposals has been the quest to (a) reduce the time it takes to collect and verify trial information, (b) simplify the collection process of trial information in hopes of increasing the accuracy of study data, and (c) reduce the resources (costs) involved in conducting trials. Only in the last few years has the technology been available to help us see how these goals might be achieved.

This chapter discusses various methods of electronic clinical trial data capture that use a variety of technologies intended to improve the clinical drug development process. In addition, consideration is given to some regulatory issues that have emerged as a result of the initiatives to integrate electronic data capture technologies into the clinical trial process.

II. HANDLING PAPER MORE EFFICIENTLY

A. Optical Character Recognition

One intermediate step in improving the efficiency of paper-based systems is to use technology to handle paper more efficiently. For example, extracting data from case report forms (CRFs) by using optical character recognition (OCR) from scanned or faxed images of CRF pages has been employed for some time. This technology allows sponsors to route, archive, and disseminate electronic versions, rather than paper versions, of the study data. However, until the last few years, the limited accuracy of OCR systems had restricted the efficiency of this process. Today, using forms designed for OCR data entry and using state-of-the-art technology, it is possible to scan data into a database with a high degree of accuracy (>99%).

However, although OCR continues to improve, as long as some error in transfer is possible, an operator will be required to oversee the product and to verify and correct questionable data. Additionally, some studies are more suitable for OCR data entry because their CRFs can be carefully designed to optimize the technology. For example, the best results can be obtained from studies whose CRFs contain a high percentage of predefined data options (i.e., check boxes) and limited requirements for hand-written text entries. Various vendors now offer systems employing form, fax, and OCR database entry for use in clinical trials. (A fairly comprehensive source of information technology [IT] vendors for clinical trials is available in the annual IT Solutions of the journal *Applied Clinical Trials*.) Although these systems are not perfect, they represent a relatively inexpensive technological investment, and they can be readily integrated into traditional paper-based trial management systems.

B. Bar Coding

Another time-consuming yet critical aspect of paper-based systems is tracking the source documentation pages of original data or data changes. Traditionally, this task has been done by some system of numbering CRF pages and other study documentation. These numbers must be accurately applied to each document and then placed in the study database as indication of the source of information entered. A filing system must then be maintained that allows retrieval of each page.

Paper systems are cumbersome to maintain and are difficult to manage, particularly when questions arise about the study data.

A technology that has shown promise to improve this system is bar coding. Applying such codes to documents provides quick and highly accurate coding of trial data and obviates the need to code each study document manually. Again, this technology is relatively cheap, available, and in the case of most industry-sponsored trials, is likely to be used within the quality and manufacturing operations of the trial sponsor.

III. REMOTE DATA ENTRY AND ELECTRONIC DATA CAPTURE

The delay between the patient visit and the time the data are entered into the sponsor's database is a problem inherent in paper-based study data collection systems. If CRFs are collected by the sponsor when the patient completes the study, then, in a year-long study, at least a year will have passed between the patient's first visit and the time the data are entered into the database. Most sponsors increase the efficiency of their process by requiring that CRF data be submitted to a central data management center at specified intervals during a patient's progress through the trial. The advantage of such a procedure is that questionable or invalid data can be identified and data issues can be resolved on an ongoing basis. However, in practice, it is often difficult for clinical sites to keep up with the sponsor's expectations for the prompt and accurate completion and submission of CRF data. In addition, when the sponsor receives the CRF data, it takes some time before it can be screened and entered and items can be identified that need to be returned to the site for resolution. During this time, the site personnel may be unaware that the sponsor has issues with the site's interpretation of the study protocol or completion of the CRFs, and the particular problem may continue unchecked.

One way industry has tried to decrease the time between the investigator's evaluation of the patient and entry of that data into the database is by implementing remote data entry (RDE) systems. In an RDE system, data entry and capture capabilities are provided at each study site. Personnel at each site are trained to enter the data upon completion of the CRF or after each patient visit. In this way, the data, although not necessarily checked by the clinical monitor, are available to the sponsor in a more timely manner. After entry, the data can be sent to the sponsor by upload over a modem connection or by mailing removable storage devices (e.g., floppy disks, CDs). Therefore, data questions from the sponsor can be posed earlier in the process, when the site is still familiar with the patient.

Although RDE systems have been used successfully, many problems exist with the overall strategy. RDE requires additional work at the site because data must be recorded on paper CRFs before being entered into the RDE system. Because the requisite computers are usually provided by the study sponsor, that company will likely limit the use of the RDE computers to only their study. Therefore, the company imposes upon the study site additional space requirements for a dedicated computer required for each RDE study being conducted at that location. In addition, because RDE systems are not standardized, the site personnel probably will also need extensive training on each system; this is further complicated by study site staff turnover. Once implemented and implemented correctly, RDE systems can provide quick turnaround and review of the study data. Realistically, however, they provide only minimal advantage over simply faxing completed CRFs (or completed portions of CRFs) promptly to a data management group.

However, the data entry process can be shortened by one full step if, using those same data entry and data capture systems, the CRF data are entered directly into a digital format (electronic data capture [EDC]) rather than first being transcribed by the site onto written CRF pages. This saves the laborious process of data entry of the CRFs either at the site or back at the sponsor's location.

In addition to CRF data, other information that might be electronically captured (digitized) at a clinical site and transmitted to the sponsor includes the following:

Study documentation (investigator's agreements, CVs, contracts, investigational product accountability, etc.)
Study data (CRFs, adverse experience reports, imaging and other assessment records, etc.)
Patient-initiated records (study diaries, event reporting, remote sensing records such as Holter Monitoring readings)
Study data queries and their resolution

Until recently, the implementation of remote data capture systems was significantly hindered by issues related to the regulatory standard that all information from trial sites be attributed to an individual qualified to certify the accuracy of the data. Traditionally this standard had been fulfilled by a qualified investigator or designee who signed and dated a form. Because there was no alternative to the written signature, data submitted electronically by the site at some point still had to be printed and sent back to the investigator for review and signature. In effect, the signature process negated some of the efficiency gained through remote data entry. However, in 1997, a Food and Drug Administration ruling (1) recognized the validity of electronic records and electronic signatures. Title 21 of the *Code of Federal Regulations*, Part 11, represents a significant step forward in electronic data capture and submission of clinical data.

IV. ELECTRONIC DATA CAPTURE SYSTEMS

With the range of technologies available today, a variety of systems exists for the remote electronic data capture of trial data into the sponsor's central database, and the workflow from EDC systems can be fairly uncomplicated. Site personnel enter study data directly into the EDC system instead of first transcribing the information onto paper CRFs. To reduce data queries, logic checks can be built into systems so that inconsistent or out-of-range values can be flagged at the time they are entered. This allows erroneous data to be corrected before it is committed to the trial database, and it prompts for additional explanatory information that may assist in interpretation of the data submitted.

Alternatively, the data may be entered into a locally stored database and then transmitted to the sponsor's database, where it is edited. At some point during the entry process, the system should provide for site review and certification that the information being submitted is consistent with the source documentation (e.g., patient records). For information derived from source documentation at the site, monitoring will still be necessary to verify that the submitted information matches the source database and to reconcile any discrepancies—the same as in paper-based systems.

EDC systems for clinical studies can be categorized as offline or online, differentiated by whether or not an active connection to the study's central database is required. Each type of EDC system is discussed below.

A. Offline EDC Systems

Offline EDC systems with local data capture and transmission to the sponsor's database can have various configurations. Generally, all involve some hardware that allows data entry into a configuration defined by the study protocol (e.g., CRF page formats). The system may involve a sponsor-supplied database to be run on the site's personal computer (PC), or a turnkey system provided by the sponsor (i.e., hardware [PC] and database). Advantages of the turnkey configuration are that the site database (and PC) can be supplied in a validated state and data can be edited against protocol requirements as it is entered. Accepted data can be transmitted in batch mode to the sponsor via modem (telephone) upload, or sent on some type of removable medium (floppy disks, CDs, etc.). Although this configuration for managing data from multicenter trials was described more than 20 years ago, it is only with the recent drop in PC prices and the availability of reliable off-the-shelf software that such configurations have become attractive.

A more sophisticated configuration of direct input into the sponsor's study database involves "thin" client configurations. In these systems, the site need have only a simple PC equipped with a browser and a modem. Data entry from the site is accomplished by dial-up to the sponsor's database so that the data entry formats are communicated from the central database to the browser. Screen entry of data by the site goes directly into the central database with no information stored on the local PC. In this configuration, data may be edited, queried, and accepted or rejected during the entry process or at the end of a data entry session. Some advantages of thin client solutions are the low cost, the flexibility regarding the PC configuration at the site (only the compatibility of the browser influences compatibility with the sponsor's database), and the availability of thin client software (products from Microsoft and Citrix are the most commonly used). Because these systems do not require a high-quality phone connection, a powerful PC, or additional validation, sites almost anywhere in the world can participate in trials using this technology. An added security advantage exists for the trial sponsor in that the data are never stored outside the central database. Thin client technology also provides the sponsor with numerous options for performing data entry. For example, the sponsor may choose to offer RDE capability to some sites, while using its own staff to perform the data entry activities on behalf of other sites.

B. Online EDC Systems

Online EDC systems require users to establish and maintain an active connection with a central server or at least have the capability to log into a Web site. This is the model on which most Internet-based clinical trial systems are structured. The data reside on a central server that users access via the Internet. In these systems, the site must have appropriate access to a PC and an Internet connection consistent with the trial requirements. Although this technology seems readily available, it is sometimes a problem for the participating clinical sites to access the Internet as required by a study. The central database is maintained on a server connected to an Internet gateway. Although it is possible for the sponsor to maintain a Web site to support clinical trial protocols, it is now both cost-effective and highly reliable to place the study database on a server through an Internet service provider who maintains such applications. These "server farms" support continuous online availability of the database and have highly developed security systems assuring that access is appropriately controlled.

As these "e-trial" systems have developed, some firms have emerged that will develop databases for Internet-connected servers and manage the connectivity portion of the trial. These firms are sometimes referred to as application service providers (ASPs). Besides providing Internet technology expertise, using these firms has proven to be an entry point into EDC-based trials that do not require large technological commitments. This strategy has proven particularly attractive because of the rapid evolution of Internet technology and the difficulty of making a technology investment in this environment. However, most of these ASPs are venture capital-funded start-ups that emerged in the mid- to late 1990s. With the recent downturn of the equity markets in developed countries, several of these firms have abruptly gone out of business. This trend has been sufficiently worrisome to the U.S. Food and Drug Administration (FDA) that the Agency has recently reminded trial sponsors that they are responsible for the integrity of trials: the failure of an ASP does not relieve the sponsor of its obligations to assure that all Current Good Clinical Practice requirements are met regardless of the need to make abrupt changes in mode of data capture in the trial. Again, because no standardization of e-trial systems exists, sites participating in trials with multiple sponsors are likely to have requirements for training their staff on multiple systems.

The development of Internet sites to support RDE trials has moved in the direction of providing fairly complete Web-based trial management systems. For instance, the Web site can maintain a bulletin board for sponsor communication with the clinical sites, other sponsor sites that are participating in the trial, or local monitors. Information on the status of the trial, such as enrollment, can be posted, and access can be controlled through passwords. Although some of these systems have become quite elaborate, it is probably too early to decide whether they add much value or are largely embellishments.

C. Advantages of EDC Systems

In principle, EDC systems can provide the sponsor with more rapid access to study results and, by providing continuous monitoring of data, decrease the volume of study data queries, resulting in reduced study costs, less frustration at the study sites, and more rapid data lock when compared with paper-based systems. Although extravagant claims have been made about the increased efficiency of EDC-based trials, the results to date have been mixed. It is clear that to incorporate EDC technology efficiently into trial systems, sponsors must adapt their procedures and department organizations to accommodate the IT support and the changes in staff roles. In some cases, it may be that the database itself becomes the source document (e.g., patient diary data uploaded through a browser with associated patient electronic signature). However, in most cases, just as with paper CRF submission, site visits to monitor protocol compliance and verification of data will still be required.

A major issue for manufacturers and contract research organizations is the acceptability of EDC systems by FDA-reviewing divisions. This point has been discussed in a variety of forums; agency spokespersons have not raised particular concerns, but have noted that any EDC system used must meet the requirements of the agency's guidance document for Computerized Systems Used in Clinical Trials (2). However, as this chapter is written, no marketing applications have been submitted to the FDA in which pivotal trials employing a strict EDC-based process of data collection were included. This may be attributable to industry caution when it comes to incorporating new technology into the high-stakes marketing application process, more than it reflects on the immaturity of EDC technology.

V. REVIEW

In a recent survey (3), EDC appears to be gaining acceptance by the industry. Most (78%) of the respondents (a mixture of personnel from clinical sites, pharmaceutical companies, and contract research organizations) viewed their EDC experiences in a positive or neutral way. Respondents cited the primary advantages of working with an EDC system as earlier and continuous data collection, less paper, savings in cycle time, reduction in errors, and facilitation of query resolution. Included in the responses, when asked what they liked least about an EDC system, were insufficient support, excessive downtime, increased training time for sites, too many bugs in the applications or systems, and lack of user friendliness.

VI. CONCLUSIONS

The technologies employed in EDC systems for clinical trials are now fairly well established and are evolving rapidly. The business argument for improved data quality and the associated reduction of study cycle time using these technologies seems both rational and compelling. The difficult decisions for trial sponsors relate to technology choices and how to integrate new study management and data capture technology into ongoing clinical trial programs. It is fair to say that, to date, the early adopters of these technologies have not gained an obvious advantage over those organizations that stayed with traditional paper-based CRF systems. However, going forward, it is difficult to imagine that EDC will not dominate the clinical trial data management process.

REFERENCES

1. 62 Fed Reg 13429 (1997) (Electronic Records; Electronic Signatures; Final Rule. Codified at 21 CFR § 11).
2. U.S. Food and Drug Administration. Guidance for Industry. Computerized Systems Used in Clinical Trials. April 1999.
3. Feller RE. Electronic data capture: survey 2000. Association of Clinical Research Professional publication. The Monitor, Spring 2001; 14:37–43.

9
Providing Patient Access to Promising Investigational Drugs

Peggy J. Berry
Dey Laboratories, Napa, California

Allen Cato
Cato Research Ltd., Durham, North Carolina

I. INTRODUCTION

While enrolling subjects into a well-controlled clinical study, it is certain that some patients, although they have the disease or condition being studied, will have to be excluded from the study in compliance with certain criteria defined in the clinical protocol. The exclusion may be due to any number of reasons, from age to disease state to personal history or habits (such as smoking cigarettes or drinking alcohol). In most of these situations, even though the patient has been excluded from the clinical trial, the standard of care for the given disease—that is, the marketed prescription or over-the-counter drugs or combinations of such drugs or other means of clinical management of the condition, such as diet modification—is still an option for the patient and is not less desirable for the management of the patient's health. However, what happens when patients are excluded from clinical studies of investigational drugs and no clinical management technique is known to be effective or no other marketed drug is available to treat the disease or condition? Or what if the patient has already failed to respond to available marketed drugs for the disease or condition? If an investigational drug exists that may provide necessary relief to the patient by reducing or curing the symptoms of the disease or that may provide hope of increasing the life of the patient, is it unethical to refuse or withhold treatment to the patient? The answer to these questions and the resulting important issues and considerations are discussed in this chapter.

II. EXPANDING PATIENT ACCESS

Until recently, the use of investigational drugs outside the scope of well-controlled clinical studies was almost nonexistent. Patients who were not eligible for ongoing clinical studies were not given access to some potentially promising drugs that might have made a positive difference in their quality or length of life.

As a result, awareness began to emerge that patients with certain diseases or conditions who were afforded a limited number of, or often no, treatment options or who were unresponsive to all available treatments, would likely be willing to accept much greater risks when being treated if it was possible that they would receive some benefit from the treatment. A recognized need led to the development of a mechanism that would allow these patients access to otherwise unavailable investigational drugs.

In developing a mechanism for patient access to therapy, many issues had to be considered. First, it would be imperative for a physician to recognize the need for treatment with the investigational drug. Second, the physician would have to be willing to accept the responsibility of using an investigational drug and monitoring the patient at closer and more controlled intervals than might be necessary with marketed drugs. Third, to avoid compromising the scientific study of the safety and effectiveness of investigational drugs through well-planned, well-controlled clinical studies, the patient must be deemed ineligible for all ongoing clinical studies with the drug. The result was a compassionate-use exception, granted upon documented justification, for investigational drugs to be used to treat an individual patient. By identifying an individual patient's need, contacting a drug company to confirm availability of the drug, and submitting a case study and other documents to and receiving approval from the Food and Drug Administration (FDA) and the Institutional Review Board (IRB), the physician could treat the patient with the investigational drug. The physician was obligated to become familiar with the investigator's brochure for the product and to report back to the FDA and the drug company sponsor on the results of the treatment.

A few years' experience reviewing and granting compassionate-use exceptions made clear the need for more definitive regulations. It was believed that not all patients were being given the opportunity to receive promising new therapies when their condition could benefit from early treatment. In addition, it was noted that in some cases, after a drug had been demonstrated to be effective and safe in at least one clinical study but was not yet approved by the FDA or in wide distribution, patients with severe diseases who could benefit from treatment with the drug were not being given access to the treatment. The FDA required physicians providing investigational drug access to patients on a compassionate basis to submit separate paperwork for each patient. Each case was then reviewed individually and subject to approval by the FDA before such an allowance could be made.

Recognizing that the process was cumbersome and significantly time consuming, and realizing that patient access to promising therapies could be expanded without compromising the development program of the product, the FDA changed the law to provide for the use of investigational drugs in the treatment of an individual patient or small group of patients in a managed way. The original considerations of physician involvement and patient management remain; however, the way in which permission is received from the FDA is more clearly defined and somewhat different. Three distinct mechanisms exist for treating patients. The first is called the single-patient-use protocol, formerly referred to as the compassionate-use protocol. This protocol may be submitted by an investigator (in the form of an Investigational New Drug Application [IND]) to the FDA to treat between one and five patients (as specified in the protocol). Additional patients may be added to the protocol by filing an amendment to the IND.

The second mechanism is called a *treatment protocol*. The treatment protocol is a protocol submitted by the study drug sponsor to provide broader access to an investigational product before receiving approval from the FDA to market the product. The protocol typically allows for the treatment of tens to hundreds of patients under the care of any interested physicians who wish to treat patients with the product. Physicians gain participation in the protocol by directly contacting the study drug sponsor and completing a small number of regulatory documents. The necessary documents are then filed by the study drug sponsor as an amendment to their IND.

The third mechanism is called *emergency use*. This mechanism is used only when no other alternative exists. If an investigator determines that a subject must be provided with an investigational drug immediately (i.e., within 30 days) and the study drug sponsor does not have a treatment protocol open, the investigator may request the investigational drug from the study drug company and may treat the patient with the drug if the following conditions are met:

The patient's condition is severe or life-threatening.
No other treatment option exists for the patient, or all other treatment options have been tried and have failed.
Delay in treatment with the investigational drug could be fatal to the patient.
There is not sufficient time to prepare and submit to the FDA the necessary documents for a single-patient-use protocol.
Notification is provided to the FDA by rapid communication (fax, telephone), indicating the urgency of the request.

The IRB is notified and provides approval of the emergency treatment (approval by the full committee is not required—the committee chairperson may make approvals for emergency treatment, if the institution's procedures so allow).

Within 1 week after the emergency use, the investigator must file documentation to the FDA along with all completed regulatory forms. Emergency-use treatments with an investigational drug must be documented fully and completely and are subject to Good Clinical Practice (GCP) regulations.

These expanded-use protocols not only afford the patient access to promising investigational drugs, they also provide the sponsor with an opportunity to study the drug in a broader population. These studies provide useful data for premarketing surveillance and may serve as a natural transition to the observational surveys that characterize Phase III and Phase IV development.

Along with the decision to proceed with the expanded use of the investigational drug, numerous important issues must be considered, including the issues resulting from the decision itself.

III. REGULATORY AND LEGAL ISSUES

Expanded-use protocols are conducted through cooperation between the sponsor, the investigator, and the FDA to achieve the primary objective of getting drugs to patients who need them as early as possible. Although the primary reason for conducting these protocols is treatment of the patient, expanded-use trials that are properly conducted and well managed have many more benefits. Expanded-use protocols contribute to academic, medical, and scientific education, foster the cooperative effort between the sponsor and the FDA, and allow the sponsor to obtain additional information on long-term safety in a cost-effective manner.

As clinical development progresses with an investigational drug, the question arises about whether an expanded-use program should be initiated and, if so, when (during the course of late Phase II or during Phase III). An expanded-use protocol cannot be considered unless the FDA agrees that such a study is warranted. This agreement is obtained through submission of an IND just as it is for well-controlled studies. The protocol must also be reviewed and approved by the IRB and is subject to the same informed consent documentation and Good Clinical Practice regulations as are well-controlled investigational studies.

For the expanded-use protocol to be justified, sufficient information regarding the efficacy and short-term safety of the drug should already have been established. However, the drug still has not completed the necessary rigorous testing to ensure safety and efficacy. Therefore, the expanded-use protocols are generally limited to diseases that are life-threatening or severely debilitating and to patients who have no alternative therapy. What liabilities do the drug company, investigator, and FDA assume when treating patients under this instrument?

A. Legal Issues

Can a patient sue the FDA or the drug company for access to an investigational or nonmarketed drug? Once given access, can the patient sue the investigator, the drug company, or the FDA for damages sustained while taking the drug under expanded-use protocols? The answer to both questions is yes. The patient has the right to sue or to pursue other available avenues (such as petitioning Congress or the FDA) to demand access to a drug that he believes he needs. The patient does not give up any legal rights at any time before, during, or after participation in a typical or expanded-use clinical study and therefore may seek legal remedy to any damages he alleges.

Patients have applied public pressure through visible campaigns to gain access to drugs whose distribution may have been discontinued or strictly limited. One such example, pimozide (Orap®), was provided to patients with Tourette's syndrome (an orphan disease). Public pressure from orphan-disease groups and a visible public education campaign coerced McNeil into continuing its supply of the drug after the company had decided to quit producing it (1).

Political and public pressure can influence decisions of the FDA and of independent advisory committees. A recent example was spurred by a debate over experimental gene therapy. A politically well-connected 51-year-old female presented with Grade 4 glioblastoma (2). After the patient underwent brain surgery twice, radiotherapy, chemotherapy, and an experimental radioactive monoclonal antibody treatment, a San Diego physician proposed, as a last recourse, providing her with an experimental vaccine treatment with interleukin-2. The treatment was presented for compassionate approval to the National Institutes of Health's (NIH) Recombinant DNA Advisory Committee (RAC) and to the FDA. The RAC did not have policies in place to review expeditiously the treatment and safety issues and to respond to requests for compassionate use of gene therapy. Lacking substantial information on the use of gene therapy and lacking formal procedures for review of such requests, the RAC determined that the experimental gene therapy treatment was not yet developed enough to be used in compassionate requests. The request for use was denied at least until the RAC could discuss its policy for handling gene therapy requests, scheduled for the next meeting—3 months later.

After the denial, Senator Tom Harkin (D, Iowa) wrote a letter persuading the RAC chairperson to seek a temporary solution to the problem of policy until the issue could be further discussed and to give timely consideration to individual requests for compassionate use from terminally ill patients. Review by the FDA was occurring in parallel to review by the RAC. The FDA's review of the gene therapy protocol resulted in its agreement to the treatment. With the FDA's agreement to the treatment, the chairperson of the RAC overturned the decision made by the full committee and granted approval for the use of gene therapy in this case (3).

The literature and news media are unrelenting in exposing side effects and multimillion-dollar lawsuits stemming from side effects not observed during the controlled trials of the drug. This type of legal action is becoming increasingly common in controlled clinical trials and, despite the image of the expanded-use protocol as a humanitarian effort by the drug company, will probably also find its way into the expanded-use study.

A company may be liable in cases where physicians enter inappropriate patients under an expanded-use protocol. These physicians may not be familiar with the clinical research process, and thus the drug may be inappropriately monitored. Although the physician is advocating in the patient's best interest, patients may be given the investigational drug even though they are responding to another drug or when they have a condition other than the indication targeted for the investigational drug. Sometimes drugs in expanded use receive large amounts of publicity or are used frequently enough that they acquire a reputation for effective treatment of a plethora of problems (the panacea principle). The misapplication of the drug not only increases the company's liability, but also potentially may contribute negatively to the safety and efficacy database.

B. Regulatory Issues

1. Drug Availability

The availability of the drug may lag far behind demand for the drug, and this factor can temper the motivation of the FDA to approve its use. The lack of commercial amounts of drug supply or the expense of obtaining raw materials to make the drug could also lead to use of the drug under conditions similar to expanded use.

The synthesis of a compound may entail many steps in a small laboratory and be quite time-consuming and expensive. The initial scale-up to commercial production may leave impurities and, because the process changes, stability data may not be available. Lack of supply poses a difficult problem. If the drug is for use by patients who have incurable diseases and no alternative treatment exists, the sponsoring drug company must decide whether to institute an expanded-use protocol. If a protocol is employed, a decision must be made to determine how patients will be selected, because insufficient supply exists for all patients with the disease or condition. This was an especially troublesome problem in the trial of potential medications for AIDS (4). When treatments are offered that have even the smallest potential for effectiveness, patients with devastating illnesses and their families are willing to take enormous risks with virtually untested therapies.

2. Paperwork, Monitoring, and Control Responsibility

The expanded-use protocol does have some regulatory benefits. Because multiple INDs can drain FDA resources that would otherwise be dedicated to the approval of drugs, most expanded-use studies are required to be carried out under the supervision of the sponsor's IND. This procedure removes the FDA from any direct responsibility for monitoring the appropriate conduct of the study protocol and study sites. This procedure places the responsibility for monitoring study conduct and verifying, tabulating, and reporting the data to the FDA with the study drug sponsor. FDA maintains direct responsibility for the emergency-use protocols and the single-patient-use protocols submitted by investigators.

3. Package Insert

Marketing approval may be facilitated by the increased number of patients exposed to the investigational drug under an expanded-use protocol. Labeling of new drugs is typically conservative until the drug has been marketed and used in larger numbers of patients and on a long-term basis (if required by the indication). By employing the expanded-use protocol, which would include broader patient populations and variations of the indication, the sponsor may gain more liberal labeling from the increased exposure. However, by attempting to achieve more liberal labeling, the sponsor runs the risk that a delay in marketing approval could occur if difficulties develop in the interpretation of the data from an expanded-use study.

Side effects and drug interactions observed during the expanded-use study are required to be included in the package insert (which will generally increase the incidence of the side effect). By admitting patients who would be excluded from the controlled clinical study, the chance also exists that side effects and drug interactions that were not observed during the tightly controlled premarketing studies will be reported. These effects and interactions will require further characterization by the drug company and may need to be included in the package insert. In a severely ill population where the course of the disease is poorly understood, it may be difficult to ascribe causality to either drug or disease. A well-designed expanded-use protocol and study controls help to minimize the speculation that accompanies causality of adverse events during clinical trials.

During an expanded-use study (5) of FK 506 in liver transplant patients presenting with dysfunction who had failed previous treatment, it was concluded that the incidence of side effects observed during the expanded-use study was higher than in controlled trials. It was reported that the difference in serious adverse events "may be related to the poor condition of the patient"; however, the labeling for the product had to include all incidences. The study was valuable in suggesting that FK 506 be used as an initial treatment for liver transplant patients, potentially allowing future trials and final labeling to be more precise.

Conversely, an expanded-use study of ondansetron (4) in chemotherapy patients with uncontrollable nausea and vomiting who had failed to respond to standard antiemetics were shown to respond favorably to ondansetron. This study, conducted in 190 patients, confirmed the effectiveness of ondansetron as an anti-emetic, allowed for broader labeling for the approved product, and offered hope to patients with no other alternative.

C. Drug Development Issues

In addition to the areas described above that relate to drug development, the expanded-use protocol provides an excellent substrate for training and education. Because the drug is being administered to a more heterogeneous population, the monitoring of the study may require more depth of knowledge about the product and its metabolism. These studies closely simulate the actual use of the drug once it becomes available on the market, so the study drug sponsor can gain experience and insight into postmarketing conditions.

As indicated previously, these expanded-use conditions often foster the recognition of adverse events and drug interactions that would not be recognized during the more restrictive controlled trials. The expanded-use protocol is complex and demanding. It increases the company's demand for monitoring resources because the sites are often scattered across the country, and each might enroll only a few patients, either because the number of eligible patients is limited or because the sites conducting the expanded-use protocols may not be experienced in conducting investigational drug trials and may not enroll larger numbers.

IV. ADVANTAGES AND DISADVANTAGES FOR THE PATIENT

The introduction of a new chemical entity into the New Drug Application (NDA) process often heralds the formulation of a unique mode of therapy for patients with a specific diagnosis. During clinical development, the patient populations identified in protocols are rigorously defined and screened under stringent inclusion/exclusion criteria. This is done to minimize "background noise" in clinical studies, making the results easier to interpret and side effects easier to identify and analyze. An expanded-use protocol is generally designed to circumvent these criteria and to provide select patients with a therapeutic advantage not otherwise available to them. Patients enrolling in expanded-use studies typically do not qualify for any of the controlled studies with the drug. These patients also generally have no other treatment available to them or were nonresponders to or nontolerators of alternative treatments.

Expanded-use protocols are often instituted during late Phase I or early Phase II, before the toxic effects are adequately characterized and certainly before efficacy has been demonstrated. By initiating an expanded-use protocol in a serious illness where few if any alternatives exist, efficacy is implied and may therefore generate a great demand for the product before controlled trials are completed. In some cases, initiation of such a protocol can make it difficult to complete controlled trials.

By extending the patient population outside the boundaries defined in the original protocol, the statistical likelihood of side effects increases, as does the potential that a side effect will present itself that can lead to a new indication or formulation of the drug. Many new indications have been discovered by investigating the side effects reported during clinical testing of a new chemical entity.

The expanded-use protocol can provide for those patients who responded to the investigational drug in early controlled trials to continue to receive the drug until it becomes commercially available. Patients who cannot tolerate the long-term effects of currently marketed drugs may also be eligible for this type of study. Patients who were nontolerators, nonresponders to alternative treatment, and certain patients who could possibly benefit from the use of investigational drugs are other common benefactors of the expanded-use protocol. It is not appropriate to enter those patients who respond to current available therapy unless some clinical advantage is especially desirable and can be justified given the limited knowledge about side effects.

V. ADVANTAGES AND DISADVANTAGES FOR THE SPONSOR

For the expanded-use study to be cost-effective for the sponsor, little or no funding should be expended for patient expense reimbursement or for investigators who desire to prescribe the investigational drug to their patients. However, it is the sponsor's responsibility to provide clinical trial material (investigational study drug) with appropriate labeling and instructions for use (including but not limited to the investigator brochure), appropriate recording instruments, and the medical, scientific, and monitoring expertise to conduct the trials in accordance with the expanded-use protocol and the current FDA regulations and guidelines.

A. Marketing Issues

The expanded-use protocol is a good selling tool. It allows the physician to become familiar with the drug before its actual marketing. However, it also creates the opportunity for overly enthusiastic drug representatives to try to sell the physician on the drug before FDA approval to market the drug and approval of the final package insert text. This may appear to be advertisement for the drug before its approval, which is prohibited by FDA regulations and, as such, would be subject to legal action by the FDA. It may also create a false sense of hope and security among patients and physicians and flood the sponsor with expanded-use requests for a compound that is in limited supply.

During the expanded-use protocol, the drug is generally provided free to patients even though the regulations do provide for the possibility of payment. Offering the drug at no charge fosters a positive and benevolent image of the company. Conversely, charging patients for a drug before marketing it can create an equally negative public opinion of the company. Preexisting marketed drugs may also face competition from unapproved agents sold under a large expanded-use IND program, despite the lack of evidence to support safety and efficacy. Charging for the drug under an expanded-use program requires prior approval, by the FDA. The charge for the drug may not exceed the cost of developing the drug, which may further put the sponsor at risk for negative publicity after approval when patients learn the difference between preapproval costs and retail costs.

B. Ethical and Practical Issues

Decision points are reached during the course of an expanded-use trial that bear on both practical and ethical reasoning.

Difficulties arise in informed consent because adequate clinical data are not usually available and patients (often desperate for therapy) are willing to enter expanded-use studies under any circumstances with the hope of obtaining a therapeutic solution to their illnesses. If a drug demonstrates efficacy in an individual patient during a short-term clinical trial, is it ethical and practical to continue that patient on the test drug without the benefit of accurate data on the long-term effects and toxicology of the compound? Is payment to the investigator or patient considered coercion in an expanded-use trial (or in any trial)?

Limiting participation in the expanded-use protocol to those patients who have participated in previous studies with the drug is an additional consideration for the sponsor. The patient who was not fortunate enough to meet the rigorous criteria defined in the previous Phase II–III studies may be denied access to a promising compound. Should patient enrollment be limited at each center, or should the protocol be opened up for all patients who would benefit from treatment?

Company resources and drug supply considerations can weigh heavily in these decisions.

The supply of drug is limited by what the sponsor is able to produce, and using the drug in an expanded-use protocol places a great strain on the supply available for conducting controlled trials. This is especially important when therapy is long-term and demand is great. How are patients selected to receive the drug? If the compound is in short supply, how will those seeking expanded use be excluded from the study? Companies often question the risk versus benefits of providing high-cost, long-term drug in an expanded-use protocol to patients who ultimately provide little or no helpful study data while potentially excluding patients from the controlled studies with the drug. For example, 2000 patients are enrolled in studies, 1500 in controlled trials lasting 6 weeks and 500 under expanded-use protocols (which will continue until approval) with one tablet that is administered four times a day. The controlled studies will require 252 tablets per patient or 63,000 tablets for the controlled study. The 500 expanded-use patients will require 730,000 tablets for the first year, at least a 10-fold increase in resources. The company must continue to supply drug to patients under the expanded-use protocol long after the controlled trials have ended and the NDA has been submitted. This is a large commitment of drug to a relatively small component of the study population.

If a drug company makes a decision to begin limiting the number of patients in an expanded-use program, they may be met with public protest. When Glaxo (now GlaxoSmithKline) was conducting an expanded-use study (6) with their drug 3TC (lamivudine), they announced that supplies of the drug were running low and planned to decrease the number of new patients entering the study. This announcement came when it was also revealed that controlled studies with the drug looked promising. Several weeks later, after tremendous pressure from the AIDS community and doctors, Glaxo announced that after final inventory review, supply of the drug was not as low as they had initially thought. They nearly doubled their new patient entry for the study.

C. Monitoring

These nonpivotal studies provide a base from which research personnel can be trained and educated. Because few formal training programs in clinical research are available, more direct exposure and interaction can be established between the sponsor and investigators interested in drug development. This exposure helps prepare both investigators and industry personnel in clinical development, providing more cost-effective expertise in the development of future NDAs while improving the quality of scientific interactions.

Monitoring is especially tenuous under these expanded-use protocols, and the data obtained can often be difficult to interpret. No matter how simplistic a protocol may appear to be or how late in the process of the clinical development of the drug it is implemented, the sponsor and the investigator may strive to maintain the highest clinical research standards but be unable to wade through the many variables that are added by the expanded-use studies. Lack of close scrutiny may lead to improper use of the drug in the field because of the physician's unfamiliarity with the product. Although most companies are reluctant to devote resources to the long-term follow-up of these patients, that may be the best way of obtaining information about the long-term safety of the drug under the conditions of routine clinical practice.

VI. STUDY DATA FROM THE EXPANDED USE

As safety is the primary concern in the introduction and maintenance of any drug in the commercial marketplace, the expanded-use protocol provides an opportunity for obtaining long-term data not captured in the shorter and more expensive efficacy and safety trials. Most important, the opportunity to gain insight into any possible unpredicted toxicity not evident in the controlled clinical trial program could emerge early to enhance acceptable balances of benefit and risk. Side effects can also reveal themselves that could lead to a new indication for the compound or modification of its use. Although the number of patients participating in an expanded-use protocol would not approximate the larger number of patients involved in the Phase IV epidemiological studies, information on previously unseen risks can be extrapolated so that the safety parameters that protect the consumer can be anticipated.

It is the rare patient who suffers from an isolated disorder and takes only a single medication. In the expanded-use protocol, much information can be gained by evaluating potential drug interactions with the current medications the patient may be taking. Frequently, this information has tremendous impact on the overall therapeutic efficacy of the investigational drug and its risk and benefits when given with other forms of therapy.

It is a distinct advantage to the sponsor to limit the number of centers to include only those investigators who have had previous experience with the drug. Such action may succeed in carefully controlling the information and data being obtained during the monitoring of these studies, but it does not fulfill the overall obligation of implementing this type of protocol.

With the initiation of the expanded-use protocol, the sponsor must construct a safety data management program within the home facility or with a contract organization so that the sponsor can fulfill its reporting obligations to the FDA. In data management, because of the expanded-use, uncontrolled nature of the studies, efficacy data may be of academic value only, but all information (both safety and efficacy data) must be appropriately tabulated for reference. Negative efficacy data, even in this small population, could be of substantial value, while positive efficacy data may be insightful, but is usually difficult to interpret.

VII. THE ROLE OF THE FDA

The lag in NDA approval has long been known to be an aggravating and expensive proposition for both the FDA and sponsors. These investigators' IND requests can be eliminated by referring the investigator to the sponsoring company for the supply of clinical material and an appropriate protocol under which to conduct their clinical studies, which are filed under the sponsor's IND. Thus, investigators who would normally apply for their own IND would save the FDA, sponsor, and themselves excess paperwork and would still be able to conduct the investigational study. Although a company may not wish to support a full expanded-use program, it may consider supplying the drug to investigators who wish to pursue their own IND. Submission of numerous INDs of this type, however, may drain the FDA's and the sponsor's resources.

Also, when side effects do occur with the investigational drug, it allows the sponsor to effectively channel this information to the FDA rather than having individual reports trickle into the regulatory agency. Furthermore, these studies allow the sponsor to obtain early cost-effective safety data (while substantiating efficacy data) that will ultimately benefit the patient. This type of collaborative effort, coordinated by the sponsor, could foster a closer network among the FDA, investigator, scientists, and patients. This strategy could substantially ease the FDA workload and expedite approval of the NDA for the benefit of everyone involved.

The FDA has developed regulations for the treatment, use, and sale of investigational drugs (7). The regulation states that an investigational drug may be used to treat patients outside a controlled clinical trial if the disease is "serious" or "immediately life-threatening," if no satisfactory alternative drug/therapy is available, if the drug is currently being investigated in a controlled clinical trial under an IND, and if the sponsor is actively pursuing marketing approval of the drug. The FDA commissioner can deny a request for use if insufficient evidence exists of safety and effectiveness to support its use. The regulations further provide safeguards for placing a treatment IND on clinical hold and a mechanism for obtaining prior FDA approval for the sale of an investigational drug during a clinical trial. Many companies, rather than filing a formal treatment protocol, will conduct an expanded-use, single-patient-use, or "continuation" or "extension" protocol under their IND. Although these other types of protocols are not defined in the regulations, a provision exists for the single-patient-use protocol (which is the same as the expanded-use protocol). If the company decides to allow expanded-use type of enrollment only to those patients who have been enrolled in former clinical studies with the drug, this can be done through a continuation or extension protocol.

VIII. CONCLUSIONS

The expanded-use protocol, when initiated with careful scientific thought and when appropriately managed, can be an extremely important instrument for obtaining cost-effective information for the FDA, the scientific/medical/academic communities, and the patient. It can provide a training ground for enhancing the quality and cost-effectiveness of future clinical trials. Most important, those patients who have been nontolerators or nonresponders to alternative treatments, those who have responded well in the controlled clinical trials of the investigational drug, and those who are in life-threatening situations can benefit tremendously and are the primary motivation for this protocol. During the course of the drug development of any compound, a balance must be struck between the risks and benefits of initiating the expanded-use protocol. The high standards applied to the early development of the clinical study must not be compromised during the conduct of the larger, open study. It is the responsibility of the investigator, the sponsor, and the FDA to maintain a collaborative environment so that these studies can serve a patient population in need of the drug before its approval and marketing.

REFERENCES

1. Myers AS. Orphan drugs and orphan diseases: the consumer's viewpoint. In: Brewer GJ, ed., Orphan Drugs and Orphan Diseases: Clinical Realities and Public Policy. New York: Liss, 1983:147–157.
2. Thompson L. Gene therapy. Harkin seeks compassionate use of unproven treatments. Science 1992; 258(5089):1728.
3. Healy B. Remarks for the RAC Committee meeting of January 14, 1993, regarding compassionate use exemption. Hum Gene Ther 1993; 4:195–197.
4. Berry WR, House KW, Lee JT, Plagge PB, Meshad MW, Grapski R. Results of a compassionate-use program using intravenous ondansetron to prevent nausea and vomiting in patients receiving emetogenic cancer chemotherapy. Semin Oncol 1992 Dec; 19(6 Suppl 15):33–37.
5. Murio JE, Balsells, J Lazaro JL, Charco R, Margarit C. Compassionate use of FK 506 in liver transplantation. Transplant Proc 1995; 27(4):2336.
6. Tastemain C. Confusion reigns over compassionate use of AIDS drug. Nat Med 1995 Oct; 1(10):986.
7. Department of Health and Human Services. Investigational New Drug, Antibiotic, and Biological Product Regulations: Treatment Use and Sale. Fed Reg 1987; May 22, 52:19466.

10
Issues in the Review of Clinical Drug Trials by IRBs

Dale H. Cowan
Cleveland Clinic Foundation, Cleveland, Ohio

I. INTRODUCTION

Clinical drug trials represent research with human subjects. All research involving human subjects that is supported by the U.S. federal government or the results of which are to be used in applications for drug or device approval must be conducted in accordance with regulations promulgated by the U.S. Department of Health and Human Services (HHS) (1) and the U.S. Food and Drug Administration (FDA) (2). The regulations of both the HHS and the FDA require that an Institutional Review Board (IRB) ''shall review and have authority to approve, require modifications in (to secure approval), or disapprove all research activities covered by [the] regulations'' (3).

The review of clinical drug trials by IRBs raises a number of interesting and difficult issues. These relate to the origin and sponsor of the proposed trial, the nature of the institution the IRB serves, and the manner in which the norms for determining ethical conduct in clinical trials can be applied to specific trials.

This chapter will review the ethical principles underlying research involving human subjects, the legal authority for IRBs, and the regulatory requirements affecting the operations of IRBs. It will then discuss the role of IRBs in reviewing clinical trials by examining how IRBs can assess the scientific design of trials, the competency of the investigator, the manner of selecting subjects for the trial, the balance of risks and benefits, informed consent, and provisions for compensating for research-related injuries. The chapter will conclude with observations regarding the role of the lay members of IRBs, problems of reviewing multi-institutional trials, and how to monitor the conduct of trials that are approved.

149

II. ETHICAL PRINCIPLES UNDERLYING RESEARCH INVOLVING HUMAN SUBJECTS

Among the basic ethical principles that are generally accepted in our cultural tradition, three are particularly relevant to the ethics of research involving human subjects (4). These are the principles of respect for persons, beneficence, and justice.

A. Respect for Persons

The principle of respect for persons was formally stated by the philosopher Immanuel Kant: "[P]ersons should always treat each other as autonomous ends and never merely as means to the ends of others . . . persons are rational agents of unconditional worth who must not be treated merely as conditionally valued things incapable of choosing for themselves" (5). This principle incorporates two moral requirements.

One requirement is to acknowledge the autonomy of individuals, their right to self-determination. This formulation of the principle of respect for persons finds expression in American jurisprudence in the statement written by Judge (later Justice) Benjamin Cardozo: "Every human being of adult years has a right to determine what shall be done with his own body" (6). This interpretation of the principle underlies the concept of informed consent. Its application demands that human subjects participate in the research voluntarily and with adequate information about the potential benefits and risks to make an informed decision regarding their participation.

The second requirement is to protect individuals with diminished autonomy. An autonomous individual is one who is capable of deliberating about personal goals and of acting under the direction of such deliberation. Not every individual is capable of self-determination. Individuals who are immature or who, having once attained maturity, have lost their capacity for self-determination wholly or in part due to illness, mental disability, or circumstances that severely restrict their liberty, may require protection while they are immature or while their are incapacitated (7).

Although some individuals may require protection even to the point of excluding them from activities that may harm them, overprotection may be dehumanizing and represent a lack of respect. Thus, a balance must be struck between protecting the welfare of individuals and not repudiating their autonomy.

B. Beneficence

The principle of beneficence states that "we . . . have a moral duty to weigh and balance possible benefits against possible harms in order to maximize benefits and minimize risks of harm'' (8). The concept that physicians have a moral duty to promote the welfare of their patients can be found in Western writings as early as the Hippocratic oath: ''I will apply dietetic measures for the benefit of the sick according to my skill and judgment; I will keep them from harm and injustice'' (9). The aim of the relationship between physicians and patients is to benefit the patient.

There are, then, two complementary formulations of the principle of beneficence. These are (a) maximize possible benefits and minimize possible harms, and (b) do not harm (10).

The obligations that derive from the principle of beneficence affect individual research projects and the research enterprise in general. In the case of individual research projects, investigators are obligated to design studies so that benefits to both subjects and society at large are maximized and the risks to the subjects are minimized. With respect to research in general, physicians need to recognize the long-term benefits and risks that may result from the generation of new knowledge and the development of new medical therapies. Additionally, it may be argued that the principle of beneficence obligates physicians and society to pursue investigative activities, improve medical care, and thereby benefit society.

As with the principle of respect for persons, implementation of beneficence in human research can lead to difficult choices in specific situations. An example is participation of individuals with diminished capacity to give informed consent—e.g., children—in research that presents more than minimal risk without immediate prospect of direct benefit to the individuals themselves. Resolution of such conflicts requires a careful analysis and balancing of the complementary formulations of the principle of beneficence.

C. Justice

The principle of justice represents the concept of fairness. It requires that the benefits and burdens of any activity, such as participation in clinical trials, be distributed equitably across the population. In short, it states that equals should be treated equally.

The Belmont report identifies five widely accepted formulations of just ways to distribute benefits and burdens. These are (a) to each person an equal share, (b) to each person according to individual need, (c) to each person according to individual effort, (d) to each person according to societal contribution, and (e) to each person according to merit.

Historically, the burdens of serving as research subjects fell largely upon socially and economically disadvantaged individuals, whereas the benefits tended to accrue to the more affluent members of society. One of the most flagrant examples of this inequity was the Tuskegee syphilis study, in which disadvantaged, rural black men were used (without their consent) to study the course of a disease affecting the entire population and were deprived of effective treatment in order not to disrupt the project long after such treatment became available.

The obligations of the principle of justice require that research subjects be individuals who are representative of the population that is at risk for the condition or disease being studied. This means that individuals should not be selected as research subjects because of "their easy availability, their compromised position, or their manipulability, rather than for reasons directly related to the problem being studied" (11). Additionally, it requires that care must be taken to avoid selecting "undesirable" individuals for research that entails risk and reserving participation in potentially beneficial research to individuals who are viewed more favorably.

III. LEGAL AUTHORITY FOR IRBs

The legal authority for IRBs derives from two parallel sets of federal regulations. One set of regulations was promulgated by the Department of Health and Human Services and implements the 1974 amendments to the Public Health Service Act (12). These regulations are codified in Title 45 of the *Code of Federal Regulations* (CFR), Part 46. The second set of regulations was promulgated by the FDA under the Federal Food, Drug, and Cosmetic Act (13). These regulations are codified in Title 21 of the CFR; regulations pertaining to IRBs are in Part 50 and those pertaining to informed consent are in Part 56.

A. HHS Regulations

The HHS regulations cover research supported or conducted by the Department of Health and Human Services. They represent the basic policy of HHS for protecting human research subjects. The applicability of the regulations is restricted to those activities that meet the definition of research: "a systematic investigation designed to develop or contribute to generalizable knowledge" (14). Although the regulations technically apply only to those research projects that are conducted or funded in whole or in part by HHS, virtually all public and private granting agencies require that all research they sponsor that involves human subjects be conducted in accordance with the HHS requirements.

Subpart A of the regulations specifies that each institution "covered by th[e] regulations shall provide written assurance to the Secretary (of HHS) that it will comply with the requirements set forth in th[e] regulations" (15). The regulations further specify the minimum elements for such assurances. Additionally, they specify requirements for IRB membership, function, and operation, and the criteria according to which approval may be given for conducting research. Finally, the regulations set out the general requirements for informed consent.

Subparts B, C, and D set out additional protections that apply, respectively, to research, development, and related activities involving fetuses, pregnant women, and in-vitro human fertilization, biomedical and behavioral research involving prisoners as subjects, and those applying to children as subjects in research.

B. FDA Regulations

The FDA has the legal authority to regulate clinical investigations in the United States when the investigational products move across state or national boundaries. Under FDA regulations, review and approval by an IRB is required for any experiment that involves a test article and one or more human subjects, either patients or healthy persons, and that is subject to the requirements for prior submission to the FDA (16). Such review is also required for any experiment the results of which are intended to be submitted later to, or held for inspection by, the FDA.

The regulations of the FDA are identical or similar to those of HHS in nearly all essential respects. Such differences as do exist reflect the different statutory authority under which the separate sets of regulations were promulgated and the difference in mission between the FDA and the National Institutes of Health (NIH), the agency within HHS charged with overseeing the implementation and enforcement of the HHS regulations. The difference in mission between the FDA and the NIH is reflected in the FDA's approach to compliance with its regulations utilizing its traditional tools of inspections and audits. The NIH, as noted previously, relies on the assurance mechanism.

The FDA regulations, like the HHS regulations, specify requirements for IRB membership, function, and operation, and the criteria according to which approval may be given for conducting research. Since these requirements are similar, a single committee can be established to undertake the activities required by both sets of regulations. Additionally, the FDA regulations allow a wide variety of ways in which private practitioners not affiliated with an institution can obtain necessary IRB review of their clinical research activities. These include review by an institutional IRB that agrees to assume this additional function or by IRBs formed by a local or state health agency, a medical school, a medical society, a state licensing board, or a nonprofit or for-profit independent group. All IRBs, regardless of sponsorship, that are assuming responsibilities for reviewing and approving clinical research protocols subject to FDA authority must comply with the IRB regulations set out by the FDA.

IV. REGULATORY REQUIREMENTS

The FDA and HHS regulations specify the duties and membership requirements of IRBs and the criteria for approving research. Since the two sets of regulations are similar, these will be reviewed by reference to the HHS regulations.

A. Duties of IRBs

IRBs are required to review and have the authority to approve, require modifications in, or disapprove all research activities covered by the regulations (17). They must require that information given to subjects as part of informed consent is in accordance with the general requirements for informed consent that are set out in the regulations. Additionally, they may require that other information be given to subjects when they judge that such information would further protect the rights and welfare of the subjects (18).

IRBs must require documentation of informed consent in all studies except those specified in the regulations in which documentation may be waived (19). Clinical drug trials are not among the classes of studies in which documentation of informed consent may be waived.

IRBs must provide written notification to investigators and institutions of their decisions to approve, require modifications in, or disapprove proposed research activities (20). Decisions to disapprove proposed research proposal must be accompanied by a statement of reasons for the decision and provide the investigator an opportunity to respond in person or in writing (21).

IRBs must conduct continuing reviews of research they approve at least once each year. More frequent reviews may be required if the risk of a particular research project so warrants (22). IRBs have the authority to suspend or terminate approval of research that is not being conducted in accordance with their requirements or that has been associated with unexpected serious harm to subjects. Such action must be accompanied by a statement of reasons for it and be communicated to the investigator, appropriate institutional officials, and the Secretary of HHS (23).

The regulations require that IRBs must follow the written procedures that are set out in the assurances they have filed with HHS (24), review proposed research at convened meetings at which a majority of IRB members are present, vote approval by a majority of members present at the meeting (25), and be responsible for reporting to the appropriate institutional officials and the Secretary of HHS "any serious or continuing noncompliance by investigators with the requirements and determination of the IRB" (26).

Institutions that are cooperating in multiinstitutional studies, such as clinical drug trials, must each review and approve the proposed studies. Such institutions may, however, use joint review, rely on the review of another qualified IRB, or utilize similar arrangements to avoid duplication of efforts (27).

B. IRB Membership

The regulations require that ''[e]ach IRB shall have at least five members, with varying backgrounds to promote complete and adequate review of research activities commonly conducted by the institution. The IRB shall be sufficiently qualified through the experience and expertise of its members, and the diversity of the members' backgrounds . . . to promote respect for its advice and counsel in safeguarding the rights and welfare of human subjects. In addition to possessing the professional competence necessary to review specific research activities, the IRB shall be able to ascertain the acceptability of proposed research in terms of institutional commitments and regulations, applicable law, and standards of professional conduct and practice. The IRB shall therefore include persons knowledgeable in these areas'' (28).

Additional requirements specify that IRBs may not consist entirely of men or women or members of one profession (29), must include at least one person who is a nonscientist (30), and must include at least one individual who is otherwise not affiliated with the institution (31). Finally, the regulations expressly forbid members participating in an initial or continuing review of a project in which the member has a conflicting interest (32).

The requirements for IRB membership have particular relevance to the manner in which they carry out their assigned functions.

C. Criteria for IRB Approval of Research

The regulations specify that ''[i]n order to approve research . . . IRB[s] shall determine that all of the following requirements are satisfied:

1. Risks to subjects are minimized: (i) by using procedures which are consistent with sound research design and which do not unnecessarily expose subjects to risk, and (ii) whenever appropriate, by using procedures already being performed on the subjects for diagnostic or treatment purposes.
2. Risks to subjects are reasonable in relation to anticipated benefits, if any, to subjects, and the importance of the knowledge that may reasonably be expected to result.
3. Selection of subjects is equitable.
4. Informed consent will be sought from each prospective subject or the subject's legally authorized representative. . . .
5. Informed consent will be appropriately documented'' (33).

Additional requirements are that adequate provisions exist for monitoring the data collected, that adequate provisions exist to protect the privacy of subjects and maintain the confidentiality of the data, and that appropriate safeguards are included to protect the rights and welfare of subjects who are "vulnerable to coercion or undue influence . . . or persons who are economically or educationally disadvantaged" (34).

V. THE ROLE OF IRBs IN REVIEWING CLINICAL DRUG TRIALS

Having reviewed the ethical principles underlying research with human subjects, the legal authority for IRBs, and the regulatory requirements affecting IRB activities, it is useful to consider the manner in which IRBs can carry out their responsibilities in reviewing clinical drug trials.

A. Assessment of Scientific Design

IRBs are established to safeguard the welfare of the subjects of research and not to provide rigorous peer review of the scientific merits of a proposed study. Nevertheless, the norm of sound scientific design, based as it is on the ethical principles of beneficence and respect for persons, and the statement of policy that flows from it, require that IRBs review the scientific basis for proposed clinical trials and assess the scientific and statistical design of the trial. Among the information needed for this review and assessment are (a) the results of animal studies and of previous clinical studies or experiences in humans, (b) whether there are similar studies currently underway elsewhere, (c) the scientific rationale for the study being proposed, and (d) the statistical basis for constructing the trial.

The manner in which an IRB processes relevant information is illustrated in the following example. A cardiologist wishes to evaluate a new antiarrhythmic agent. An IRB reviewing the proposed study should ask whether the drug has been previously tested in animals or humans and, if so, under what circumstances and with what results. The IRB should also inquire whether similar trials are presently being conducted elsewhere and whether all patients in the proposed trial will receive the drug or patients will be randomly allocated to receive either the drug being evaluated or current standard therapy. If the trial is designed as a randomized clinical trial, the IRB should satisfy itself that it is constructed in a manner allowing for the accrual of sufficient numbers of patients and allocates subjects between the proposed treatment and the standard therapy in a manner that allows the investigators to draw conclusions regarding the relative effectiveness of the two treatments.

A thorough analysis of these matters generally requires substantial medical and statistical expertise. It is to be remembered that the federal regulations require that the membership of IRBs not be drawn exclusively from one professional group, e.g., physician-investigators. Rather, IRB membership should include representatives of a variety of disciplines and professions in order to reflect more appropriately the values of society at large. Given their composition, how can IRBs exercise their responsibilities for review of research design?

It is suggested that one of two approaches may be adopted by those IRBs lacking the requisite expertise to assess research design. One approach, which may be particularly suitable for IRBs in community hospitals, is merely to accept the information included in the project proposal as providing an adequate basis for justifying the study and a suitable design for achieving its purposes. This approach might be acceptable in the case of a multi-institutional clinical trial conducted under the sponsorship of one of the National Institutes of Health. Such trials have had the benefit of outside review groups such as the National Heart, Lung, and Blood Institute and the FDA during their development and prior to their submission to IRBs for approval.

In the development of the proposal, the investigators responsible for the study would have addressed the specific issues of scientific rationale and statistical design. These individuals or others with whom they might have consulted would presumably have the training and experience in the disease being treated and in statistical methods. The design of the proposed trial would be reviewed by personnel from the sponsoring Institute and, in the case of trials involving investigational new drugs, by the FDA. The proposal submitted to the IRB would have had the benefit of an analysis with respect to research design substantially more extensive and more sophisticated than that which could be undertaken by most IRBs. Under these circumstances, it would be appropriate for an IRB to take cognizance of the prior review and not proceed with an independent analysis of scientific design. Indeed, it could be argued that an additional review of scientific design by an IRB lacking the expertise available to a scientific peer review group would not contribute further to safeguarding the welfare of the subjects.

This approach would not be acceptable in the case of a clinical trial proposed by an individual investigator that had not been exposed to review by outside agencies. In the case of such proposals, IRBs have a quasi-peer review role in assessing the design of the studies. In these instances, IRBs have a relatively more significant function in safeguarding the welfare of potential subjects than when proposals have had prior outside peer review. It is unjustified to omit this assessment simply because of the practical problems in carrying it out. Additionally, to do so would result in the IRB being out of compliance with the spirit and the letter of the federal regulations.

To carry out the review of research design of investigator-initiated proposals, IRBs can adopt an alternative approach, that of soliciting the opinions of outside consultants. This approach can be utilized by university hospitals as well as by community hospitals and is applicable to the review of multi-institutional trials as well as those proposed by individual investigators. The consultants should be individuals familiar with the medical issues in question and with statistical analysis. They would determine whether suitable information exists to justify the proposed trial and whether the trial as designed would achieve its intended purposes.

The outside reviews would not be intended necessarily to determine whether the proposed trial is the best one that can be done. They could well lead, however, to improvements in the study design that would benefit both subjects and investigators. The use of consultants would thereby enable IRBs to compensate for limitations of expertise on the part of their members and allow them to meet their responsibilities for assuring satisfactory research design.

B. Competence of the Investigator

Related to the norm of good research design is the norm that the investigator should be competent. IRBs should determine that the investigators responsible for conducting clinical trials are qualified by background and experience to manage the diseases being treated and the treatment regimens being tested. This can be accomplished by confirming that the investigators have met the standards for competence established by national groups that certify medical specialists. For example, several years ago an investigator sought to undertake a study that involved the administration of insulin using an insulin pump. A review of the investigator's credentials revealed that he lacked board certification in the subspecialty of endocrinology and had no prior experience with the use of an insulin pump or with performing clinical trials. The IRB voted not to approve the proposal because of its concern that the investigator lacked the qualifications for overseeing the proposed study.

IRBs should also certify that the investigators do in fact practice in conformity with the standards of the specialty in which the investigators are members. This can be both a delicate matter for inquiry and difficult to do. The difficulty can arise from the fact that much of an investigator's clinical practice may occur in an office setting, a setting not ordinarily subject to hospital peer review. In order to fulfill their obligations to safeguard the welfare of prospective subjects of clinical trials, IRBs should inquire from others within the professional community whether a particular person is qualified to act as an investigator. This inquiry can be facilitated by asking the chairperson of the department to which the investigator belongs to confirm that the investigator is qualified to assume the responsibility to conduct the research.

In addition to certifying that investigators possess the necessary medical qualifications for conducting clinical trials, IRBs should ascertain that the investigators manifest ''a high degree of professionalism necessary to care for the subject'' (35). This determination requires an inquiry into the relationship of the investigator to the prospective subjects. Investigators can relate to subjects in two capacities: as physician and as investigator. In the traditional physician–patient relationship, the physician's primary concern is the patient's welfare. The physician acts as the patient's friend or ''advocate'' and seeks to do that which is in the best interest of the patient. In the investigator–subject relationship, the investigator has a major interest in the furtherance of the research goals. A potential conflict exists in which pursuing the goals of the research may conflict with actions that promote a patient's welfare. Although the conduct of the research is ideally a cooperative venture between investigator and subject, the physician acting as investigator has a potential conflict of interest between his or her allegiance to the patient and to the goals of the research.

An example of this conflict is a clinical trial of a new antineoplastic chemotherapeutic agent for the treatment of newly diagnosed, nonresectable, non-small-cell carcinoma of the lung confined to the thorax. The physician-investigator knows that radiation therapy is considered to be standard treatment for this disorder. However, such treatment is only rarely curative. More commonly it provides only partial, short-lasting control. He may agree that the proposed drug regimen is at least rationally based and merits testing. But he also knows that hitherto non-small-cell carcinoma of the lung has been relatively unresponsive to chemotherapy. In determining whether to proceed with radiation therapy or enlist his patient into the clinical trial, the physician has to balance his primary duty to act in furtherance of his patient's best interest against his desire to contribute to the generation of new information regarding the treatment of this disease. A potential conflict may arise that affects the recruitment by the physician-investigator of the patient-subject into the clinical trial and the ability of the latter to exercise free and informed choice with respect to his or her participation in it.

It is important, therefore, for IRBs to inquire into the sensitivity of investigators to the existence of potential conflicts of interest and to the manner in which these conflicts can be minimized or avoided so that the interest in the research does not override the interest of the patient-subjects.

C. Selection of Subjects

The norm that subjects shall be selected equitably is based on the principle of justice. The principle of justice requires that the benefits and burdens of research be distributed fairly. It is inappropriate for subjects of clinical trials to be drawn primarily from members of a specific subpopulation of the community unless the disease being treated affects only members of that group. For example, it would be inappropriate for a clinical trial of a new antiarthritic drug to be undertaken solely with individuals from lower socioeconomic groups who receive their care in municipal hospital clinics. Rather, the trial should include individuals from all socioeconomic groups and racial backgrounds. No single socioeconomic or minority group should bear the burdens of the research (36).

The recommendations of the National Commission for the Protection of Subjects of Research stated that ''the burdens of participation in research should be equitably distributed among the segments of our society, no matter how large or small those burdens may be'' (37).

To determine that prospective subjects of proposed clinical trials are selected equitably, IRBs should determine (a) the patient population from which subjects will be selected, (b) the basis or rationale for selecting subjects, and (c) the precise manner in which subjects will be selected.

IRBs should ascertain that subjects will not be selected exclusively or even primarily from groups whose dependence on the institution is such as to cause them to be reluctant to decline to participate for fear of loss of benefits. This precaution is particularly important for IRBs at Veterans Administration hospitals. IRBs at such institutions, where the majority of patients constitute potentially vulnerable populations, may have little opportunity to insist that subjects belonging to these groups not constitute the major source of participants in clinical trials. In these settings, IRBs acting on behalf of the potential patient/subjects must certify that the setting for selecting subjects and obtaining informed consent is such as to minimize to the extent possible the coercive atmosphere that potentially exists.

D. Balancing Benefits and Risks

The norm that the balance of benefits and risks be favorable rests on the principles of beneficence and respect for persons. This norm is expressed in all codes of ethics and is a specific duty of IRBs. The federal regulations state that IRBs must determine that ''risks to subjects are reasonable in relation to anticipated benefits to the subjects and the importance of the knowledge to be gained'' (38).

To balance the benefits and risks of a clinical trial, IRBs must consider the disease being treated, the specific details of each treatment regimen, and the manner and setting in which treatment will be administered and responses of patients monitored. To illustrate, consider a proposed clinical trial intended to study the effect of a new drug for the treatment of breast cancer. To date, drugs that are active in this setting can induce partial or, occasionally, complete remissions, ameliorate symptoms, and improve the quality of life of affected patients. They do not, however, cure the cancer or prolong survival.

The benefit of pursuing this trial is judged by reference to the natural history of the disease both in the absence of any therapy and with interventions using existing treatments. It is related to the estimated likelihood that the new drug will induce remissions in a greater percentage of patients than those responding to existing drugs, ameliorate symptoms more rapidly, completely, or for a longer time than existing drugs, and/or increase overall survival.

To estimate the risks that might be associated with the clinical trial, consideration must be paid to the nature and potential severity of specific side effects from drugs being tested and the possibility of less favorable outcomes in women in control groups receiving standard therapy. In this trial, the side effects include nausea, vomiting, hair loss, neurological deficits, fluid retention, and reduced blood cell counts. In addition, there could be asthenia that commonly occurs with chemotherapy, the time spent in receiving treatment, the costs of the treatment, and the side effects, time, and costs associated with administration of growth factors given to counteract the decrease in blood cell counts.

The calculus of risks must also include considerations as to whether side effects can be anticipated, detected, and treated, including whether facilities exist to treat side effects in the event they occur. For example, in the clinical trial of metastatic breast cancer, it should be confirmed that blood counts will be checked before treatment and that appropriate treatment is available in the event that severe depression of blood counts occurs. Detailed information regarding the various medical issues involved in clinical trials will likely be known only to individuals with expertise in the disease or condition being studied. IRBs will therefore have to determine from the description of how the proposed trial will be performed or from advice of consultant experts that appropriate preventive and antidotal measures are intended to be utilized when necessary.

Balancing benefits against risks is in a sense trying to compare apples and oranges. The issue comes down to the question of whether the anticipated side effects and potential harm associated with either receiving treatment or being a member of a control group receiving ''standard'' therapy or no therapy is justified on the basis of the expected benefits to be attained.

Allowing for the essential uncertainty that surrounds the calculations of benefits and risks, the task can be substantially simplified if there are complete descriptions of the pertinent information in the proposals submitted for review. Thus, members of IRBs should be able to make informed judgments regarding the relative benefits and risks of clinical trials from the information that is provided by the investigators. Although a consultant can facilitate the interpretation of the information, the need for outside guidance is less in balancing benefits and risks than in assessing research design.

E. Informed Consent

Assuring that adequate provisions exist for securing informed consent is a central duty of IRBs. The requirements for informed consent are specified in the federal regulations. These require that investigators ''shall seek such consent only under circumstances that provide the prospective subject . . . sufficient opportunity to consider whether or not to participate and that minimize the possibility of coercion or undue influence. The information that is given to the subject . . . shall be in language that is understandable to [him]'' (39). The regulations further stipulate that ''No informed consent, whether oral or written, may include any exculpatory language through which the subject . . . is made to waive or appear to waive any of the subject's legal rights, or releases or appears to release the investigator, the sponsor, the institution or its agents from liability from negligence'' (40).

The federal regulations specify the information that shall be provided to each subject:

(1)   A statement that the study involves research, an explanation of the purposes of the research and the expected duration of the subject's participation, a description of the procedures to be followed, and identification of any procedures which are experimental;

(2)   A description of any reasonably foreseeable risks or discomforts to the subjects;

(3)   A description of any benefits to the subject or to others which may reasonably be expected from research;

(4)   A disclosure of appropriate alternative procedures or courses of treatment, if any, that might be advantageous to the subject;

(5)   A statement describing the extent, if any, to which confidentiality of records identifying the subject will be maintained;

(6)   For research involving more than minimal risk, an explanation as to whether any compensation and an explanation as to whether medical treatments are available if injury occurs and, if so, what they consist of, or where further information may be obtained;

(7)   An explanation of whom to contact for answers to pertinent questions about the research and research subjects' rights, and whom to contact in the event of a research-related injury to the subject; and

(8)   A statement that participation is voluntary, refusal to participate will involve no penalty or loss of benefits to which the subject is otherwise entitled, and the subject may discontinue participation at any time without penalty or loss of benefits to which the subject is otherwise entitled (41).

In addition to these basic elements of informed consent, IRBs shall also require that information shall be provided, where indicated, to the effect that (a) the particular treatment or procedure being tested may involve risks to the subject that are currently unforeseeable; (b) foreseeable circumstances may exist under which continued participation by the subject may be terminated by the investigator without regard to the subject's consent; (c) additional costs to the subject may result from participation in the research; (d) the consequences of a decision to withdraw; and (e) significant findings that may influence a subject's continued participation will be related to the subject (42).

In addition to the elements enumerated in the federal regulations, IRBs must consider whether consent forms should include the fact of randomization in the case of prospective randomized clinical trials. Numerous arguments have been made for and against disclosing to prospective subjects the fact that their treatment will be selected by a randomization procedure (43).

Those who feel that the fact of randomization need not be disclosed to prospective subjects argue that since the alternative treatments to be tested are not known to produce significantly different results and since the physician would have to make an arbitrary selection of one treatment or the other for a particular patient, notification that selection of treatment is by computer rather than by the patient's own physician does not provide additional protection for the subjects and is unnecessary. The response to this contention is that a subject's ability to exercise full autonomy over what will be done with his or her own body is best served by notifying the subject as to how the treatment will be selected and by whom, even if the selection process is equally arbitrary whatever process is used.

The weight of the arguments favors the notion that for consent to be fully informed, subjects must be notified that their treatments will be allocated in a random manner, i.e., selected by a process other than the judgment of their own physician. The meaning of the concept of randomization and the fact that it will be the manner by which treatment is selected is therefore considered to be an important and integral part of informed consent for participation in randomized clinical trials.

Implicit in the elements that comprise informed consent for subjects participating in clinical trials is that subjects will be notified of the nature of their disease. Current bioethical thinking views this to be essential in order for patients/subjects to give legally effective informed consent. The current practice in the United States is that informed consent to participate in clinical trials requires that patients be notified of their diagnosis. Accordingly, a statement regarding the diagnosis is required in consent forms for participation in clinical trials that are sponsored by national cooperative groups. It is of interest that other Western countries do not feel that it is necessary or even appropriate to inform patients of their diagnosis as part of the consent process.

The elements listed above that need be provided for consent to be informed must be expressed in a written consent form. It is evident that a consent form with all these elements will be a lengthy one. In fact, consent forms for participation in clinical trials often run to three or four single-spaced typewritten pages. However, the anecdotal experience of those involved in clinical trials is that the majority of the patients appreciate the full explanation provided in the consent forms and that these explanations do aid patients and their families significantly in determining whether to participate. Although there was widespread concern that these detailed, extensive explanations would frighten patients and reduce the incidence of participation in clinical trials by prospective subjects, there are no data indicating that this has occurred. Rather, the evidence appears to be that the more fully informed patient is able to participate in a clinical trial in a more meaningful way, thereby making the trial a cooperative venture between the patient/subject and the investigator. IRBs should therefore not be deterred from requiring that consent forms be truly informative and should include all of the elements described above.

Two additional questions remain regarding informed consent in clinical trials. The first question is who should prepare the consent forms. Although it may be argued that a layperson, such as a lawyer, might be able to take the information provided in the clinical trial protocol and cast it into a form that would be most readily understood by prospective subjects, it is suggested here that the investigator is in a better position to perform this task. The investigator is the one who is fully informed as to the various issues that pertain to the clinical trial. Accordingly, the investigator is potentially in the best position to express the necessary information in a manner that is comprehensible to laypersons. This requires that the investigator must be capable of explaining the issues involved in terms that are understandable to the nonphysician. IRBs should insist that, if an investigator wishes to have patients participate in clinical trials under his or her authority, he or she ought to be able to explain to prospective subjects precisely what is involved in terms that subjects can understand.

The second question is whether a physician should act in the dual capacity as physician and investigator with respect to his or her own patients. Depending on the particular circumstances, IRBs may be satisfied in allowing physicians to enlist their own patients in clinical trials in which they serve as investigators and to act as the caring physician during the trial. Alternatively, IRBs may wish to require that a knowledgeable third party, for example, another physician familiar with the disease and its treatment, or a party whose concern for the patient is without any apparent conflicts of interest, such as a close family member, participate in the recruitment process and in a monitoring capacity throughout the duration of the trial.

In most university-affiliated and community hospitals, the matter should be decided with reference to the particular clinical setting for the trial, the type of patient/subject involved, and the nature of the disease entity under study. For example, in a community hospital having no medical oncologist, cardiologist, etc., other than the physician/investigator, and where the prospective subjects are all private patients of the investigator, it may be appropriate that a patient advocate in the person of a family member or a member of the nursing service be present at the time of the consent proceeding. In a municipal hospital that is university-affiliated and has specialists on staff other than the investigator, it may be appropriate for one of the other staff members to be present at the time consent is enlisted so that the coercive elements that some deem to be inherent in such settings may be minimized. IRBs have to review each proposed clinical trial and specify conditions in which informed consent will be obtained on a case-by-case basis.

F. Compensation for Research-Related Injuries

The norm of compensation for research-related injuries derives from the principle of justice. As stated by the Task Force on Compensation of Injured Research Subjects, "human subjects who suffer physical, psychological, or social injury in the course of research conducted or supported by the PHS [Public Health Service] should be compensated if (1) the injury is proximately caused by such research, and (2) the injury on balance exceeds that reasonably associated with such illness from which the subject may be suffering, as well as with treatment usually associated with such illness at the time the subject began participation in the research" (44).

The norm was initially propounded in interim final regulations in which HHS specified that the availability of compensation must be included as an element in the informed-consent form. It now constitutes a basic element of informed consent in both HHS and FDA regulations. Those regulations stipulate that informed consent must include an explanation regarding the availability of compensation and medical treatment in the event of research-related injury (45).

The application of this norm by IRBs to clinical trials can be illustrated by considering a study in which administration of streptokinase in the coronary arteries to patients with acute myocardial infarction was being assessed. In this trial, half of the patients were randomly allocated to receive streptokinase via intracoronary artery perfusion. The patients in this group had to undergo catheterization of the coronary arteries in the immediate postinfarct period. The other half of the patients were allocated to be treated in the conventional way. They did not undergo coronary artery catheterization or receive streptokinase, although they were anticoagulated with heparin. The treatment being tested could have produced complications similar to those occurring with standard treatment, e.g., bleeding, or from the disease itself. However, the investigational arm of the study could also have introduced additional risks, e.g., those arising from the coronary artery catheterization.

IRBs called upon to review a trial such as this can satisfy the norm for compensation for research-related injury in one of two ways. First, they might interpret the regulations that embody the norm strictly. They might merely ascertain that the consent form includes a statement regarding the availability of compensation, without inquiring further as to whether the investigators or the institution should provide compensation. Since schemes for providing compensation are not readily available, this approach would not impose upon the investigators or the institution requirements that they would have difficulty meeting. It would, however, serve to alert prospective subjects to the issue of research-related injury

and allow them to consider the loss from such injuries in their decision to participate trial.

Alternatively, IRBs might determine which potential complication might
arise from the disease or the standard therapy and hence would not be compensable simply because they occurred in an individual participating in a clinical trial.
They could further determine which complications, if any, could be attributable
to the investigative component of the clinical trial. The IRBs might then recommend that the investigators and/or the institution signify a willingness to compensate subjects injured as a result of their participation in the trial or provide medical
treatment without additional cost to the subject.

This approach may very well increase the cost for doing research and might
make the performance of the clinical trial unacceptable to the investigators and
the institution. IRBs do not have the authority or power to require that compensation be made available. Consequently, a recommendation by the IRB to this effect
would not be enforceable. A recommendation, however, would alert the investigator and the institution to the potential existence of a compensable injury. To
the extent that this would promote additional safeguards for preventing such injury, the patient/subject would be benefited.

It is important that IRBs keep the matter of compensation in perspective.
Many medical experts are of the opinion that the best treatment is often provided
in the course of clinical trials. The legitimate concern regarding the cost of research-related injuries to particular subjects of clinical trials should be balanced
against the benefit arising from trials to individual subjects and to classes of
subjects of which individuals may be members. It is suggested that this can be
best accomplished by IRBs ascertaining that the potential subjects of clinical
trials be notified as to the availability of compensation for research related injuries
and that they be similarly notified as to the standards that apply in determining
whether injuries are in fact research-related and therefore compensable.

VI. SPECIAL ISSUES

Five special issues arise with respect to the role of IRBs in reviewing clinical
trials. These are the role of lay members of IRBs, the review of multi-institutional
trials sponsored by national cooperative groups, the duty to monitor the trials,
the financial risk assumed by patients entering clinical trials, and adherence to
new policies promulgated by the FDA or HHS.

A. The Role of Lay Members of IRBs

Members of IRBs fall into three general classes: scientific, nonscientific professional (lawyers, philosophers, clergy), and laypersons. Although all members will

make some assessment with respect to each of the ethical considerations that enters into a decision regarding the acceptability of a research proposal, it is understandable that members having varying backgrounds and expertise will weigh differently the factors that affect the decision. The scientific members of IRBs are best able to evaluate the scientific issues of proposed clinical trials, the anticipated benefits and risks associated with the trials, and the competence of the investigators to conduct the trials. In contrast, the nonscientific professionals and the lay members on IRBs can be expected to play more prominent roles in judging the adherence of proposed clinical trials to the norms of informed consent, equitable selection of subjects, and compensation for research-related injuries. Depending on their particular training and background, nonscientific professionals analyze the issues raised by proposed clinical trials in the light of prevailing legal, ethical-philosophical, or religious standards and norms. Lay members, by contrast, presumably reflect and represent general community attitudes (46).

It is anticipated and perhaps desirable that the nonscientific members not acquire an intimate understanding of the scientific basis and methods of the proposed research. To do so may result in their identifying more with the interests of the investigators and less with those of the subjects, assuming that the two interests are not identical. It is necessary, however, that they develop sufficient understanding of the science involved so that they can, like a jury, make reasonable, informed judgments as to the several issues involved in the research proposals.

The different roles of the several nonscientific members of IRBs can be illustrated by considering how they assess the procedures proposed for selecting subjects and obtaining informed consent. Whether there is equitable selection of subjects, particularly from presumably vulnerable subpopulations, is analyzed by individuals representing different professional or community constituencies in terms of equal protection, distributive justice, or prevailing standards of fairness. The adequacy of the consent procedure—whether consent is informed—is analyzed by attorney-members of IRBs in terms of battery and negligence and the objective standard of what the reasonable person similarly situated would want to know. It is analyzed by the philosopher in terms of the ethical principle of autonomy or respect for persons. Finally, it is analyzed by the lay member in terms of what the average "man-in-the street" would want to know. The lay member is perhaps best able to act as a surrogate for prospective subjects and indicate the setting that should exist for consent proceedings as well as the particular information that should be imparted in order for the subject to decide whether to participate in the study.

This analysis of the roles of different classes of IRB members in reviewing proposed clinical trials leads to two conclusions. The first is that the different members of IRBs should be expected to represent different perspectives. Their perceptions of the relative weight to give to different factors and the manner in which they think about and judge these factors are intended to be different. This diversity of viewpoints is complementary so that the final decision represents a consensus derived from balancing competing considerations and values. The second is that the role of IRB members reviewing clinical trials is similar to that with respect to any other research proposal. The anxiety and frustration that non-scientific members of IRBs in particular experience when reviewing clinical trials (at least as seen by this writer) can be minimized if these two points are kept in mind (47).

B. Review of Multi-institutional Trials

The review of clinical trials that are sponsored by national cooperative groups and/or involve the cooperative efforts of multiple institutions can present special problems for IRBs. The federal regulations state: ''In such instances, the grantee or prime contractor remains responsible to the Department (of HHS] for safeguarding the rights and welfare of human subjects. Also, when cooperating institutions conduct some of all of the research involving some or all of these subjects, each cooperating institution shall comply with [the] regulations as though it received funds for its participation in the project directly from the Department'' (48).

The scientific background that underlies these trials and their statistical design is often complex and may not be readily understood by individuals, including physicians, who are unfamiliar with the area of medicine involved. The role of IRBs in reviewing such protocols can be determined by considering the norms that define the conditions that should exist for the ethical conduct of clinical trails.

These norms involve considerations that are scientific as well as ethical. Assessment of the scientific issues can be done by utilizing consultants, joint review, the review of another qualified IRB, or another arrangement that avoids duplication of effort.

Assessment of the ethical issues, such as informed consent and equitable selection of subjects, can be competently undertaken by all members of IRBs. There is no need to treat proposed clinical trials sponsored by national cooperative groups and multi-institutional trials differently from any other research involving human subjects.

There is, to be sure, some difference of opinion regarding whether IRBs can request changes in the study protocol without effectively disapproving the involvement of the institution in the trial. Levine has stated, ''any deviations from the protocol render useless to the cooperative study the involvement of the institution in which such deviations occur. One cannot, therefore, request changes in drug doses, inclusion criteria, and the like (49). Rather, the multi-institutional randomized clinical trial should be viewed by the IRB as a package—take it or leave it.

In contrast, Freedman asks "whether a local research review committee can fulfill its regulatory, legal, and ethical responsibility without undertaking its own active review of any research to be conducted locally. Does the integrity of the research review process allow for two sets of standards of ethics and science, one to be imposed on local research and another, more cursory set, reserved for use in multicenter trials?" (50).

Freedman answers these questions by asserting that IRBs have an obligation to review multi-institutional trials in order to exercise their responsibility to safeguard subject safety and assure scientific validity of the study in question (51). In particular, he argues that IRBs should assess the eligibility criteria used for selecting subjects for such trials and should be prepared to request, if not require, changes in these criteria, if circumstances warrant. He disputes assertions that changes in eligibility criteria requested or required by IRBs should prevent participation of the institution in the trial.

Freedman further suggests that a process should be established that permits IRBs to know the names and addresses of contact persons of the IRBs considering multi-institutional trials to facilitate communication regarding issues identified in the course of reviewing the studies (52). Ultimately, however, the responsibility for safeguarding the rights and welfare of prospective subjects of research conducted within an institution lies with that institution's IRB. That responsibility cannot be deferred or abnegated simply because the source of a proposed clinical trial is a national group or organization that exists outside the institution.

Ultimately, the responsibility for safeguarding the rights and welfare of prospective subjects of research conducted within an institution lies with that institution's IRB. That responsibility cannot be deferred or abnegated simply because the source of a proposed clinical trial is a national group that exists outside the institution.

C. The Duty to Monitor

The federal regulations state that IRBs "shall conduct continuing review of research . . . at intervals appropriate to the degree of risk, but not less than once per year, and shall have authority to observe or have a third party observe the consent process and the research" (53). Continuing review must be substantive and meaningful (54).

The regulations outline the minimum requirements for continuing review. These specify that the IRB should review "the protocol and any amendments as well as a status report or the progress of the research, including (a) the number of subjects accrued; (b) a description of any adverse events or unanticipated problems involving risks to subjects or others, withdrawal of subjects from the research, or complaints about the research; (c) a summary of any recent literature, findings, or other relevant information, especially information about risks associated with the research; and (d) a copy of the current informed consent document'' (55).

Additionally, it is required that review of the currently approved consent document must ensure that the information is still accurate and complete. IRBs must ensure that any significant new findings that may relate to a subject's willingness to continue participation is or has been provided to the subject as required in Section 46.116(b)(5) of the federal regulations.

The regulations do not provide specific instructions to IRBs on how to undertake continuing review within the framework of the regulations. A major consideration for IRBs, therefore, is how to monitor the progress of clinical trials. A related issue is whether, how, and to what extent IRBs should monitor the preliminary data being generated by clinical trials.

Arguably, preliminary data generated during the course of a clinical trial may indicate trends that may be of interest to prospective subjects deciding whether to participate. On the other hand, such trends may not hold up as the trial continues. To notify prospective subjects of trends that may be appearing in preliminary data may lead to their deciding on the basis of incomplete information not to participate in the study. This may impair the ability of the study to achieve statistical significance and to reach a definitive conclusion. However, not to notify prospective subjects of preliminary trends that may be of interest to them may impair their ability to make an informed decision whether to participate and may conceivably expose them to a greater risk of harm.

Few IRBs are in a position to monitor adequately the ongoing performance of clinical trials and the data being generated on a continuing basis. This is due, in part, to the time lag between the generation of the data and the analysis of it. It is due also to the fact that the data in many drug trials are reported to statistical offices that are remote from the local institutions. Thus, practically speaking, IRBs are not in a position to exercise their responsibility for continuing review of the outcomes of clinical trials, particularly those sponsored by cooperative groups.

The question remains, then, how can IRBs carry out their duty to monitor clinical trials? One specific action is to require the investigator to report any planned changes in the conduct of the study for review and approval by the IRB, the occurrence of specific unanticipated events that pose significant risks to subjects, new information that may affect the assessment of risks and benefits, and any change that must be implemented immediately in order to protect the subjects of the research.

Second, IRBs can require investigators to certify that the selection of subjects and the procedures used are consistent with those set out in their research protocols. Finally, IRBs can request copies of signed consent forms and/or monitor the consent process to ensure that the subjects are being fully informed as to the trial in which they are participating and that consent is being obtained consistent with the research protocol.

D. Financial Risks of Clinical Trial Subjects

Clinical research, including clinical drug trials, are most commonly sponsored by government, business, private agencies, or foundations. These organizations generally provide funding for those aspects of the clinical trials that are clearly associated with the experimental activities: drug costs, special laboratory testing, data manager support, and investigator salaries. The costs associated with clinical services that would be utilized by the patient in the course of standard practice are usually not paid for by the research sponsor. Rather, they are considered the responsibility of the patient and are expected to be paid by the patient's health insurer.

Increasingly, health insures, both governmental and private commercial payors, expressly disallow payment for medical services that are labeled experimental. Many insurers include in this prohibition all services provided to patients who are subjects of clinical trials even if much of the care provided is the same as that provided patients with similar conditions who are not enrolled in clinical trials.

Thus, patients who consent to participate in clinical trials risk losing health insurance benefits otherwise available to them because of their willingness to serve as research subjects. This loss of benefits may apply to the care provided while the patient is being treated and, in some instances, to the care that is provided to treat complications or side effects of the treatment. Stated simply, patients entering clinical trials may incur significant financial risks as a consequence of their participation in the trials.

Until recently, IRBs have tended not to address this issue. With the advent of managed care and the disinclination of managed-care organizations to pay for all services related to experimental therapy, it is reasonable and appropriate that the IRB address the financial risks assumed by patients in the course of reviewing proposed studies.

This review may vary in scope. It may consist simply of ensuring that the informed consent process and the consent form clearly identifies the potential risk for each prospective subject. Or, the IRB may wish to require that the investigator and/or institution hold the patient harmless against any costs incurred during the study that are not paid for by the patient's health insurer.

At the very least, IRBs should be prepared to address it as one aspect of their mission of safeguarding the rights and welfare of prospective subjects of clinical research (56).

E. Compliance with New Federal Regulations

To comply with the assurances filed with HHS and FDA, IRBs are required to adjust their policies and procedures to conform with newly promulgated federal guidelines and procedures. In order to do so, either the staff of IRBs or the office of legal counsel for the institution must be responsible for knowing when such guidelines or regulations are issued. The IRBs must then incorporate any such changes into their operations and advise investigators of the new requirements.

An example of one guideline of particular relevance to clinical drug trials is the *Guideline for the Study and Evaluation of Gender Differences in the Clinical Evaluation of Drugs*, which the FDA published on July 22, 1993 (57). This guideline was developed to address a growing concern that the drug development process was not producing adequate information about the effects of drugs in women. One reason for this deficiency was the 1977 FDA guideline, *General Considerations for the Clinical Evaluation of Drugs*, that excluded women of child-bearing potential from participation in early studies of drugs.

The revised guideline, adopted in 1993, withdrew the restriction on the participation of women of child-bearing potential in early clinical trials. It stated instead that, in accordance with good medical practice, women should be counseled against becoming pregnant during the trial and should be advised to take appropriate precautions to avoid pregnancies.

The FDA stated that the change in the policy set forth in the guidelines would not by itself cause IRBs to alter restrictions they might impose on the participation of women of child-bearing potential. It did state, however, that IRBs have broader discretion to encourage entry of a wide range of individuals into the early phases of clinical trials. Additionally, the FDA urged IRBs "to examine carefully study protocols to see whether entry criteria needlessly exclude women or other groups in the target population of the drugs, or set up entry criteria that are difficult for women to meet" (58).

The guidelines on the participation of women in clinical drug trials are similar to those published in 1989 to ensure that elderly patients would be included in clinical drug studies (59).

Another example of a guideline of relevance to IRBs reviewing clinical drug trials is the procedures for IRB review of National Institutes of Health (NIH) multicenter clinical trial protocols that include NIH-approved sample informed-consent documents. The procedures state:

(1) The Office of Protection from Research Risks (OPRR) now requires that each local IRB receive a copy of the NIH-approved sample consent document and the full NIH-approved protocol as a condition for review and approval of the local informed consent documents.
(2) Any deletion or substantive modification of information concerning risks or alternative procedures contained in the sample informed con-

sent document must be justified in writing by the investigator and approved by the IRB.

(3)   The justification for an approval of such deletions or modifications must be reflected in the IRB minutes. For trials sponsored by the National Cancer Institute (NCI), investigators must forward copies of such IRB-approved changes, with their justifications, to the appropriate Cooperative Group headquarters (60).

The directive quoted above, issued by the OPRR, asserts that the policy contained in it does not reflect any change in the OPRR's policy concerning the importance of local IRB review. Rather, it reiterates the requirement that "[e]ach IRB must continue to review all protocol and informed consent documents with the greatest of care, regardless of any prior review at the national level" (61).

These two examples illustrate that IRBs must remain current with federal guidelines and regulations and be prepared to implement them when they become effective.

VII.   CONCLUSIONS

The review of clinical drug trials by Institutional Review Boards can be difficult and challenging. Adequate review by IRBs requires a firm understanding of the ethical principles that underlie the participation of human subjects in research, the legal authority under which IRBs operate, and the regulatory requirements that inform IRB activities. Resolution of specific issues requires careful balancing of competing considerations. Judicious decision making on the part of IRBs can enable important research into the treatment of disease to proceed while assuring that adequate safeguards exist to protect the rights, safety, and well-being of the subjects of the research.

ACKNOWLEDGMENT

Portions of this chapter were drawn from material previously prepared by the author that appeared in *Human Subjects Research* (Plenum Press, New York, 1982), and are used with the permission of the publisher.

REFERENCES

1.   The regulations of HHS that provide for protection of human research subjects are set out at 45 CFR 46.

2. The regulations of the FDA that provide for protection of human subjects are set out at 21 CFR 56.
3. 45 CFR §46.109(a); 21 CFR 556.109(a).
4. The Belmont Report (1978). Ethical Principles and Guidelines for the Protection of Human Subjects of Research. Report of the National Commission for the Protection of Human Subjects of Biomedical and Behavioral Research. Washington, DC: DHEW Publication (OS)780012. Hereinafter, The Belmont Report.
5. As published in Beauchamp TL, and Childress, JF. Principles of Biomedical Ethics. 2d ed. New York: Oxford University Press, 1983: 60.
6. Schloendorif v. Society of New York Hospital, 211 N.Y. 125, 105 N.E. 92, 93 (1914).
7. The Belmont Report. Supra note 5, at p. 4.
8. Beauchamp and Childress, Supra note 5, at p. 159.
9. Id. App. II, at p. 330.
10. The Belmont Report. Supra note 5, at p. 4.
11. Id. at p 5.
12. National Research Act. Pub.L. 93–348. July 12, 1974.
13. 21USC §301 et seq.
14. 45 CFR §46.102(e).
15. 45 CFR §46.103(a).
16. 21 CFR §50.3, 56. 103.
17. 45 CFR §46.109(a);21 CFR §56.109(a).
18. 45 CFR §46.109(b);21 CFR §56.109(b).
19. 45 CFR §46.109(c);21 CFR §56.109(c).
20. 45 CFR §46.109(d);21 CFR §56.109(d).
21. Id.
22. 45 CFR §46.109(e);21 CFR §56.109(e).
23. 45 CFR §46.113; 21 CFR 556.113.
24. 45 CFR §46.108(a); 21 CFR §56.108(a).
25. 45 CFR §46.108(b); 21 CFR §56.108(b).
26. 45 CFR §46.108(c); 21 CFR §56.108(c).
27. 45 CFR §46.114; 21 CFR §56.114.
28. 45 CFR §46.107(a); 21 CFR §56.107(a).
29. 45 CFR §46.107(b); 21 CFR §56.107(b).
30. 45 CFR §46.107(c); 21 CFR §56.107(c).
31. 45 CFR §46.107(d); 21 CFR §56.107(d).
32. 45 CFR §46.107(d); 21 CFR §56.107(e).
33. 45 CFR §46.111(a)(1–5); 21 CFR §56.111(a)(1–5).
34. 45 CFR §46.111(b); 21 CFR §56.111(b).
35. Levine RJ, and Lebacqz K. Some ethical considerations in clinical trials. Clin Pharm Ther 1979; 25:728–741, p. 730.
36. Research Involving Children. The National Commission for the Protection of Human Subjects of Biomedical and Behavioral Research. Washington, DC: DHEW Publication (OS)77–0004, 1977: 4–5.
37. 45 CFR §46.404(a)(6) 31793, Fed Reg 1978.
38. 45 CFR §46.111(a)(2); 21 CFR §56.111(a)(2).

39. 45 CFR §46. 116.
40. Id.
41. 45 CFR §46.116(a)(1–8).
42. 45 CFR §46.116(b)(1–5).
43. Levine RJ, and Lebacqz K. Supra note 35.
44. DHEW Secretary's Task Force on the Compensation of Injured Research Subjects. Washington, DC: DHEW Publication No. (OS)77–003, 1977.
45. 45 CFR §46.116 (a)(6).
46. Ghio JM. What is the role of a public member on an IRB? IRB Rev Hum Subj Res 1980; 2(2):7.
47. Cowan DH. Scientific design, ethics, and monitoring. IRB: A review of randomized clinical trials. IRB Rev Hum Subj Res 1980; 2(9):1–4.
48. 45 CFR §46.114.
49. Levine RJ. Ethics and Regulation of Clinical Research. 2d ed. Baltimore: Urban and Schwarzenberg, 1986: 211.
50. Freedman B. Multicenter trials and subject eligibility: should local IRBs play a role? IRB Rev Hum Subj Res 1994; 16(1,2):1–6, at p. 3.
51. Ibid., at p. 5.
52. Id.
53. 45 CFR §46.109(e); CFR §56.109(e)
54. Ellis GB. OPRR Rep 95–01. Bethesda, MD: National Institutes of Health, January 10, 1995.
55. Id.
56. Lind SE. Dilemmas in paying for clinical research: the view from the IRB. Rev Hum Subj Res 1987; 9(2):1–6.
57. Fed Reg 58(139):39406–39416. (July 22, 1993).
58. Suydam LA. Letter issued by Food and Drug Administration to IRBs, 1994.
59. Center for Drug Evaluation and Research Guideline for the Study of Drugs Likely to be Used in the Elderly. Washington, DC: Food and Drug Administration, 1989.
60. Lin MH, Miller JG. Local IRB review of multicenter clinical trials. OPRR Rep 93–01. Washington, DC: OPRR, 1992.
61. Id.

11

Personal Care and Randomized Clinical Trials:

Understanding the Ethical Conflicts

Paul J. Reitemeier
National Center for Ethics, Veterans Health Administration, White River Junction, Vermont, and Department of Medicine, Dartmouth Medical School, Hanover, New Hampshire

> The moral convictions of thoughtful and well-educated people are the data of ethics, just as sense perceptions are the data of science.
> W. D. Ross, *The Right and the Good*, 1930

I. ETHICAL BASIS OF THE SCIENTIFIC IMPERATIVE

Medical researchers, their supporting institutions, and governments have long recognized an ethical obligation to develop more effective medical treatments to improve public health through improving the welfare of individual patients. This effort to constantly improve the effectiveness of medical therapies may be termed the *scientific imperative* (SI). The SI requires individual physicians to determine for a given illness which therapy among several options is the best therapy for a particular patient. For example, patients seeking treatment for cancer of the prostate might be referred to or otherwise seek the opinions of a medical oncologist, a urological surgeon, and a radiotherapist. Each specialist may recommend a different therapy with different incumbent risks as the *best* therapy for prostatic

---

The opinions of the author expressed in this essay are personal and do not reflect those of the National Center for Ethics, the Veterans Health Administration or the federal government.

cancer. Making a choice among chemotherapy, surgery, and radiation (or a combination of two or more therapies) is not something most patients are emotionally or intellectually prepared to do. Therefore, the patient may rely on his primary care physician for advice on which specialist's recommendation to take. To make this determination, physicians need to know the results of therapy comparisons. Typically this involves consulting the published reports of clinical trial comparisons of the various therapeutic options.

Ethically sensitive procedure requires that these comparison studies be designed with as little burden to subjects and as little waste of resources as possible. In this chapter, I discuss the ethical issues inherent in conducting therapy comparison trials and I examine several proposals to address the ethical issues.

A. Research Design

Two significant obstacles to comparing medical therapies are the extensive time and the large number of subjects required to complete such studies with sufficient accuracy for the results to be reliable. To minimize both the time required and the number of subjects needed, research designs have been developed that emphasize statistical power and validity. For more than 40 years, blinded, randomized clinical trials (BRCTs) have been the "gold standard" of study designs because they emphasize both statistical power and validity and provide for economy of resources. BRCTs have definitively established some treatments as effective and eliminated others as ineffective (1). Large, multicenter trials often use data monitoring boards to provide an added degree of regulatory oversight so that the safety and interests of research subjects are maximally protected (2,3). This is most common when one of the therapies is experimentally new. Therefore, the need to identify the most effective therapies as quickly as possible can best be met if researchers conduct BRCTs.

But ethical concerns in BRCT research have been raised by several commentators (4–10). Physicians who conduct BRCT research must adjust their medical treatment of enrolled patients so it accords with the research protocol requirements. Adherence to these requirements is necessary to produce therapy comparison results that will be most compelling from a scientific point of view, so clinicians are persuaded by the results and use them in selecting therapies to offer to patients in the future. Conducting well-designed comparison trials on a few patients will enable many more future patients to benefit by avoiding what the trial reveals to be the inferior therapy. The comparison process is driven and success is measured by the objective endpoints specified in the trial design. Endpoints typically include either time-to-death (survival) of subjects or a specified physiological change such as tumor shrinkage, blood-count level, or other objective measures. Trial endpoints are specified by the study investigator so analysis of aggregate subject outcomes can be measured independently of the

individual patient's subjective judgment about the therapy. Thus, the ethical justification for conducting BRCT research is outcome-centered.

It is presumed that BRCTs are conducted only by physicians and researchers who genuinely believe that, as competent scientists, they stand in clinical
equipoise in relation to other investigators considering the same therapeutic
choices for patients (11). That is, they believe the advantage of one therapy over
another is not currently known or, alternatively, that the negative effects of the
standard and experimental therapies are judged to be comparable. The crucial
feature for ethically responsible decision making in this circumstance turns on
what counts as the relevant information or knowledge needed to form a well-
considered judgment among therapeutic options (12,13). An individual clinician's beliefs about the relative merits of individual therapies often differ from
the rest of the community of informed commentators (experienced clinicians and
statisticians). Equipoise may not exist at the individual level; each specialist will
claim to know what therapy is best for his or her patients. However, different
specialists may also disagree on which therapy is best for identically situated
patients, as in the case of the patient with prostatic cancer described above. At
the level of the community of informed commentators, these individual disagreements will result in a collective conflict indicating that in the informed community, community equipoise exists (14). That is, without the results of a completed
BRCT comparing therapies, no choice among these treatment alternatives can be
known collectively to be the best therapy to the general satisfaction of well-
informed clinicians as a group. Thus, for primary care physicians to make an
ethically responsible recommendation and for patients to have the best chance
for receiving the most effective therapy under circumstances of uncertainty, enrolling in a multiarmed BRCT appears to split the difference among the conflicting recommendations from specialists.

Because of known toxicities and mortalities associated with standard and
experimental treatment options, the earlier one therapy can be known with some
confidence to be superior to alternative therapies, the better it will be for patients.
Thus, an ethical concern for clinician researchers is to reach a nonarbitrary judgment about the comparative efficacy of different therapeutic interventions as early
as possible so that further BRCT study is not required. This is especially true in
cases where the illness under study is life-threatening and the currently accepted
standard treatment is not significantly effective in most cases, such as with pan-
creatic cancer.

II. THE PERSONAL CARE IMPERATIVE

As patient advocates, physicians have an ethical obligation to recommend to patients and to help them acquire what the physician believes is the best treatment

for their illness, all things considered. This obligation is a cornerstone of the physician–patient model, which Fried has termed *personal care*, and it is the predominant model used in training new clinicians (15). Indeed, it often is described as an ethical imperative in learning the professional standard of care for clinicians. This *personal care imperative* (PCI), sometimes termed the therapeutic obligation (12,13), is grounded in the presumption that patients and physicians come together to form a highly personal relationship within which they each have discernable roles. They share some, but not all, values and principles related to the patient's care, but they both seek the same clinical outcome objectives: maximal beneficial response to therapy. Moreover, this relationship is diachronic; it persists over a period of time with multiple interactions and circumstances requiring shared decision making.

Physicians who embody the PCI acknowledge their duty to respect patients' rights, which are described by Fried as lucidity, fidelity, humanity, and autonomy (15). In a complementary way, patients are expected to participate as reasonable, if often highly vulnerable, consumers who make efforts to understand the limitations and uncertainties associated with specific medical therapies. Patients, therefore, need to be competent to give informed consent or informed refusal to the various treatment options as explained by their physician.

In contrast to the outcome-centered SI, the ethical perspective of the PCI is patient-centered; the therapeutic process is driven and success is measured according to the willful, subjective desires of the informed and consenting patient. Because these subjective desires are often idiosyncratic, patients may forego enrolling in BRCTs in favor of alternative therapies or pursue the same therapy off-protocol so as to avoid the additional research requirements. If they do enroll in research, some patients may elect to withdraw before the trial is completed. In any event, the PCI emphasis on patient preference satisfaction and autonomy does not easily accommodate the procedural requirements of many BRCTs (16,17).

III. CONFLICT BETWEEN OBLIGATIONS IN THERAPY AND RESEARCH

Clinicians typically do not have a clear choice between either a well-established and effective standard of care or perfect equipoise concerning multiple treatment options, including investigational ones. Some evidence usually exists to prefer one treatment alternative over another, even if that evidence is merely anecdotal. When analysis of aggregate study results indicates that no therapy preference can be rationally justified to the community of experts by differences in effectiveness of treatment outcomes, then collective equipoise exists. Individual practitioners may have a personal preference for one therapy over another, but the numbers of those with preferences and the reasons for their preferences may balance each other out.

At the same time, the patient's personal preferences or circumstances may contribute to the patient having a rational preference for one therapy over another.

Under the PCI, a patient's preference for therapy choice under these circumstances of collective clinical equipoise ought to be determinative unless that preference can be shown to be against the patient's true interests. Even then, it may still be ethically appropriate to support the patient's pursuit of therapy preference. Therefore, to follow a BRCT protocol and use random assignment mechanisms to determine therapy for a particular patient is to ignore the PCI and to violate the patient's rights of fidelity and humanity because the patient's particular vulnerabilities and preferences are not taken into account. Indeed, if the patient elects to enroll as a subject in a BRCT, unless clearly harmful results to the patient can be reasonably foreseen, Fried argues that patients should even be provided interim research study results* if they desire, so that continued informed consent can be assured (15). Individual patient autonomy is a prominent part of ethically valid clinical trials (15). But while they may choose to do this, it surely involves a value judgment about the seriousness of the consequences of being wrong. Moreover, it also virtually assures that patient accrual in sufficient numbers for statistical power and validity will be significantly prolonged or even precluded. Adequate subject accrual into clinical trials has been a vexing problem for researchers, especially in adult populations (16,17).

At the level of ethical theory, the conflict between obligations generated by the SI and PCI may reflect a friction between a rights-based ethical theory and a goal-based ethical theory. The PCI rights-based theory values most highly the respect for individual patient autonomy, whereas the SI goal-based theory grants primacy to discovering reliable clinical measurements with the least net harm to subjects. But neither the superiority of one ethical theory over the other nor the reconciliation of one with the other has ever been established to the general agreement of commentators from either bioethics or clinical research. This ethical conflict has proven to be very difficult, and several proposals to address it have generated considerable discussion in the professional literature (4–10).

---

* The notion of what constitutes ''information'' in this context is a long-debated issue and essentially divides along frequentist versus Bayesian lines. Clinical investigators begin by assuming protocol A is equivalent to protocol B (on whatever metric is important). Random variability, especially in the earliest stages of the study, will produce interim outcomes that look different simply by chance. However, investigators choose to assume the null hypothesis (that there is no difference) continues to be true until such time as the available data provide sufficient information to conclude they are no different. In this regard, all information short of that allowing a choice to be made is considered noninformative. [I owe this important clarification to Professor James Anderson, University of Nebraska.]

IV.   PROPOSED THEORETICAL SOLUTIONS

A.   Avoiding Conflict by Alternative Designs

A patient's rights to personal care are violated when the physician does not incorporate the patient's personal choice when making treatment decisions (15–19). BRCTs require that patients be randomly assigned to therapy options, thereby precluding the possibility of incorporating any existing personal preferences for treatment selection. Therefore, enrolling a patient in a BRCT violates, in at least some cases, the personal care imperative.

1.   Prerandomization

Zelen (20) has suggested that investigators who are in clinical equipoise with respect to multiple therapy options privately use a randomization mechanism to select the treatment option for their patients, and then inform the patient which treatment will be used if the patient consents to participate in the study. This technique is known as *prerandomization*, and two versions of it have been developed. In both versions one-half of the patients are secretly prerandomized to the standard care arm A and followed without their knowledge (or consent) of participating in a trial.* The difference between the two schemes is how the second half, those secretly prerandomized to the experimental arm B, are treated.

In version 1, the patients prerandomized to experimental arm B are informed of the treatment and then asked for consent to receive the experimental treatment B. If the patient refuses treatment B, he or she is offered the standard treatment arm A and asked to consent to be followed as part of the research study. In version 2, patients prerandomized to the experimental arm B are asked for their preference of A or B, and that preference determines which treatment they receive. To make the relevant statistical comparisons among all participants, *all* the group 2 patients (those prerandomized to the B arm and then asked to choose between A and B) have to be compared with *all* the group 1 patients (those prerandomized to A, but not asked to choose). As the group 2 patients express an aggregate preference for one arm over the other (either A > B or B > A), the total number of patients enrolled in the study must enlarge to maintain statistical validity.

The main advantage of Zelen's two prerandomization designs is that they allow investigators to accrue subjects into protocols more effectively because one-half of the subjects are ignorant of their participation (21).

---

* It may be the case that in actual clinical practice, all of these studies using prerandomization obtain consent from subjects randomized to all of the treatment arms. Accordingly, it is unclear whether the single-arm design is used, or ever has been used. [I owe this empirical caution to Professor Donald Marquis, University of Kansas.]

Critique. For subjects prerandomized to arm A, patient autonomy is violated by precluding the possibility of the patient providing informed consent to participate. Because the patients do not know about the study, they do not know about the possible experimental options. Therefore, their consent cannot be fully informed, and their autonomy is necessarily and unjustly curtailed (18,19). This is to commit the moral wrong of failure to respect the subject as a person with moral rights, especially the right of personal autonomy. In a 1990 California lawsuit, the court explicitly used both the fiduciary-duty doctrine and the informed-consent doctrine to establish a legal obligation for researchers to disclose to participants both the fact of their research participation and any economic interests the investigators may have in that research (22). This is not a new finding of responsibility, however, because the ethical—if not legal—requirement for informed consent for research subjects dates to at least the late nineteenth century (23,24).

2. Expert Selection

Before conducting a course of clinical therapy under BRCT conditions, investigators can identify an initial probability distribution for subject outcomes based on the reported prior clinical experience of patients similarly situated and treated. Kadane (25) has suggested that, as trial data accumulate, this initial probability distribution should be updated and made more accurate through regular review by a panel of experts. Over time, as improved therapies are developed, research goals can be refined and the detailed prognostic variables and determinants better identified and firmly established. As the process continues further, the experts' opinions about the relative merit of each treatment option become further refined, and computer models of the opinions are generated. Eventually, individual prognostic variables can be entered into a computer program, and a model of all the experts' opinions concerning treatment selection for a new patient can be consulted before entering the trial. At this point, a treatment may be offered to the patient if, and only if, at least one expert finds it is the best treatment for that patient. Patients are intentionally not informed of the existence of the experts' opinions for fear that patients may (erroneously) favor one expert's opinions over another's, or make their participation decision based on idiosyncratic personality factors that may influence the statistical validity of the trial results.

Critique. Failure to provide patients who are prospective research subjects information concerning the opinion of experts regarding the therapy offered to them diminishes the patient's autonomy by withholding information potentially relevant to the patient's perspective (26). The experts' opinions are directly sought by the study designers for their own purposes, so it is reasonable to assume that at least some patients also may feel these opinions are of material interest to them. To intentionally refrain from sharing the opinions of the potentially interested subject is to fail to respect him or her as a person of moral worth. The ethical analysis must conclude that the investigators' obligations of personal care toward study subjects (the PCI) have not been met using either Zelen's or Kadane's research enrollment designs.

3.   Uninformed Consent

A third approach is to either autocratically decide not to inform prospective subjects about the interim results of the different arms of the research study at all, or to mention that the data will exist, but then ask them voluntarily to waive their rights to lucidity and informed consent when they enroll in a clinical trial (27,28). This approach eliminates the need for the patient and investigator to make several important choices by eliminating all but one option for treatment, namely, the one selected by random assignment. Interpretation of interim study data about the relative efficacy of the two arms is prohibited, as is looking at interim study data about reported side effects. All subjects enrolled in the trial are followed to completion. Investigators using this approach must ask potential research subjects, in effect, whether they wish to waive their rights to informed consent and to give uninformed (or at least underinformed) consent to participating in a BRCT. In dialogue, it might sound like the following:

> We cannot conduct the best possible research if we have to tailor the therapy according to individual patients' personal preferences. Therefore, we would like to ask you to agree to be treated according to the research protocol we have designed and which you can review, but to await the results of the completed study before making any treatment decisions that are in conflict with the study being conducted.

A more coercive version of this would add a subject-nonwithdrawal-agreement clause.

   Critique. Some patients may indeed be willing to waive their right to informed consent regarding important aspects of selecting and receiving therapy for a serious illness. For many, belief that their physician is doing everything possible on their behalf is as far as they wish to investigate the nature of the research study itself. However, when patients do agree to provide uninformed consent to participate, such waivers should precipitate a very careful exploration of the patient's reasons for agreeing (29). For example, if the patient is so scared of disability or death as to be incapable of understanding relevant and material aspects of the research (e.g., treatment selection and outcome monitoring requirements), or if the patient can articulate no rational basis for weighing the anticipated balance of potential risks and benefits, such a patient is not capable of giving informed consent—or informed refusal—to participate in the research. In such cases, allowing a patient to waive informed consent is unethical because the alternative—giving one's informed consent—is not a realistic option for the patient. Only those patients who are truly capable of providing informed consent can be offered the option of waiving that right and participating as an uninformed subject.

V. ADDITIONAL CHALLENGES TO CONDUCTING BRCTS

In addition to the ethical concerns raised in regard to subject autonomy, Rabeneck et al. (1, p. 511) have described procedural and conceptual problems in the conduct and analysis of BRCTs. The authors write:

> Clinical medicine is inherently an interactive process in which the patient and physician continuously modify treatment. This dynamic process of clinical care cannot usually be captured by the inflexible rules of traditional RCT analysis.

As a result of this tension between serving the patient's needs for personal care (the PCI) and the study design's needs for careful protocol adherence (the SI), changes in the physician's intention to treat the patient frequently arise after the occurrence of certain events. Such events include partial adherence to protocol, withdrawal of subject participation, errors in following the protocol, changes in the subject's clinical state, changes in dosages in response to hematological or other changes in the subject, and discontinuation of the study as a whole. Rabeneck (1, p. 509) argues that changes in the physician's intention to treat a study subject is a problem in clinical research is because:

> . . . [a]ny treatment changes that occur after randomization are ignored and all outcomes are charged to the originally assigned therapy. This intention to treat policy (ITT) protects the validity of the answer because it is assumed that no adequate adjustment for bias is possible after the subjects have been randomized to the treatment groups.

In direct contrast to the ITT method, alternative policies involving subject removal have been developed that allow the extracting and discarding of data for all subjects whose treatment is modified relative to the research protocol design (1, p. 509).

> This [removal] policy attempts to answer the question of the effect of treatment *as taken* [italics added]. However, as with the ITT policy, it fails to reflect the entire clinical experience in all patients and again limits the scope of the trial's results. . . . [But] when there are significant modifications of the randomly assigned treatments, clinical treatment of patients is not advanced by either the policy of entirely excluding treatment changes from

consideration in the analysis or the policy of excluding the subjects who experience those changes.

This dilemma between the all-inclusive versus the all-removal policies appears to create an ineliminable conflict of interest for the BRCT physician-researcher, and a conflict of interest, by its very nature, threatens the professional integrity of the physician-researcher. Purtillo (30, p. 4) has noted that

> . . . [t]he scientific ethos is a social contract setting in which members voluntarily chose to participate and therefore there is a responsibility on the part of the members to either follow the rules or make rules that are more consistent with the appropriate ends of the group. . . . Virtues or character traits that are ascribed to "good" researchers include integrity and constancy, exactitude or attention to detail, trustworthiness, curiosity, and rigor. The "telos" or end toward which the community rightfully strives is the discovery of truth.

VI. AN APPARENT IMPASSE

At what cost to current research subjects' welfare can scientific certainty and the benefit to future patients be pursued ethically? Can we continue to conduct BRCTs in the face of their assault on subject autonomy in deference to the scientific imperative? On the other hand, can we afford not to conduct BRCTs in light of their superior economic ability to establish statistical power and validity in comparing different therapies' benefits to subjects with the least overall risk to current subjects?

Attempts to resolve the conflict between the obligations of the PCI and those of the SI have been made from three different approaches, each without success. First, resolving the conflict at the level of ethical theory is not possible unless and until general agreement is reached on which overarching fundamental ethical theory is best for purposes of clinical research: a duty- and rights-based, patient-centered theory or a goal-based, outcome-centered theory. Prospects are not promising for such an agreement to emerge in the near future. The second approach, exemplified by Zelen's prerandomization alternatives and Kadane's Bayesian study designs, do not resolve the conflict, but only supplant it with other difficulties, most notably deception of subjects through nondisclosure of research participation and the risk of misrepresentation of scientific uncertainty to patients. The third approach, asking subjects to waive informed consent or to provide underinformed consent to the risks inherent in BRCT participation, may provide a solution at the theoretical level, but in practice, patients and physicians do not behave as purely rational, intentionally uninformed agents. They do not select medical treatment, especially in cases of serious illness, from behind a veil of ignorance. In addition, patients are more likely to withdraw early from a study in which they can see little chance of direct personal benefit and have little or no control of decision making. This risk of interrupting clinical trials through subject withdrawal may be increased by the skepticism patients may have of the trial succeeding if they are informed of the concerns Rabeneck and others have raised concerning scientific uncertainty (1). Moreover, even many well-educated subjects cannot understand clinical designs, and others are too dependent on their physicians to decide for them which treatment to undergo (18,19) and consequently may feel less obligated to remain in the study if continued participation becomes at all burdensome.

Thus far, this discussion has emphasized the ethical primacy of subject autonomy in deciding whether to enroll and remain in a BRCT. Now we turn to consideration of whether patients may have particular responsibilities to participate in clinical research as part of an ethical obligation to support the SI.

VII. SUBJECT OBLIGATIONS TO PARTICIPATE IN CLINICAL RESEARCH

Many more patients are treated off research protocols than are treated on them. Taylor et al. (31) reported a 1993 study in which 80% of the study subjects were enrolled by 10% of the more than 1700 physician members of an oncology cooperative study group. All respondents of the study indicated they had a "systematic pattern of patient preselection for entry onto trials beyond the formal inclusion/exclusion trial criteria." Eighty-three percent defined randomization and adherence to trial protocol as serious challenges to their ability to make individualized treatment decisions.

A. The Argument from Fairness over Time

Whenever two groups of similar patients are under a physician's professional care, other things being equal, it is discriminatory and, therefore, unjust to consistently serve the interests of one patient group over the interests of the other group. Depending on the exact nature of the relationships between the physician and patients and the role responsibilities entailed by those relationships, at least some of the time the interests of each patient group must be acknowledged and promoted. This is especially true if the net trade-off between the two sets of interests is roughly equivalent; that is, if the interests of individual patients in each group are either promoted or hindered by the (same) physician's actions to the same degree.

This analysis becomes considerably more complicated, however, when the two patient groups are the current and future patients of individual physician-investigators. The therapy interests of future patients require that prior efforts at developing effective therapies be optimally pursued so the treatment options available to them (in the future) are the best possible. This implies that at least some BRCTs should be conducted on prior (i.e., current) patients. Accordingly, the proper research question for clinicians is not *whether* BRCTs should be done, but *what safeguarding conditions* are needed to conduct BRCTs with one's current patients in as ethical a manner as possible. However, more needs to be said about the obligation of physicians to serve the interests of their future patients.

Having an interest in X is not the same as having a rights claim to X. Without establishing a rights claim to having one's interest served, there is little basis for recognizing a correlative duty on anyone else to serve that interest. For example, I may have an interest in having highly detailed maps available to enable me to navigate remote areas of wilderness for recreational camping purposes, but that interest does not encumber anyone else with a duty to provide those maps for me. Therefore, we must find a connection between future patients' interests in having optimal medical treatments options available and their having a right to have that interest served by current physicians and their current patients. If the important ethical rights and interests of current research subjects are abrogated, then no possible scientific outcome leading to future therapeutic benefit can, retrospectively, legitimize those research methods. Therefore, future patients' interests in having available optimally effective medical therapies cannot entail that current researchers and subjects may behave immorally to bring about those therapies. Consequently, we must become clear on what sort of obligations and duties present researchers and subjects have, if any, in serving the future interests of future patients.

Critique. The two types of rights claims made in the fairness-over-time argument have important differences. Current patients who claim the right to personal autonomy and the right to decline or to withdraw from BRCTs make that claim to their actual physician in the present. If the rights claims of current patients are respected and subject accrual in BRCTs is thereby slowed or even rendered insufficient to complete the clinical trials, then scientific progress will not advance as quickly as it would if BRCTs were conducted more quickly. But future subjects' interests in having the best possible therapy available can be optimally satisfied only if the best testing and confirmation methods are conducted in the present. And that seems to require conducting sufficient BRCTs now so as to maximize the rate of progress in developing effective therapies. Thus, future patients can be assured their interests in effective therapy will be optimally respected only if current patients' interests in autonomy and personal care are compromised and their medical therapies are determined by random assignment in a BRCT. In effect, serving the interests of future patients (now) requires not maximally serving the interests of (at least some) current patients and vice versa.

But what sort of a right is the right to have medical research previously conducted so that one may benefit now from its results? And against whom is this right directed so that they have a correlative duty to produce such research? Such a right perhaps is best understood as an opportunity right. An opportunity right is a right to have in place certain structures and processes in society so one may have an equal opportunity to pursue the good life when compared with other persons. For example, we have opportunity rights of access to good schools and teachers and roads so our individual potentials to flourish in society are not abrogated by avoidable obstacles. Equality of opportunity has long been one of the touchstones of the American way of life and serves as a moral beacon for the judicial branch of U.S. government.

Persons with serious illness are often effectively prevented from pursuing their own conception of the good life unless they can receive effective medical therapy for their illness. If effective therapy is not currently available, then a choice between the best therapy available (which may not be very effective) and the possibility of enrolling in a clinical research trial to improve therapeutic options in the future will provide them the greatest opportunity to pursue the good life. Using analogous reasoning, we can argue for construction of schools and roads and the training of teachers and other professionals so as to benefit future members of the community. It is hard to object, then, on ethical grounds, to a claim that medical research should be conducted so that optimally effective therapies as pathways to the good life exist in the present or, if such research previously was not done, that it be begun now. Unless compelling reasons exist to the contrary, it seems the rights claim to have both prior medical research conducted and current research opportunities available, understood as opportunity rights, is well grounded.

However, to ensure that current research efforts produce the necessary range of effective therapies that will be desired in the future, certain obligations on current researchers are logically entailed. Even if we agree that an equal opportunity to benefit from medical research is the ethical minimum below which no member of our society should be allowed to fall, because such opportunities define a level of functioning beneath which a minimally acceptable life is not possible, no theory of ethical rights can support entitlement or opportunity claims that engender unreasonable burdens on others or that are impossible to fulfill. A sense of balance must be struck among all the competing claims for medical research among all known illnesses. Microallocation decisions about the effort and resources devoted to various research initiatives are always required. Respect for future patients' opportunity-rights claims for effective therapy must be balanced with consideration and pursuit of other relevant goals of medical research.

Rights claims by future patients are not the only relevant rights or necessarily even the most powerful rights claims to obligate current researchers and patients to participate in medical research.

B. Sorting out Duty to Patients: Here and Now Versus There and Then

Leaving aside considerations of current patients who will continue to be patients in the future, it is not possible for a physician-investigator to have a personal relationship in the present with a future patient. Therefore, future patients' (future) claims that their interests were frustrated by the earlier actions of physicians must be understood correctly. Today the interests and lives of future patients are statistically real projections of future realities. It is reasonable to presume that in the future some patients' interests in maximally effective therapy will be measured in terms of duration of life. But it is also reasonable to presume there will be other patients whose therapy interests focus primarily on having pain-free mobility, intact cognition and memory, etc., rather than, perhaps even in exchange for, a maximal length of survival. The former group of patients' interests are best served by conducting BRCTs now so as to produce the most effective therapy possible for, maximal length of survival. The latter group of patients' interests, however, are best served by developing effective pain-relief methods without, at the same time, encumbering cognition or memory or producing unpleasant side effects. Thus, because individual investigators can only do a limited amount of research, and resources are finite for all types of clinical research, investigators now cannot act so that both sets of interests are simultaneously equally maximized. Therefore, when investigators consider their professional obligations to act in the interests of their future patients, they must recognize that they will frustrate some future patients' interests and enhance other future patients' interests *whatever action they take now.*

Morally reflective physician-investigators who are cognizant of these coexisting and mutually exclusive obligations must decide what approach to take toward communication and decision making with each of their current patients. The most important ethical conclusion that can be drawn is that physician-investigators cannot presume to know what is in the best interests of any particular patient without discussing all of the options with the patient. Risks and benefits of all alternatives must be discussed, but the patient's duties and responsibilities should also be discussed.

C. Patients' Obligations to Participate in BRCTs

Two related arguments from social justice can support the conclusion that patients who are suitable candidates in BRCTs have an ethical obligation to seriously consider participation. Similarly, the physician has a corresponding ethical obligation to offer patients the opportunity for research trial participation when they are eligible to participate.

1. The Argument from Social Duty

Among our moral convictions are that certain responsibilities are owed to fellow community members by virtue of shared community fellowship and that those responsibilities are reciprocal. This principle was stated in its most general form by the legal theorist H. L. A. Hart: "When a number of persons restrict their liberty by certain rules in order to obtain benefits which could not otherwise be obtained, those who have gained by the submission of others to the rules are under an obligation to submit in their turn" (32). Individual responsibility to participate in medical research, therefore, arises from a complex social and ethical structure of shared fellowship and common response to challenge.

Insofar as we have benefited individually, either directly or indirectly, from the voluntary participation of other subjects in prior medical research, including the training of our current medical practitioners, and insofar as we desire those benefits to exist in our future and in the futures of our loved ones and their loved ones, then to that degree, we have an obligation to participate in medical research when the opportunity is presented. To fail to fulfill one's ethical responsibilities arising out of a shared community and mutual challenge is to fail to contribute to the moral improvement of our community and to fail to contribute to that community for the prior sacrifices of those who made our current well-being possible.

For example, consider the increase in student fees to defray the costs of a new library building on campus. Those who pay the fees will be long gone before the building is ready for use. On the other hand, they have been using buildings that were paid for with fees from earlier students, who never had an opportunity to use them. In the longitudinal picture of community, justice and morality combine to require a communitarian orientation where community includes members whose lives span at least one generation ahead and one generation behind our own.

Patients' consideration of their duty to benefit the future human community should be facilitated by their physicians who have to consider the interests of their patients in the future as part of their current and future professional responsibilities. Patients also have personal responsibilities to their children and indirectly to personal intimates of their children, all of whom likely will be medical patients at one time or another. Patients who are candidates for BRCTs should consider their capacity and opportunity to contribute to the improved welfare of future patients out of recognition of their social duty to benefit the future community. To fail to address this consideration is to fail to be a contributing member (perhaps even to refuse to consider oneself as a member) of an ongoing moral community of interdependent persons of equal moral worth.

2. The Argument from Reciprocity

According to the *argument from reciprocity* (AR), insofar as current patients benefit from access to more therapeutically effective medical treatment than would be the case if there had been no prior clinical research, then to that degree such patients have an obligation to participate in the continuation of that research effort out of consideration of reciprocal fairness. Virtually all persons currently under medical care have experienced such benefits either through direct improved welfare or the avoidance of harms that prior research prevented from becoming available, such as thalidomide and Laetrile.

Critique. Because an ineliminable disconnection exists between most research participants and the future beneficiaries of that research, the ethical persuasiveness of AR relies on the view that all beneficiaries of therapy developed from prior clinical research share a common dependency on, and therefore a moral debt to, prior research subjects. The ethical question is whether and to what degree this dependency and debt requires reciprocal participation in clinical research. In medical care and research, if person A voluntarily participates in a BRCT whose results lead to an improved therapy, but not until after A has died, A's participation makes the larger domain of clinical research more efficient, and medical care for the future human community is thereby enhanced. Similarly, if current patients desire to have competent care providers and effective therapies both in the present and in the future for themselves, their loved ones, and their loved ones' loved ones, they must recognize the need to participate in the training of student professionals and in the conduct of clinical research when those opportunities arise.

We must carefully examine the relationship between ethics and justice in this context because, although they are intimately related, they are not identical nor are they coextensive. Multiple ethical theories exist, as do multiple conceptions of justice operating in different spheres of social living and decision making. What is just in regard to the provision of public education or roads and utilities may not be just in regard to environmental protection or divorce proceedings or medical research. Particular conceptions of justice and just relationships may exist and operate in separate spheres (33).

Just acts are not always ethically right; sometimes the just act will result in great harm to innocent others, in which case it should be foregone and the unjust action done. For example, sacrificing animal subjects to the goals of medical research may be unjust, but without doing so, many thousands of human lives would be lost that otherwise could be saved. Moreover, the just act—refusing to sacrifice animals and requiring the use of only human volunteers for every stage of research—would result in avoidable harm occurring to humans, which is unethical. Therefore, the ethically right thing to do is the unjust thing. We can try to minimize the injustice of sacrificing animals by requiring specific standards of care for them, but we will never eliminate the injustice completely, no matter how successful we are in animal husbandry. That ineliminable conflict between ethics and justice in certain contexts is what fuels the debate about many aspects of medical research. Neither political nor ethical theory alone can solve these questions because no theory can go all the way down to the local data of individual lives and relationships, which is where one needs to think about actual conflicts in the duties and rights of the affected parties.

So now we must turn to the question of assessing how compelling is this ethical obligation to participate in medical research. What if someone refrains from participating? Two types of moral consequences result from not dutifully participating in medical research. A direct consequence is that one suffers the loss of benefits and avoids the potential harm that would have occurred from participating in the research itself. Depending on the nature of the research and the likelihood of benefits and risks to the subject, this loss of benefit or avoidance of harm may be significant. An indirect consequence is the foregoing of an opportunity to benefit others. That is, by refraining from participating, one contributes to bringing about a future that lacks more effective medical treatment as a result of under-researched medical conditions and illnesses.

Consider the case of human blood and plasma. Most persons are unlikely ever to need a transfusion, so failure to donate blood is unlikely to result directly in a net loss of personal benefit. However, at the same time, we must acknowledge that we already have benefited from many types of research conducted on previously donated blood from other community members. If we refuse to participate in blood collection efforts, we will be morally culpable in failing an important ethical responsibility of reciprocity to the larger community by knowingly, intentionally, and therefore selfishly seeking to gain a net advantage from earlier blood donors. By failing to participate when offered the opportunity, we should foresee that we will be contributing to bringing about, even if we do not always directly intend it, a future with less effective medical treatments. That future will contain risks to both ourselves and to all of our loved ones to whom we have moral responsibilities of safekeeping.

In failing others in regard to this duty we also may be failing ourselves. Part of the moral life is the recognition, acceptance, and fulfillment of one's duty toward others. Intentionally refraining from fulfilling that duty, or being prevented from fulfilling it, can lead to a diminishment of our own moral capacity, and consequently, to our humanity. William May (34) has argued the following:

> Medical ethics concentrates exclusively on the ethics of the caregiver, but not those of the care receiver. It emphasizes the patient's rights, but not the patient's duties. We may subtly dehumanize patients when we do not take seriously the question of their virtues and vices, the nobility or meanness of their responses to ordeal. We act and reflect as though the patient does not have a moral life.

With the moral life comes both moral tragedy and moral responsibility. If we do not wish to surrender our personalities and lives when under professional care, we must assure we have both a reasonable opportunity to, and the expectations of our care providers that we will, fulfill our moral duties as patients or research subjects.

Participation in medical research can be viewed as an ethical responsibility in the same way donating blood is an ethical responsibility. Both obligations arise from our membership in a social community with shared challenges and desires for continued and increased benefit in the future. This responsibility also arises as a clear opportunity to make reciprocal contributions to the public good for benefits we have already received from the prior participation of other community members. Like opportunity-rights claims, the ethical responsibility to participate must be balanced against other worthy social responsibilities. Not every eligible prospective subject must participate in medical research, but all who refuse the opportunity must provide an ethical account of their reasons to decline. Similarly, physicians who do not discuss research opportunities with their study-eligible patients have an ethical obligation to account for that decision.

Participation in medical research can be construed as an ethical duty, but only in the very limited predictive sense of duty describing what we can expect if we collectively fail to fulfill our responsibility to participate. We can expect not to have the same rate of development of effective treatments to benefit ourselves and our loved ones in the event of serious medical illness in the future. We have the moral duty now to reflect on the fact that our failure to participate helps to bring that darker future into being. Ethical rights and their correlative duties that are unsupported by coextensive legal rights and duties exist only by virtue of the power of persuasion among persons who share similar interests in bringing about a common ethical objective. But the parties to this shared objective do not have to have a personal relationship to have a personal duty or right with respect to each other. For example, the authors and the readers of this book share the common ethical objective of having accurate and useful information. One group's interests are as producers, and the other group's interests are as consumers of that information. In pursuing that common interest, the authors have a duty to the readers to follow the usual standards and procedures of checking facts, citing original sources, etc., and the readers have the correlative right to expect these duties will be fulfilled by the authors. None of the parties needs to have any personal relationship to any other for the correlative duties and rights to exist. Thus, future patients have at least ethical interests in and possibly a weak form of rights to having well-researched, optimally effective medical therapies available. Similarly, current researchers have at least ethical interests in and possibly a weak form of duty to producing those therapies for use in the future.

VIII. THE REEDUCATION OF PHYSICIANS AND PATIENTS

The traditional view of the relationship between individual physicians and their patients has been characterized by Katz (35) as follows:

> Physicians have esoteric knowledge . . . which patients are incompetent to understand . . . so patients must trust physicians' altruism, and . . . allow physicians authority over them.

More recently, however, alternative characterizations of this relationship have been offered seeking to empower patients as coequals in shared decision making (36). This difference is of ethical importance in how it affects the process of decision making regarding medical therapy choices. Potentially beneficial alternatives to any medical treatment course almost always exist. Patients and physicians are presumed to have some differences in their personal values, plans, and preferences and will make different judgments about their relative importance. Therefore, in circumstances of uncertainty or conflict, the patient's perspective ought generally to rule the way treatment decisions are made unless the physician can provide compelling reasons why the patient's choices do not, in fact, reflect the patient's own acknowledged best interests. The primacy of enabling patient-desire satisfaction (sometimes interpreted as autonomy) then becomes the ethical guide for resolving treatment conflicts between the dictates of the therapeutic imperative and the patient's personal desires.

Though failure to respect a patient's personal selection and idiosyncratic ranking of values and preferences in medical care violates that patient's autonomy, to abandon one's patient amidst a set of almost incomprehensible technical therapy choices is also to violate the patient's autonomy. It is to withhold intentionally the physician's highly valued skills of scientific interpretation and explanation from a patient struggling amid the uncertainties of medical practice and science.

The physician-investigator is recognized as *an authority* in medical science because of specialized knowledge and skill, but is not *in authority* over patients in the sense of being one who commands obedience (37). Therefore, the primacy of informed consent and shared decision making as the determining influence in therapy choices remains the investigator-subject model most widely taught and promoted. Despite this prevailing pedagogy, its wide acceptance in practice has been slow to emerge, and many authorities recognize that it does not exist in practice in most situations. If truly informed consent and refusal were to begin to occur on a wide basis in nonresearch clinical situations, the ethical problem of consent in experimental clinical trials would be more easily resolved. But until that occurs, the "informed-consent solution" will be merely a theoretic solution and likely will not be effective at the level of practice.

REFERENCES

1. Rabeneck L, Viscoli CM, Horwitz RI. Problems in the conduct and analysis of randomized clinical trials: are we getting the right answers to the wrong questions? Arch Intern Med 1992; 152:507–512.
2. Smith MA, Ungerleider RS, Korn EL, Rubenstein L, Simon R. Role of independent data-monitoring committees in randomized clinical trials sponsored by the National Cancer Institute. J Clin Oncol 1997; 15(7):2736–2743.
3. Walters L. Data monitoring committees: the moral case for maximum feasible independence, Stat Med 1993; 12(5–6):575-580.
4. Koppelman L. Randomized clinical trials and the therapeutic relationship. Clin Res 1983; 31(1):1–25.
5. Miller B. Experimentation on human subjects: the ethics of randomized clinical trials. In: VanDeVeer D, Regan T, eds. Health Care Ethics: An Introduction. Philadelphia: Temple University Press, 1987:127–159.
6. Beecher HK. Ethics and clinical research. N Engl J Med 1966; 274:1354–1360.
7. Passamani E. Clinical trials: are they ethical? N Engl J Med 1991; 324(22):1589–1592.
8. Schafer A. The ethics of randomized clinical trials. N Engl J Med 1982; 307:719–724.
9. Hellman S, Hellman DS. Of mice but not men: problems of the randomized clinical trial. N Engl J Med 1991; 324(22):1585–1589.
10. Applebaum PS, Roth LR, Lidz CW, Benson P, Winslade W. False hopes and best data: consent to research and the therapeutic misconception. Hastings Cent Rep 1987; 17:20–24.
11. Friedman B. Equipoise and the ethics of clinical research. N Engl J Med 1987; 317:141–145.
12. Gifford F. Community equipoise and the ethics of randomized clinical trials. Bioethics 1995; 9(2):127–148.
13. Gifford F. The conflict between randomized clinical trials and the therapeutic obligation. J Med Philos 1986; 11:347–366.
14. Friedman B. A response to a purported ethical difficulty with randomized clinical trials involving cancer patients. J Clin Ethics 1992; 3(3):231–234.
15. Fried C. Medical Experimentation: Personal Integrity and Social Policy. New York: American Elesevier, 1974.
16. Ellenberg S. Randomization designs in comparative trials. N Engl J Med 1984; 310:1401–1408.
17. Smith M, Simon R, Cain D, Ungerleider RS. Children and cancer: a perspective from the Cancer Therapy Evaluation Program, National Cancer Institute. Cancer 1993; 71:3422–3428.
18. Marquis D. Leaving therapy to chance. Hastings Cent Rep 1983; 6:40–47.
19. Marquis D. An argument that all prerandomized clinical trials are unethical. J Med Philos 1986; 11:367.
20. Zelen M. A new design for randomized clinical trials. N Engl J Med 1979; 300:1242.

21. Truog R. Randomized clinical trials: lessons from ECMO. Clin Res 1992;40(3): 519–527.

22. Moore v. Regents of the University of California. Supreme Court of California, 51 Cal. 3d 120, 271. Cal. Rptr 1990; 146, 793 P.2d 479.

23. Vollmann J, Winau R. Informed consent in human experimentation before the Nuremberg Code. Br Med J 1996; 313:1445–1449.

24. Vollmann J, Winau R. The Prussian Regulation of 1900: early ethical standards for human experimentation in Germany. IRB Rev Hum Subj Res 1996; 18:9–11.

25. Kadane JB. Progress toward a more ethical method for clinical trials. J Med Philos 1986; 11:385.

26. Brody H, Campbell M, Faber-Langendoen K, Ogle KS. Withdrawing intensive life-sustaining treatment—recommendations for compassionate clinical management. N Engl J Med 1997; 336(9):652–657.

27. Tobias JS, Souhani RL. Fully informed consent can be needlessly cruel. Br Med J 1993; 307:1199–1201.

28. Tobias JS, Houghton J. Is informed consent essential for all chemotherapy studies? Eur J Cancer 1994; 30A(7):899–900.

29. King N. Patient waiver of informed consent. N C Med J 1990; 54(8):399–403.

30. Purtillo R. Editorial. Fulcrum, MGH Institute of Health Professions 1991; 2:1–4.

31. Taylor K, Feldstein ML, Skeel RT, Pandya KJ, Ng P, Cabone P. Fundamental dilemmas of the randomized clinical trial process: results of a survey of 1,737 Eastern Cooperative Oncology Group Investigators. J Clin Oncol 1994; 12(9):1796–1805.

32. Hart HLA, quoted in Benn SI. Rights. In: Encyclopedia of Philosophy. New York: Macmillan and Free Press, 1967:195–199.

33. Walzer M. Spheres of Justice: A Defense of Pluralism and Equality. New York: Basic Books, 1983.

34. May WF. The Physicians' Covenant: Images of the Healer in Medical Ethics. Philadelphia: Westminster, 1983.

35. Katz J. The Silent World of Doctor and Patient. New York: Free Press, 1984.

36. Brody H. The Healer's Power. New Haven, CT: Yale, 1990.

37. Engelhardt HT. Bioethics in pluralist societies. Perspect Biol Med 1982; 26:64–78.

12

Informed Consent in Clinical Trials:
Emerging Issues

Cheryl K. Fiedler
SCIREX Corporation, Hartford, Connecticut

H. Russell Searight
St. Louis University School of Medicine, St. Louis, Missouri

I. INTRODUCTION

Research informed consent is developed in a parallel, yet distinct, manner from its clinical counterpart. While clinical guidelines have largely been shaped by the courts, informed consent guidelines for clinical research have been developed through ethical principles governing the professions, federal regulations, and administrative policies of specific institutions or networks, such as the Veterans Administration (1).

Informed consent regulations in research are usually traced to the Nuremberg war trials tribunal. During the trials, it became apparent that many concentration camp internees and prisoners had been subjected to cruel experimental procedures including irradiation of the gonads and extended immersion in cold water. These procedures were conducted without subjects' informed consent and often were not guided by any clear scientific rationale (2). The American physicians who served as expert witnesses at the Nuremberg tribunal were asked to describe basic ethical standards for conducting human research. The resulting principles included required voluntary consent before a procedure is implemented, prior investigation with animals, and proper medical supervision of the experimental procedure (1).

In the early 1960s, research in the United States was almost exclusively regulated by non-binding ethical codes (1). By the mid-1960s, several controversial discoveries raised serious questions about the protection provided by existing principles. The birth defects associated with thalidomide were well publicized in the United States. Additionally, the anesthesiologist Henry Beecher published a provocative article detailing ethical violations in studies published in major medical journals. It became increasingly apparent that clinical ethics were often not applicable to the research setting. The roles of physician and investigator as well as that of the patient-subject were governed by divergent agendas (3).

The U.S. government articulated clear standards for research consent in 1966. An international consensus code for research ethics, the Declaration of Helsinki, was established in 1967 (1). The U.S. guidelines, developed by the Food and Drug Administration (FDA), were largely based on the Declaration of Helsinki and Nuremberg Codes. By 1978, with the Belmont Report, a detailed research policy emerged. The Belmont Report, published by the U.S. Department of Health, Education and Welfare (now the Department of Health and Human Services) was founded upon three fundamental ethical principles: (a) respect for persons—individual well-being and autonomy takes precedence over research objectives; (b) beneficence—benefits should be maximized and harm avoided; and (c) justice—benefits and personal costs of research should be equitable (4).

With these newly established principles, external review of research was also initiated. Institutional Review Boards (IRBs) provided prospective analyses of research procedures to assure that they were in conformity with federal guidelines.

The basic principles of informed consent include: (a) a description of the study, its purpose(s), and a clear labeling of the project as research; (b) risks or reasonably foreseeable adverse effects; (c) description of possible benefits; (d) availability of alternative treatments; (e) confidentiality of data and description of the parties having access to subjects' data; (f) availability of compensation in case of injury; (g) contact person for questions about the study and responsible party in case of adverse event; (h) statement that participation is voluntary and that the subject may withdraw at any time without penalty (1,4).

Studies are often categorized according to the level of risk involved. These categories are: "(1) research involving more than minimal risk; (2) research involving more than minimal risk but with potential for direct benefit; (3) research involving a slight increase over minimal risk without direct benefits; and (4) research not otherwise approvable." (5, p. 274). This risk:benefit ratio becomes particularly important when research is conducted with vulnerable populations. Examples of these groups include children and the frail elderly.

There are additional elements of disclosure left to the discretion of Institutional Review Boards. Among these include statements of unforeseen risks, conditions for terminating subjects' participation, consequences of early withdrawal from a study, and the impact of new findings about study procedures on continued participation (1). The IRB can modify or waive the basic informed consent elements as necessary—particularly in research posing minimal risk and/or prior to participation. In this latter case, subjects should be provided with relevant information as soon after their participation as possible.

II. INFORMED CONSENT: OVERVIEW OF RESEARCH

The federal requirements for the type of information that must be present in an informed consent document are presented above. While there are specific requirements regarding the content of the informed consent document, there is no accompanying mandate to ensure patient comprehension of the information. If the goal of the informed consent process is to allow the patient to make a truly "informed" choice, every effort must be made to assure patient understanding of the information presented to him or her. Sorrell (6). has suggested that, to promote subject comprehension, the informed consent document should be as brief as possible, direct, not complex, and written at a grade level commensurate with the subject's reading ability (generally eighth grade or less). The information must be presented, preferably by a professional directly involved in the research, in a nonthreatening manner; the ideal is to present the information verbally to supplement the written document. Patients must also be allowed to ask questions (1,7).

Even when all the above measures are undertaken (which may be seldom), research has shown that subjects' memory of information provided to them during the informed consent process is fragmentary; some information is retained while other material is either never comprehended or forgotten, either completely or "selectively." When this occurs, the question of whether informed consent has been obtained is often raised. Ethicists would argue that, to be truly informed, subjects must not only be given information at the outset of the study, but the information must be retained and used on an ongoing basis for decision making (7). Historically, research in the area of retention of information during the informed consent process has focused on the subjects' ability to recall or recognize specific study information given to them during the consent process (7–11). This research is typically conducted by a test, written or otherwise, that is given to the subject at a predesignated time after signing the informed consent document. While results may vary among studies, specific patterns have emerged.

When interviewing a large number of cancer patients, Cassileth et al. (12) found the amount of information (as perceived by the study subject) contained in the informed consent document was positively associated with scores on a recall-type quiz. This test was given to the participants a short time after the informed consent document was signed, and then patients were asked to rate the amount of information as "just right," "too little," or "too much." Patients who perceived that the amount of information presented to them was "just right" had significantly higher scores on the test than did patients who perceived the amount of information was either "too little" or "too much."

The degree of complexity of an informed consent document with respect to reading difficulty level may also influence comprehension or understanding. Consent form readability has been the subject of empirical study. Investigators have relied on two formulas—the Fry Readability Scale (13) and the Flesch Readability Formula (14). The Fry system involves a syllable count as well as a computation of the number of sentences in a 100-word passage. The result is expressed as a grade-level equivalent. In the Flesch method, data are referenced according to the level of a particular publication type (e.g., comic book, scientific journal) as well as according to grade level.

In a study by Grundner, surgical consent forms from five different major medical facilities were analyzed (15). The forms were found to be ''more difficult to read than materials in the popular press and slightly less difficult than articles founds in medical journals.'' Riecken and Ravich studied consent forms at four Veterans Administration (VA) hospitals and found they required college-level reading ability (16). This despite the fact that only 27% of the patients interviewed had more than a high school education. Even if consent forms are at an ''acceptable'' grade level for most research subjects, this does not assure comprehension of the information presented. A study by Mariner and McArdle found that while the reading level of a consent document used in childhood immunizations was appropriate for most of their research subjects (i.e., twelfth grade), few subjects were able to answer correctly more than 4 of 10 factual questions regarding the study (17). Of particular interest is a recent direct comparison of two research consent documents—one written at the seventh-grade level with the other form requiring twelfth grade reading skills (18). While participants rated the seventh-grade version as easier to read, comprehension did not differ between the two forms. Comparison rates were slightly below 60% for both versions (18). When taken together, these studies seem to suggest that readability is just one component of comprehension and must not be used alone to assess comprehension. Nevertheless, the reading ability of the research subject should not be ignored. In a study using a validated tool to measure comprehension, Miller (Fiedler) et al. found a moderately positive correlation between the subjects' scores on the comprehension test and their reading ability, as assessed by the Wide Range Achievement Test—Revised (WRAT—R), a standardized measure of reading vocabulary (19).

A remaining question centers on the criteria for determining the adequacy of consent form comprehension. Redish and Selzer (20) note that a common criterion for readability is the level at which half of the sample comprehends half of the printed material. While this standard may be acceptable statistically, it raises practical dilemmas. How much of the consent form should be comprehended before a signature for study participation is considered valid? As noted earlier, informed consent is obtained much like any medical procedure. Subjects assent to their participation but are not required to demonstrate their understanding underlying the decision being made.

There are suggestions that consent form readability is enhanced by a writing style with active versus passive voice and relatively short sentences (21). Compound sentences and those with embedded clauses should be used only when related concepts are presented together to enhance understanding (20). Word familiarity appears to be more important than number of syllables (20).

Many researchers have studied the effect of time on memory and/or comprehension of the consent document information. In a study of hypertensive patients entering a controlled clinical trial, patients were given a multiple-choice test regarding the information presented to them during the informed consent process (22). The percentage of correct answers on the test given 2 hours after the informed consent document was signed was approximately 72%; the percentage of correct answers 3 months later was 60%. In a similar study, subjects were given a recall/recognition test within 60 days of obtaining informed consent (23). Recall of specific information regarding the study was exceptionally low on some items, leading to speculation that the long time interval between obtaining informed consent and the interview was likely to have compromised participants' recall. Additionally, in a subsequent study by the same researchers using a validated tool for measuring comprehension, the change in comprehension over time was positively associated with declining scores on the comprehension test (19). While studying patient retention of information over long intervals of time may initially appear nonapplicable or unimportant, it must be remembered that many clinical trials are months or even years in duration; a considerable length of time may exist between obtaining informed consent and completion of the trials. In these studies, participants are expected to retain specific information about diet, dosing schedules, and medication side effects for the duration of the study. They also must be aware of possible side effects and risks that may occur for which medical attention may be required. Therefore, patient knowledge of the informed consent material may be just as important during the study as it was at the time of study enrollment (20).

Other factors identified as contributing to decreasing retention and/or memory of the consent document information include increasing age (9,24,25), acute illness (26,27), and lower education levels (16,28). However, these issues do not entirely account for the apparent inability to retain or recall information. In a study evaluating research subject retention and recall of information presented in the consent form process, Miller (Fiedler) et al. tested over 150 patients who had completed an over-the-counter analgesic study (23). The patients were not acutely ill at the time of study enrollment and all were given the same information both verbally and in writing via a standardized presentation. Subjects had a mean education of more than 12 years and were generally college-age. Subjects were contacted with 60 days of participation in the study and asked a series of questions regarding the information presented to them and their participation in the trial. Almost 100% of the subjects remembered participating in the trial and signing the informed consent document. The study purpose was accurately stated by approximately three-fourths of the subjects. However, when asked to name the two study medications, fewer than 20% could do so correctly, and an almost equivalent number were unable to recognize either drug from the list. This despite the fact that the study participants were almost unanimous in reporting they "thoroughly" understood the study and that the consent form accurately represented the actual conduct of the investigation. In a subsequent study by the same authors using a validated tool to measure comprehension rather than recall or recognition, study subjects comprehended approximately 70% of the information presented to them (19).

Finally, research has shown that medical patients as well as research subjects selectively block out or "forget" threatening or unpleasant information (18,11,22). Examples include information regarding possible side effects of the medications or treatment and the possible risks of a study. In the study by Miller (Fiedler) et al., over one-half of the patients could not recall a single medication side effect (23). When given a list of possible correct answers, only 5% correctly identified one-half or more of the side effects. Bergler found that only 2 hours after signing the informed consent document, less than one-third of the patients were aware of the side effects (i.e., wheezing and slow pulse) which had been described to them (22). When given the same multiple-choice test 3 months later, only one subject recalled both potential side effects. Many other researchers have found similar information regarding patients' recall of threatening information. In a study by Schultz et al., 50 patients were tested regarding their understanding of the informed consent document (29). Of all areas included in the test, the questions related to risks were answered appropriately less than 20% of the time. Robinson and Merav studied patients 4–6 months after the informed consent process (27). Although recall in general was inadequate, the recall of potential risks and complications was exceptionally low (10%). Finally, Muss interviewed 100 cancer patients to assess understanding of their chemotherapy regimen (30). Approximately 49% of the patients were unaware of the potential lethal complications of infection and bleeding. Although the authors felt this might be due to lack of clarity in the consent document, it is also possible that the patients selectively "forgot" this unpleasant information.

Often, investigators or ancillary study personnel are uncomfortable with discussing the potential untoward effects of a clinical study. This discomfort may lead them to minimize, downplay, or completely omit this type of information from their verbal presentation of the consent document. There may also a fear on the part of the researcher that full disclosure of all potential side effects might lead to a biased sample, with only those subjects who are not anxious about the possibility of risks consenting to participation.

It has also been suggested that patients who do not, at least initially, experience a side effect of a study drug may forget the negative information and dismiss it as something that does not apply to them (8). And finally, patients may decide that the potential benefits are worth the risks and, because the patients desire to participate in the study, they "forget" the negative information (8).

Although there is a large body of research regarding comprehension and retention of study information, many of the studies vary in methodology or have limitations that prevent drawing clear, generalizable conclusions. Many studies in the area of informed consent involved patients of insufficient numbers to yield statistically meaningful results. The type of subjects studied has also varied. Memory impairment, such as that seen in many geriatric or psychiatric patients (9,24,25), may affect retention or comprehension of the consent material. Time periods between initially providing participants with informed consent information and subsequent assessment have varied from several hours to over a year.

Perhaps the greatest concern is the definition of exactly what is being measured in any given study. Many investigations have employed recognition and recall tasks interchangeably as measures of comprehension, without an appreciation of these two memory processes as distinct (10). Research tools such as multiple-choice, true–false, and lists of items from which to choose measure predominately recognition rather than comprehension. One study by Miller (Fiedler) et al., which addressed this problem, involved the development of an open-ended questionnaire given in both written and verbal form to the subject (19). The test was validated using a known standard for assessing verbal skills, the vocabulary subtest of the Wechsler Adult Intelligence Scale—Revised (WAIS—R).

III. RESEARCH VERSUS CLINICAL CARE: DO SUBJECTS MAKE A DISTINCTION?

Patients consenting to medical treatment at the suggestion of a personal physician enter into this agreement with the expectation that the therapy, whether palliative or curative in nature, will be of direct benefit. Although there may be inherent risks with the treatment or procedure and no guarantee of success, the intent is to provide individual care that will ultimately improve the patient's health and/or quality of life. In contrast, when signing an informed consent document to participate in a research study, the subjects cannot assume the choice of treatment is made with their best interest in mind. Many study designs mandate that treatment be assigned in a random, blinded fashion; often the possible treatments include either no intervention or placebo. Therefore, the goals of research are very different from that of general medical care. The intent of research is not to benefit any individual patient, but to use the patient to generate data and obtain generalizable knowledge. While the ultimate outcome of a study may benefit society as a whole, there is no guarantee this outcome will happen or that subjects will not be harmed during the process.

Although research subjects are informed of the possible risks associated with a study, some do not make the distinction between usual medical care and research. This phenomenon has been labeled by Appelbaum as the "therapeutic misconception'' (31). Because research is often carried out in a medical clinic or hospital and involves numerous evaluations and tests, many subjects incorrectly assume that they are receiving care that is superior to that rendered by their private physician. From this process, they may also surmise that the research study is of direct benefit and decisions are being made with their best interest in mind.

Several aspects of methodology have been identified which may play a role in the therapeutic misconception. These include the use of placebos, control groups, random assignments to treatment, and blinding of treatment regimens. Research has shown that patients may distort, deny, or fail to hear what has been told to them regarding elements of study design. In a study of psychiatric patients participating in a research study, patients were informed that one of three groups would receive usual hospital care (i.e., no treatment intervention) rather than social skills training (31). However, when interviewed later, 10 of 13 subjects believed that all participants would receive social skills training. In a similar study, subjects were explicitly told that they would receive placebo or an inactive medication. When interviewed later, 16 of 18 subjects indicated that they knew some subjects would be receiving placebo; however two of these thought it would be used only in those who had no need for medications. Two other patients were completely unaware that a placebo was being used.

Park and Covi reported on 15 patients who were told they would be treated with placebo. Of these, only three indicated they were aware of the possibility of placebo treatment one week later; six of these patients believed that they had been treated with active medication (32). This phenomenon of apparent distortion of study facts was also noted in a study of 14 research subjects who were interviewed after completing participation in one of two ambulatory clinical research studies (8). While most participants could provide a reasonable definition or description of a placebo, and all patients recognized that placebos had been used, a number of them volunteered that they ''were sure'' they had received the active treatment.

Blinded randomization to study treatment or intervention is commonly employed in research studies as a means of minimizing patient and investigator bias. In contrast to usual medical care, randomization deprives the patient of individualized treatment, since doses and active versus inert treatments are chosen randomly rather than based on patient or disease characteristics. However, patients may not understand or choose not to believe the possibility exists that the dose of medication used may not be the optimal or safe dose for them as an individual. One study found that approximately 70% of subjects in a clinical research trial did not understand the double-blind randomization process even though they had been informed of the possibility that treatment would be randomly assigned (31). One subject, when asked how the investigators decided which drug to give him, indicated that he supposed they would take his condition into consideration and thus choose the best drug for him. This response indicates the presence of the therapeutic misconception and the lack of understanding of study methodology or research goals. In contrast, in a study by Searight and Miller (Fiedler), all participants demonstrated an understanding of randomly assigned treatment (33). Subjects generally described the process as "the drug company rolls the dice," or "it was random; depends on who walks through the door next." It is important to note that these patients received a verbal as well as written presentation of the information contained in the informed consent document. Phrases such as "rolls the dice" were quoted verbatim from this presentation. Although not scientifically proven, verbal presentation in lay terminology of complex research concepts may be beneficial when explaining such material to the patient.

Previous research has also revealed that patients often believe that they understand information presented to them when, in fact, they may not. In an earlier study, we found that almost all patients rated their understanding of the informed consent document as "thorough" and the consent form as "highly accurate" with regard to explaining study procedures. However, less than 1% of the respondents could name all three parties that had access to their study records and over one-half failed to name any possible side effects of the study medication (23). It is unknown whether the patients actually perceived themselves as informed or were reluctant to admit to the investigators that they lacked knowledge concerning the study. When studying patient perceptions of research, Searight and Miller (Fiedler) noted that a number of patients viewed the consent form as a tool for protecting the investigators and drug company from legal liability (33). It is disturbing that these patients who otherwise exhibited a high degree of knowledge about often complex study issues (e.g., randomization, blinding), viewed the informed consent document primarily as a legal tool designed to prevent litigation. There appeared to be little, if any, educational value placed on the document or the consent process.

IV. IS CONSENT REALLY INFORMED?

Institutional Review Boards focus their attention almost exclusively on the consent form itself. Relatively little attention is devoted to whether subject recruitment is actually carried out as described and whether protection of participant's rights follows established guidelines (1). For practical purposes, the informed-consent document has become the focus for external review of a study's ethical appropriateness.

Oral presentations are a helpful adjunct to the written form but may not be required. More brief consent documents with accompanying oral presentations may be permitted under certain conditions such as when obtaining consent from minors. From the subject's perspective, a signature on a consent form appears to have similar status as a signed contract. In our qualitative study, research subjects emphasized that the consent document was for the investigator's legal protection (33). It appears to be viewed similarly to signing a contract to purchase a house or car. Despite the written protection that subjects may withdraw at any time, it is likely that the signed consent has an implication of irrevocability to the research participant. From a regulatory perspective, the signed consent form is "proof" that the subject has voluntarily agreed to participate in the study.

The consent process emphasizes protection from coercion and deception. However, little attention is paid to subjects' understanding of this information. Current regulations provide no criteria for determining the adequacy of subjects' knowledge of relevant ethical or study information (1). There is also no guidance for investigators when subjects' understanding appears to be deficient. For example, a 25-year-old male with a high school diploma is provided with a consent form and a verbal explanation for a double-blind placebo trial involving a new analgesic. After being presented with the information, the investigator asks the subject if he has any questions. The subject responds, "I'll get real medicine, right?" The investigator tries to clarify: "We don't know if you'll get the real medicine or the placebo." The subject nods and, while signing the consent form, says, "Well, you are all doctors. I know you would not give me any pills that wouldn't help me." Although the subject's statements suggest that he does not fully understand that he may receive a placebo with no direct benefit, available regulations provide no clear guidance for the investigator in this situation. From a strictly regulatory perspective, the subject's signature on the consent form would allow him to be enrolled in the study.

In cases where a patient is determined incompetent, a legally authorized representative may consent on the patient's behalf (1). Surrogate decision makers are determined by state law. There are several areas of ambiguity surrounding patients with possible impairment in decision-making capacity. First, the majority of subjects who exhibit questionable decision-making capacities have not been determined legally incompetent. Eliciting consent from a patient who exhibits signs of impaired decisional skills in a clinical context typically involves seeking treatment authorization from the next-of-kin. However, until a *legal* decision has been made by the courts rendering the patient incompetent and a second legal decision has established a surrogate decision maker, the surrogate's authorization is invalid (34). The process by which treatment authorization for a patient with apparent cognitive impairment is automatically sought from a family member is commonplace in acute hospital settings. However, this common automatic process may not be legally sound.

The authority of a legally recognized surrogate decision maker to consent to treatment decisions may not extend to research. The applicability of a surrogate's authority would be even more questionable in a placebo control condition and/

or clinical trial in which little direct benefit is likely to accrue to the individual subject. More troubling would be a surrogate's authorization to withdraw a patient-subject from moderately effective drug to initiate a new experimental treatment with less well established efficiency.

Decision-making capacity is usually cast as a dichotomous choice—the patient *is* or *is not* competent to decide. Most clinicians will recognize, however, that many geriatric patients often demonstrate fluctuating levels of decisional skills. These capacities may vary according to time of day, surroundings, or effects of psychoactive drugs (35). While these circumstances frequently arise in "real life," there are no guidelines for clinical investigators. Caplan suggests that in cases of fluctuating competency, family members may function as "amplifiers" of subjects' wishes (35).

V. SPECIAL ISSUES: THE ELDERLY OR DEMENTED PATIENT

When examining the issues surrounding comprehension and informed consent, special consideration must be given to populations who have either lost or who have diminished capacity to make informed decisions. Included in this group are the elderly and/or the otherwise demented patient. The number of elderly people in the United States is growing and will continue to grow in the coming years (36). As such, the number of therapeutic agents used to treat diseases associated with aging (e.g., Alzheimer's disease) is also increasing. Because of the growing number of elderly and their obvious impact on the health care system, the number of social, behavioral, and quality-of-life studies in this population is also increasing. For these reasons, the elderly, many of whom are unable to understand the study information, weigh the risks and benefits, and make an informed, voluntary decision whether to participate, are being recruited for these clinical trials.

The Belmont Report identified three important elements with regard to informed consent: providing adequate information to the subject, comprehension of this information by the subject, and voluntariness on the part of the subject to participate in the research (4). As age increases, often the subject's ability to comprehend the information decreases, which calls into question the ability of the elderly to comprehend sometimes technical information regarding a research study.

Therefore, if one cannot assure the information presented to a potential study subject was understood, comprehended, and used in the decision-making process, then voluntary participation cannot be guaranteed.

When faced with the situation in which a study subject is unable to give valid informed consent, the researcher has two options. The first is to exclude the patient from the study altogether. While this decision may be one of frustration for the investigator, it seems the most conservative way to proceed to assure the patient incurs no unforeseen risks; on the surface, no harm is done if the subject is not entered into the study. However, as will be addressed later in this section, this may not necessarily be the case, especially if the treatment being studied is unique (i.e., no current therapy for the disease exists), potentially life-saving, or able to improve the quality of life. Additionally, if a behavioral or social study reveals information about the subject of which others may have been unaware (i.e., caretaker abuse), then denying the patient entry into the study may not have been in the subject's best interest.

The second option when a study subject is unable to give informed consent is to obtain permission from another party, or "proxy." A proxy is a third party, either a legal guardian, durable power of attorney, or a family member or friend, who acts as a surrogate decision-maker for the one deemed unable to make decisions for himself. The "ideal" proxy would be one who knows the wishes of the patient before he can no longer make decisions for himself. Although it seems that consent by proxy would be an alternative that would allow ethical research to be conducted in the elderly, several potential problems exist.

The most frustrating issue for researchers is that many elderly and/or demented patients have no court-appointed or legally designated proxy or guardian. In a recent study involving patients with dementia, one-third of the potential subjects did not have a legally appointed surrogate (37). In clinical practice, when medical or other basic care decisions must be made, these choices are often automatically made by a relative, usually a spouse or adult child. Many elderly patients or their families do not take the steps necessary to have a legal guardian appointed by a court for all decision making for that family member. This seems to be less of an issue, however, with the medical community in general. When a patient requires medical care, including surgery or hospitalization, often the next-of-kin will be required to sign consent for this to be performed. This is deemed acceptable even if the next-of-kin is a distant relative (e.g., nephew) or even unrelated to the patient (i.e., friend or acquaintance). While it is desirable to obtain permission from a legal guardian for medical care, most institutions accept the consent of a relative or friend, especially if the outcome would clearly be worse if treatment was withheld from the patient (e.g., surgical removal of a ruptured appendix). However, Institutional Review Boards often do not view research in the same context as medical care. Unless the compound under study is a life-saving alternative or a "last-ditch" effort to save the patient, it cannot always be assured that including a patient in a clinical study is in the patient's best interest. Therefore, many IRBs require the investigator to obtain consent of a legal guardian and/or durable power of attorney to allow the patient to participate. Of particular concern is Baskin and colleagues' recent finding that 18% of surrogates were determined to exhibit impaired capacity themselves and could not meaningfully consent to their ward's study participation (38).

A common scenario is one like that of an elderly nursing home resident (MB) who was transported to the hospital for surgical debridement of a pressure ulcer. The attending physician wanted to enroll MB in a research study involving the use of an investigational antibiotic, and sought consent from his wife, who had accompanied MB to the hospital and had already given consent for his surgery. However, MB's wife was not designated as his legal guardian or durable power of attorney, and the IRB was unwilling to allow her to consent to his participation in the study. The study drug was similar in antimicrobial spectrum to the control agent, which had previously been approved for general use by the FDA. The patient also would have received, among other benefits, free medical care for the ulcer as well as free cultures and laboratory tests. The IRB ruled that since there was approved therapy available and MB had no legal guardian or durable power of attorney, risks to him should be minimized by treating him with a known, FDA-approved agent.

Consistent with the IRB's stance is a recent New York court ruling that potential subjects exhibiting impaired decisional skills could not be enrolled in studies that included a nontherapeutic element (39). This decision has been criticized on several grounds. First, it could result in depriving individual's with certain conditions such as Alzheimer's from participation in treatment research for the condition itself. Hainowitz and colleagues note that if the proposed study includes a procedure such as a PET scan that has a minor risk, Alzheimer's patients would not be able to participate in a project otherwise of potential direct benefit (39).

Time may be a critical factor in situations where consent from a legal guardian is required of a patient to participate in a research study. A recent example is that of a study for an investigational agent for the acute treatment of stroke. The nature of the disease requires that the investigational drug be administered within 6 hours of the patient presenting with signs of a stroke. Often elderly patients, especially nursing home residents, will be transported to the emergency room unaccompanied by a family member or legal guardian. In many instances, a family member has signed, in advance, permission for care to be rendered in case of emergency. This permission typically does not apply to participation in research studies. If a proxy for the patient cannot be located in a timely fashion, the subject may be denied entry into the trial. In this example, there are no approved agents that slow or arrest an evolving ischemic process. However, the investigational agent may have unforeseen risks and it is possible that its use may result in more harm than no treatment at all. Again, the risks and benefits must be weighed, and IRBs are typically unwilling to allow the patient to proceed without the consent of a proxy and possibly even a court-appointed guardian. Indeed, if the compound proves effective, this patient may be denied therapy that might have improved her medical status, quality of life, and save substantial health care dollars. In situations where a drug is not available for treatment or cure of a disease state, it may be argued that the patient is receiving a disservice by not being allowed to participate in the trial.

Even if the IRB approves of consent by a proxy who was not appointed by the courts, the proxy may be unwilling to allow the patient to participate in an investigational protocol (36,40). One study evaluated the decisions made by proxies for nursing home patients about whether to permit patients' participation in a relatively low-risk study (36). The initial study involved looking at the morbidity from the long-term use of urinary catheters among nursing home patients. One hundred patients (50 with long-term use of catheters and 50 without) were required for the study. Required study procedures (i.e., phlebotomy and x-rays) were minimal with respect to risk to the patient. Of the 168 proxies approached for the purpose of obtaining informed consent, 78 (46%) refused to grant consent for the patients' participation in the study. Subjective characteristics, such as those based on the proxy's believes, perceptions, and attitudes, were helpful in determining why many of the proxies refused participation. When asked open-ended decision questions about why they refused, the following were reasons given: "She's been through too much already," and "I don't want her to go through more than she really has to." The four factors most commonly given as important in the proxies' decisions to refuse consent were the belief of the proxy that the patient "had already been through too much" and the fact that the proxy "didn't want the patient disturbed," "didn't want the patient upset," and thought the patient was "too sick." Additionally, many of the proxies were uncomfortable making that type of decision for the patient, and many stated that the patient's advanced age was an important factor in their decision. This stance was taken despite the fact that most proxies were not inherently opposed to medical research in general. Of all proxies, 96% thought research in general was important for medical care, and 83% thought that elderly people should participate in research. Obviously, the proxies were uncomfortable making this decision for another person, and it may have been easier not to decide and thereby forfeit the patient's participation in the trial.

An ongoing issue in the area of proxy decision making is who should be designated as a proxy for a patient who is unable to make choices for himself (41). How does one assure that the proxy will make ethical decisions that are in the best interest of the patient? Research and common sense tell us that we cannot assume that a proxy, even if she is a close relative who has assumed the responsibility of care for another individual, would always put the patient first when deciding what is best (41). One disturbing finding from the previously cited study was that one-third of the proxies who believed the patient himself would not have consented to participation in the research study consented to the patient's participation anyway (36). Clinical studies often offer substantial incentives that may be attractive to the guardian and influence his or her decision-making. Benefits offered to study participants at no cost often include medical care, physician evaluations, procedures (e.g., x-rays, CAT scans), laboratory testing, and study medication. If the patient can obtain all these at no cost through a research protocol, this may well translate into monetary savings for the patient and, ultimately, the legal guardian. In addition, study patients are often paid substantial cash stipends for participation in a research protocol. An obvious conflict of interest exists if the legal guardian stands to gain monetarily by the patient participating in a research study.

Although a number of unresolved issues are associated with proxy consent, some guidelines which should be considered by researchers and/or IRBs when conducting research with elderly or incompetent patients are available (40–43). Certainly, the known risks of the study should be taken into consideration when deciding the "level" of proxy consent required (i.e., legal guardian versus family member). IRBs might relax their proxy requirements if the risk to the patient is minimal and confidentiality issues have been addressed; examples of this include retrospective chart reviews or quality-of-life surveys. A second situation where legal consent might not be obtained is when the investigational drug has potential to be life-saving or superior to the current standard of care. This issue is dealt with more extensively in the critical-care research literature.

If the wishes of the patient prior to the loss of cognitive ability are know by the proxy, these should always take precedence over the decision or feelings of the proxy or the investigators. Among Alzheimer's dementia patients, obtaining informed consent and appointing a guardian can in most cases occur during the early stages of the disease, when cognitive deficits are relatively mild (37). The concept of "substituted judgment" is also helpful (42,43). According to this principle, the proxy should decide the way the patient would have decided if he or she had been able to do so. Sometimes this is the best point of reference by which a proxy can make a decision. Substitute judgment also speaks to the need for someone closely associated to the patient to be designated as proxy.

Finally, if the patient herself refuses participation in a research study, even if the patient is deemed incapable of making such a decision, the wishes of the patient should always be respected (36). Investigators should consider all consent by the elderly or demented patient a "temporary consent," meaning that the patient is asked before every procedure, questionnaire, etc., if she still wants to participate in the trial. If she declines, she is not forced to continue at that time. The investigator may return later or the next day to see if the patient has changed her mind.

VI. SPECIAL ISSUES: CHILDREN AND ADOLESCENTS

Minors constitute another "vulnerable" population. The research consent issues are somewhat different than with the elderly. Definitions of "adult" and "minor'' are largely determined by state law, with the vast majority of states using age 18 as the criterion for ''adult'' status.

With some exception, most persons aged 17 and under do not have the legal right to independently seek medical care or enter into research without a parent's or guardian's approval. Some states do allow minors to receive contraception, substance abuse treatment, or mental health services without parental authorization or notification (1). Most states also recognize ''emancipated minor'' status, which is determined by the courts or can be established though marriage, child bearing, or entry into the military.

With respect to research participation, there are suggestions that many adolescents do not differ cognitively from adults in their capacity to provide informed consent. Results of several studies suggest that by age 14 or 15, adolescents of average intellect are as able as adults to understand legal aspects of treatment consent and the elements of research consent (5,44).

A useful distinction in research with minors is ''assent'' versus ''consent.'' ''Consent'' implies comprehension of the conditions of one's research participation. ''Assent'' sets the lower standard of the ''child's agreement to participate in research'' (45). Developmentally, children aged 6 and up can usually meaningfully assent to their research involvement if information is presented appropriately. Even with parental authorization, children who refuse to agree or who voice reservations should not be enrolled. Minors should also sign the consent document along with their parent or guardian.

Another dimension used to determine childrens' research participation is the degree of risk involved and potential benefit to be derived. Ethicists have presented three key criteria for enrolling children in research that does not have potential for direct therapeutic value to the participant: (a) minimal risk of adverse events; (b) some anticipated benefit with slightly more than minimal risk; and (c) societal benefit with ''not more than a minor increment over minimal risks'' (46, p. 352).

Voluntariness and coercion are issues with minors as well as with elderly subjects. In studies involving financial compensation, parents may enroll their child without serious reflection about risks and benefits in order to receive remuneration. However, at the same time, many conscientious parents would have reservations about young children receiving a significant financial sum (e.g., $100.00) without parental control over its use. To our knowledge, there are no well-established guidelines around paying minors for research participation. The situation may arise when a minor wishes to be in a study and the parent refuses participation. With older adolescents, this conflict raises ethical issues regarding the limits of autonomy. However, from a legal perspective it would be unwise to enroll a minor in a study without signed parental approval. At the time of this writing, federal legislation is being debated about whether adolescents should continue to be able to participate in a low-risk anonymous survey research without parental consent. Teenagers had been able to complete surveys about issues such as drug/alcohol use and sexuality with parental notification only. Parents who did not wish their teenagers to complete the study could inform the investigators of their desire for their child not to participate. In the absence of parental refusal, however, adolescents could complete the study. This policy is currently undergoing review by Congress because of concerns about invading family privacy and usurping parental authority. If these restrictions are passed, it is likely that survey pools will shrink dramatically and become less representative.

Standards for enrolling adolescents as research subjects may be more stringent than legal requirements for independently seeking medical treatment. However, two general guidelines are employed to determine the appropriateness of enrolling adolescents without parental consent. First, the study should involve no more than minimal risk. Second, adolescents who do volunteer should be cognitively mature enough to comprehend the study's purpose and other informed consent elements. The adolescent should ideally be assisted by a clinician who has no vested interest in the research project and who can assist the teenager with decision making (13).

In involving adolescents in a clinical trial, a further qualification is that the "risk benefit ratio must be at least as favorable as that presented by available therapeutic alternative" (5, p. 267). This guideline would prevent enrollment of minors into randomized, placebo-controlled trials in which there are effective, established alternative treatments. With illness involving an experimental treatment with no established standard of cure, cognitively mature adolescents who do not have an available legal guardian probably should be able to provide independent consent (47). However, investigators should be certain that involvement of minors in research with more than minimal risk is consistent with state law.

VII. FULFILLING THE OBJECTIVES OF INFORMED CONSENT: RECOMMENDATIONS

Our research suggests that well-educated clinical trial participants appear to comprehend about 70% of the standard consent material. Among the basic informed consent dimensions, risks and possible adverse events may be less well retained or comprehended (23). One strategy to improve subjects' understanding would be repeated testing with a structured interview or written test such as the Deaconess Informed Consent Comprehension Test (DICCT). The DICCT is a 14-item structured interview test that assesses subjects' comprehension of the informed consent material. The questions are based on the informed consent elements included in the Belmont Report (14). Subjects are instructed to respond in their own words. Each DICCT question is scored on a 0, 1, 2 scale depending on the quality of the reasoning demonstrated. Our early studies with the DICCT indicated that the test could be scored by more than one person with a high degree of agreement. In addition, the DICCT's validity is suggested by moderate correlations with established measures of cognitive and academic functioning (19). The DICCT items can be adapted for a variety of investigatory protocols. The DICCT and other such instruments could be employed "diagnostically" to determine specific areas of weakness in comprehension. Based on this information, investigators could then highlight deficit areas in a subsequent presentation of the consent elements. Multimodal presentations including flip charts featuring key points, as well as video tapes added to verbal and written presentations, could further improve comprehension.

Given current concerns about institutional liability and periodic reports of maltreatment of research subjects, it is unlikely that consent forms will be significantly reduced in length. Instead, these documents, emphasized by IRBs as the primary vehicle for educating subjects about a clinical trial, are likely to become even more detailed. Since increased consent form length is associated with decreased comprehension, adjunctive procedures will become even more important for clinical trials participants to be adequately knowledgeable. Educational research suggests that periodic testing—particularly with clear objectives—will also improve subjects' comprehension of study information.

Results of our qualitative study suggest that while subjects may understand basic elements such as purposes, procedures, and confidentiality, important contextual dimensions may not be readily grasped. The distinction between medical procedures conducted as part of a research study and personal medical care does not seem to be understood. This difference is not customarily highlighted in clinical research (1). It is assumed that participants implicitly understand that medical treatment received through a research protocol may not be of direct personal benefit. Though our respondents demonstrated knowledge that their study was randomized, double-blind, and placebo-controlled, they continued to believe that they would receive direct treatment through the protocol. There seems to be a disjunction such that study participants can correctly define "randomized placebo" as a concept but do not recognize what this condition means for them, personally. To assist understanding, subjects could be explicitly told, "Half of the people in this study will receive a placebo—a sugar pill; the other half will receive the experimental drug; we do not know if you will receive the real medicine or the sugar pill. There is a 50% chance of receiving the sugar pill."

Appelbaum and colleagues point out that in medical research, subjects make inferences that are based on clinical care (1). There is minimal expectation that procedures will not be harmful, and a common perception that the subject will receive immediate benefit. This "therapeutic misconception" can be corrected by making a clear distinction between research and customary clinical care: "Because this is a research project. . . we will be doing some things differently from what we would do if we were simply treating you for your condition" (1, p. 251). "It is possible that you won't receive any direct treatment for your illness from being in this study." If strict adherence to a protocol is part of the study, this aspect should also be made explicit: "Ordinarily doctors change the amount of medication according to how their patients are doing. Here, in order to test the usefulness of the medications we are trying out, we will leave your dosage at the same level for 4 weeks—unless you suffer a severe reaction to it" (1, p. 2521).

When there is the option of established medical treatment outside a research protocol, this option should be clearly communicated to potential subjects. In addition to conveying a clear distinction between research and clinical care, subjects' understanding of study information will likely be enhanced if a "process" versus "event" approach is employed (1). Subjects in studies requiring multiple visits could be provided with descriptive material at each contact with encouragement to ask questions (1). Investigations which include these additional safeguards more closely capture the genuine intent of informed consent as a principle for promoting individual autonomy.

VIII. CONCLUSION

There is a growing body of research indicating that the ethical and educational objectives of informed-consent are incompletely realized. Subjects do not appear to retain and/or comprehend important aspects of the information that they are given at a study's outset. Our research with the DICCT suggests that about 30% of relevant study information is not comprehended and/or retained over a 1-hour period. More disturbingly, under current consent procedures, subjects do not make the important distinction between personal medical care and their research participation.

These findings leave a number of potentially disturbing implications for the clinical investigator. How much knowledge about a study should a potential research study be able to demonstrate? Is 70% adequate? 60%? 90%? Even if screening tests were employed as a prerequisite to enrolling study participants, the absence of a clear quantitative standard for adequate performance prevents these measures from having practical utility. A process-oriented approach to informed consent could address this issue. Repeated testing about a study's purposes, etc., with further review of failed areas for retesting until a specified criterion is reached could better assure subject comprehension. For studies involving multiple contacts, investigators, together with IRBs, could agree on a core body of information that subjects must know at enrollment, with additional information presented at later visits. This sequential presentation would likely optimize acquisition of information.

From the perspective of enrolling the maximum number of subjects, investigators have probably benefited from the therapeutic misconception. If subjects are explicitly told that medical procedures within a research study are not necessarily of direct benefit, there is a very real risk of a greater refusal rate. However, the consumer rights movement that has made patients more skeptical of all professionals will also continue to be directed toward medical research. While the number of ethical safeguards that biomedical researchers have been required to adopt has dramatically increased over the past 30 years, there are suggestions that these guidelines may become even more demanding. Clinical investigators should be preemptively considering ways to improve the informed consent process and be developing efficient, practical procedures toward this end.

REFERENCES

1. Appelbaum PS, Lidz CW, Meidel A. Informed consent: legal theory and clinical practice. New York Oxford University Press, 1987.
2. Rothrnan D. Strangers at the bedside. New York: Basic Books, 1991.
3. Beecher H. Ethics and Clinical Research. N Engl J Med 1966; 274:1354–1360.
4. Department of Health Education & Welfare: The Belmont Report. Washington, DC: U.S. Government Printing Office, 1979.
5. Santelli JS, Rosenfeld WD, DuRant RH, Dubler N, Morreale M, English A, Rogers AS. Guidelines for adolescent health research: a position paper for the Society for Adolescent Medicine. J Adolesc Health 1995; 17:270–276.
6. Sorrell JM. Effects of writing/speaking on comprehension of information for informed consent. Western J Nurs Res 1991; 13:110–122.
7. Hamilton MP. Role of an ethicist in the conduct of clinical trials in the United States. Control Clin Trials 1981; 1:411–420.
8. Silva MD, Sorrell JM. Enhancing comprehension of information for informed consent: a review of empirical research. IRB 1988; 10:1–6.
9. Taub HA, Baker MT. The effect of repeated testing upon comprehension of informed consent materials by elderly volunteers. Exp Aging Res 1983; 9:135–138.
10. Taub HA. Comprehension of informed consent for research: issues and directions for future study. IRB 1986; 8:7–10.
11. Hassar M, Weintraub M. "Uninformed" consent and the wealthy volunteer: an analysis of patient volunteers in a clinical trial of a new anti-inflammatory drug. Clin Pharmacol Ther 1976; 20:379–386.
12. Cassileth BR, Zupkis RV, Smith KS, March V. Informed consent—why are its goals imperfectly realized? N Engl J Med 1980; 302:896–900.
13. Fry EA. A readability formula that saves time. J Reading 1968; 11:513–516.
14. Flesch R. A new readability yardstick. J Appl Psychol 1948; 32:221–233.
15. Grundner TM. On the readability of surgical consent forms. N Engl J Med 1980; 302:900–902.
16. Riecken HW, Ravich R. Informed consent to biomedical research in Veterans Administration hospitals. JAMA 1982; 248:344–348.

17. Mariner WK, McArdle PA. Consent forms, readability, and comprehension: the need for new assessment tools. Law Med Health Care 1985; 13:68–69, 71–74.

18. Davis TEL, Holcombe RF, Berkel HJ, Pramanik S, Divers SG. Informed consent for clinical trials: a comparative study of standard versus simplified forms. J Natl Cancer Inst 1998; 90:668–675.

19. Miller (Fiedler) CK, O'Donnell DL, Searight HR, Barbarash RA. The Deaconess Informed Consent Comprehension Test: an assessment tool for clinical research subjects. Pharmacotherapy 1996; 16:872–878.

20. Redish JC, Selzer J. The place of readability formulas in technical communication. Tech Commun 1985; 4:46–52.

21. Schwartz R. Effects of test-retest on comprehension, recall and retention of written consent in a drug trial study. Unpublished Masters' thesis, 1995.

22. Bergler JH, Pennington AC, Metcalfe M, Freis ED. Informed consent: how much does the patient understand? Clin Pharmacol Ther 1980; 24:435–440.

23. Miller (Fiedler) CK, Searight HR, Grable D, Schwartz R, Barbarash RA. Comprehension and recall of the informational content of the informed consent document: an evaluation of 168 patients in a controlled clinical trial. J Clin Res Drug Dev 1994; 8:237–248.

24. Taub HA, Baker MT. A reevaluation of informed consent in the elderly: a method for improving comprehension through direct testing. Clin Res 1984; 32:17–21.

25. Morgan LW, Schwab IR. Informed consent in senile cataract extraction. Arch Ophthalmol 1986; 104:42–45.

26. Priluck IA, Robertson DM, Buettner H. What patients recall of the postoperative discussion after retinal detachment surgery. Am J Ophthalmol 1979; 87:620 623.

27. Robinson G, Merav A. Informed consent: recall by patients tested post operatively. Ann Thorac Surg 1976; 22:209–212.

28. Taub HA, Baker MT, Starr JF. Informed consent for research: effects of readability, patient age and education. J Am Geriatr Soc 1986; 34:601–606.

29. Schultz AL, Pardee GP, Ensinck JW. Are research subjects really informed? Western J Med 1975; 123:76–80.

30. Muss HB, White DR, Michielutte R, Richards IIF, Cooper MR, William S, Stuart JJ, Spurr CL. Written informed consent in patients with breast cancer. Cancer 1979; 43:1549–1556.

31. Applebaum PS, Roth LH, Lidz CW. The therapeutic misconception: informed consent in psychiatric research. Int J Law Psychiatr. 1982; 5:319–324.

32. Park LC, Covi L. Nonblind placebo trial: an exploration of neurotic outpatients' responses to placebo when its inert content is disclosed. Arch Gen Psychiatry 1965; 12:336–345.

33. Searight HR, Miller (Fiedler) CK. Remembering and interpreting informed consent: Results of a qualitative study. J Am Board Fam Pract 1996; 9:14–22.

34. Searight HR, Barbarash RA. Informed consent: clinical and legal issues in family practice. Fam Med 1994; 26:244–249.

35. Caplan AL. Let wisdom find a way: The concept of competency in the care of the elderly. In: Caplan AL, ed. If I were a rich man I could buy a pancreas and other essays of the ethics of health care. Bloomington, IN: Indiana University Press, 1992.

36. Warren JW, Sobal J, Tenney JH, Hoopes JM, Damron D, Levenson S, DeForge BR, Muncie HL Jr. Informed consent by proxy: an issue in research with elderly patients. N Engl J Med 1986; 315:1124–1128.
37. Dukoff R, Sunderland T, Durable power of attorney and informed consent with Alzheimer's disease patients: a clinical study. Am J Psychiatr. 1997; 154:1070–1075.
38. Baskin SA, Morris J, Ahronheim JC, Meier DE, Morrison RS. Barriers to obtaining consent in dementia research: implications for surrogate decision making. J Am Geriatr Soc 1998; 46:287–290.
39. Haimowitz S, Deluno SJ, Oldham JM, Uninformed decision making: the case of surrogate research consent. Hastings Center Rep 1997; 27:9–16.
40. Sachs GA, Stocking CB, Stern R, Cox DM, Hougham G, Sachs RS. Ethical aspects of dementia research: informed consent and proxy consent. Clin Res 1994; 42:403–412.
41. Kapp MB. Proxy decision making in Alzheimer disease research: durable powers of attorney, guardianship, and other alternatives. Alzheimer Dis Assoc Disord 1994; 8(Suppl 4):28–37.
42. Dubler NN. Legal judgments and informed consent in geriatric research. J Am Geriatr Soc 1987; 35:545–549.
43. Franzi C, Orgren RA, Rozance C. Informed consent by proxy: a dilemma in long term care research. Clin Gerontologist 1994; 15:23–35.
44. Weitholm LA. Childrens' capacities to decide about participation in research. IRB 1983; 5:1–5.
45. Mammel KA, Kaplan DW. Research consent by adolescent minors and institutional review boards. J Adolesc Health 1995; 17:323–330.
46. Gordon V, Bonkovsky FO. Family dynamics and children in medical research. J Clin Ethics 1996; 7:349–354, 362–364.
47. Levine RJ. Adolescents as research subjects without permission of their parents or guardians: ethical considerations. J Adolesc Health 1995; 17:287–297.

13

Orphan Drug Development:
David and Goliath

Allen Cato
Cato Research Ltd., Durham, North Carolina

Susan L. Watts
Family Health International, Research Triangle Park, North Carolina

Lynda Sutton
Cato Research Ltd., Durham, North Carolina

Marlene E. Haffner
United States Food and Drug Administration, Rockville, Maryland

I. INTRODUCTION

Orphan products, which include drugs and biologics, are an often-neglected area of clinical research. Orphan products are used to treat rare diseases or conditions that by definition, affect fewer than 200,000 people (or up to 1 in 1300) in the United States. Approximately 5000 orphan diseases have been identified, most of which lack effective drug treatment (1).

The names of some rare diseases have become familiar. For instance, amyotrophic lateral sclerosis (ALS), commonly known as Lou Gehrig disease, is an orphan disease affecting between 20,000 and 40,000 people in the United States. ALS is one of the 40 neuromuscular diseases supported by the Muscular Dystrophy Association, the highly visible national organization behind the annual Labor Day telethon for muscular dystrophies. Then there is Huntington's chorea, a rare disease that affects a population of 14,000 to 20,000 and became widely recognized after claiming the lives of folksinger Woody Guthrie and boxer Izzard Charles. Other well-known orphan diseases include Tourette's syndrome (affecting

100,000 Americans) and sickle cell anemia (affecting approximately 70,000 Americans of various ethnic origins). And although the number of people who meet the Centers for Disease Control and Prevention's definition for AIDS exceeds 200,000, fewer people are affected by each of the various opportunistic infections associated with AIDS, which permits some manifestations of the disease to be classified as orphan under the Orphan Drug Act.

For each familiar rare disease, however, many others are much less well known, such as Gaucher's disease (affecting 30,000 Americans), Turner's syndrome (affecting 60,000 U.S. females), acute graft-versus-host disease, acute (adult) respiratory distress syndrome (13,000 to 27,000 cases annually), and Paget's disease of bone (estimated to affect 100,000 or more Americans). Indeed, no telethons are held for von Hippel-Lindau disease or myelodysplastic syndrome, and no hospital wings have been dedicated to the study of epidermolysis bullosa. Whether such diseases are less "glamorous" to study or are victims of the drug manufacturing system, orphan drug development presents a peculiar quandary that pits human welfare against government regulation and industrial development—David versus Goliath.

Pharmaceutical firms traditionally have had little interest in developing drugs with a sales potential of less than $20 million because of the high costs associated with developing, manufacturing, and marketing drugs. Today, many large pharmaceutical companies avoid developing drugs that have less than several hundred million dollars in potential yearly sales because sale of those small-market drugs typically just do not recoup the companies' developmental costs (see Chapter 1). In the early 1990s, an estimated $290 million was required to bring a new drug to market (2). By the late 1990s, that price tag had risen to $500 million (3). It should be noted, however, that these development-cost figures actually reflect the costs of maintaining a company's entire research effort. Most companies can reap larger profits by investing in the development of more lucrative drugs. Even "super" drug manufacturers have limited resources to commit to drug development, so the most obvious choice from a financial viewpoint is for them to pursue drugs with a reasonable chance of success—drugs with annual sales potential of at least several hundred million dollars—rather than pursuing several drugs with only $20 million potential in sales. Because of the rarity of patients with orphan diseases, orphan products suffer from a limited commercial market that lacks a cost-effective benefit to the company developing that product.

A. Varying Perspectives

The government, academicians, individual patients, and industry present different perspectives regarding orphan drug development. The government—with a responsibility to maintain the public's health and welfare—is ethically bound to mandate that the patients with rare and debilitating diseases have access to effective treatment equal to that of those with more common ailments. There should be no favoritism.

Academicians may synthesize new compounds by accident or for treatment of those patients whose diseases are recalcitrant or without alternative therapy. In return, the academician receives public recognition, publication, career enhancement, and greater credibility in obtaining grants and equipment for research. Drug development is an extensive and arduous process, and the major disadvantage for academicians involved in this process is that they are often removed from mainstream research, and their already shrinking time and resources are expended.

Patients with rare diseases have a personal investment: they need treatment for diseases the general population is usually unaware of. But no matter how rare the disease, that disease is a very real issue for the patients who have it and for their families.

Industry is motivated to develop orphan drugs for scientific and medical research reasons. Seemingly little financial incentive exists (except tax credits granted by federal law and User Fee exemptions), and most companies view "service drugs" and companies serving in the public interest as echoes of a bygone era.

B. Special Groups

Although orphan drugs conjure up images of isolated populations of suffering patients overlooked by mainstream medical science, there are also three rather large groups of patients for whom few drugs are being specifically developed: children, the elderly, and pregnant women. Most prescription (and nonprescription) drugs contain warnings against prescribing them for children; nonetheless, many of these drugs are used to treat children. Such warnings—usually found in the official labeling or package insert of the drug—are necessary because insufficient clinical study data in pediatric use prevent the sponsor from making appropriate recommendations (see Chapter 7).

Elderly patients also metabolize drugs differently than younger adults—something for which drug formulations do not always account. Although children and elderly patients are routinely treated with nonrecommended drugs, most pregnant women are advised not to take any drugs at all for the duration of their pregnancy because of unknown risks of drug teratogenicity.

It is curious to consider that, in the face of medical and drug therapy advances, pregnant women have lost medications once employed to help them with some of the more unpleasant and health-threatening side effects of their condition. Heightened coverage by the media and the ensuing liability trials buried Bendectin and thalidomide. Bendectin (doxylamine and vitamin B_6) fell victim to nonscientist jurors who had to make decisions that extended beyond their understanding and that were based more on emotion than on scientific fact (4). Enormous liability settlements exacted large sums from the manufacturer, and the drug combination was removed from the market in 1983. These court settlements were reached despite independent reviews presenting overwhelming scientific and medical evidence that Bendectin is a safe combination drug and not teratogenic (5). Similarly, thalidomide was removed from foreign markets; at the time, however, it had never been marketed in the United States. On July 16, 1998, the U.S. Food and Drug Administration (FDA) approved thalidomide as a treatment for erythema nodosum leprosum, a severe and debilitating condition associated with leprosy. Researchers are also assessing thalidomide as a potential treatment for other indications, including some of the opportunistic infections associated with HIV infection, various forms of cancer, and chronic graft-versus-host disease after bone marrow transplant. But no inroads have been made in drugs for pregnant women.

II. HISTORY

The first major attempt to address the special needs and inadequate resources for particular patient diseases was the 1972, voluntarily initiated Department of Health, Education and Welfare Interagency Committee on Drugs of "Limited Commercial Value." This committee outlined all the legal and insurance roadblocks and recommended removing them. Furthermore, it identified the availability of governmental and industry support and the need for incentives to stimulate interest. It also recommended further study.

A new task force was convened in 1978 with broader representation and considerable input from special-interest groups. The Office of Technology Assessment of Congress and a special commission appointed by the Secretary of Health, Education and Welfare contributed additional data and clarification of issues; in addition, professional staff in the executive office of the White House participated.

III. THE ORPHAN DRUG ACT

These earlier efforts culminated in the Orphan Drug Act, which was initially introduced in the House in 1981 by Representative Henry Waxman, then chair of the Subcommittee on Health and the Environment of the House Committee on Energy and Resources. After several amendments by both Houses, the bill finally passed in December 1982 and was signed into law by President Ronald Reagan in February 1983.

The Orphan Drug Act enables the FDA to provide specific recommendations for the animal and human toxicity studies that would be necessary to approve a drug that has achieved orphan status. This greatly streamlines the development process and minimizes the anxiety and guesswork in applying to the FDA for approval of these products. There have been some cases in which the FDA's Office of Orphan Products Development (established in 1982) assembled information for evaluating orphan drugs, solicited orphan drug applications, and even offered to perform the laboratory animal toxicity and reproductive studies.

The Orphan Drug Act also provided several incentives for pharmaceutical companies to develop drugs and recover their costs. A 50% tax credit was offered for certain clinical trials; and for those drugs not patentable, the act provided for a 7-year period of exclusive marketing rights. Four million dollars a year for the ensuing 3 years was requested for orphan drug research. The money, however, was not appropriated until 1985, when the act was reauthorized by Congress.

When the act was reauthorized, amendments to it extended the authorization for research grants, expanded the market protection to a full 7 years after FDA marketing approval for patented and unpatented drugs, and established the 20-member National Commission on Orphan Diseases to evaluate government research on rare diseases. Again, $4 million was appropriated for each of the ensuing 3 years to fund grants for drug research for which the FDA could not find a sponsor. This money was now also available to support animal testing.

In 1988, another amendment to the act established that the orphan drug application had to be made before the submission of an application—New Drug Application (NDA) or Product License Application (PLA)—for marketing approval. To qualify for the incentives, the drug in question must not have been previously approved under an NDA or PLA for a specific orphan disease and must have had an adequate pharmacological basis for being considered an orphan product. Orphan status applies only to that disease or condition. To receive orphan status, a drug company must submit a "Request for Designation of a Drug as an Orphan Drug" application to the FDA (6).

Despite the success of the Orphan Drug Act, more amendments were considered in 1990 and were passed by Congress only to be vetoed by the president. These amendments tried to address products with high revenues and, presumably, high profits. Amendments were again introduced in 1991 to establish a sales cap for orphan drugs beyond which the drug developers would lose exclusivity, but these changes were not voted on.

In 1992, the FDA issued final regulations for orphan drug development. The regulations outline the process by which the FDA provides written recommendations for the nonclinical and clinical studies required for approval of a marketing application for an orphan drug, designate what an orphan drug is, encourage sponsors to make orphan drugs available for treatment under an "open protocol" before the drug is approved for general marketing, and provide exclusivity for 7 years after the date of the drug's marketing approval (7). Exclusivity, which is awarded when the NDA or the PLA is approved, provides a 7-year license to market the product to the first sponsor developing an orphan drug approved for a specific indication. Identical drugs, however, can be approved for other indications.

The act authorizes the U.S. Congress to appropriate funds for grants and contracts to physicians and companies developing orphan drugs. In fiscal year 2001, these funds totaled $12.5 million. Grants may cover up to $150,000 for Phase I studies or up to $300,000 for Phase II/Phase III studies. Grant money may be applied toward the direct clinical development costs for up to 3 years for new products or for unapproved new uses of marketed products. Each year the FDA issues a request in the *Federal Register* for applications for orphan drug development. These applications are then reviewed by a panel of experts from outside the FDA and are funded based on a priority score.

In addition, because of the continuous and rapid evolution of molecular biology, the regulations help clarify the criteria for determining whether two similar drugs are different for the purposes of marketing. According to the FDA, two drugs are considered the same if the principal, but not necessarily all, structural features of the two drugs are similar. For micromolecular products, the FDA considers two drugs to be the same if the active moiety is the same. For macromolecular products, two products are considered to be the same if the principal molecular structural features, but not necessarily all structural features, are the same. In addition, if a drug can be shown to be clinically superior (i.e., provide greater efficacy or greater safety, or offer a major contribution to patient care) to a similar drug with orphan exclusivity, it will be considered different. Drugs with significantly improved safety profiles also might qualify for this designation if they produce fewer side effects (8).

The regulations address the issue of medically plausible subsets of patients—that is, when a drug might be beneficial for a subset of patients and not all patients with the same condition. A subset is defined by the disease process (e.g., petite mal seizures would be a subset of seizures), the characteristics of the therapy (e.g., toxicity limiting the use of a drug), and special characteristics of the patient population (e.g., pediatric patients).

Another result of the act was the creation of the National Organization for Rare Disorders (NORD), a voluntary group of national health agencies and support groups that helped pass the act. NORD provides information on orphan diseases, clinical trials being conducted for various diseases, and other help to people with rare diseases (9).

According to the FDA's Office of Orphan Products Development, in 1983, when the Orphan Drug Act was passed, only 10 orphan drugs were on the market. Within 2 years after passage of the act, 90 drugs and biologics had been designated orphans and were under development or were approved. At the end of

1998, 15 years after the act was established, 184 orphan products had market approval, benefiting a potential patient population of approximately 8 million people. Today, 221 orphan products have been approved, with a potential patient population of 10 to 11 million (Marie L. Moses, OOPD [mmoses@oc.fda.gov], e-mail, January 30, 2001). These drugs include a significant number to treat illnesses found in children and a smaller number used to treat illnesses associated with the elderly. Obviously, the act has stimulated the industry to develop hundreds of orphan products that for many years may have languished in a laboratory. Consequently, the patients with the many rare diseases and conditions targeted by these products can lead better lives.*

IV. ORPHAN DRUGS VERSUS NON-ORPHAN DRUGS

The images of philanthropy and the political advantages of offering orphan compounds are often motivation enough for a company to pursue orphan drug research and development. Because of the tremendous resources and expenditures necessary for drug research, pharmaceutical companies tend to be the only facilities capable of developing drugs. Therefore, these companies have an ethical obligation to promote and support the research necessary for the development of these compounds. Industry, unlike academia or private enterprise, has the unified communications network crucial for the investigation, data collection, interpretation, and reporting of the information gathered during the characterization of a new chemical entity (see Chapter 2). For industry to ignore this obligation, seeking only the most profitable "Goliath" drugs, is unacceptable indeed, and potentially shortsighted, as discussed previously.

Considering the incentives provided by the Orphan Drug Act to pharmaceutical companies, it is surprising that more companies have not aggressively pursued orphan drug development. This lack of activity may stem from a fear of stigmatizing a drug as an orphan, thereby limiting its sales potential.

Orphan drugs, in theory, undergo the same rigors of testing and development to which drugs with more widespread application are subjected. Pharmacological, safety, and efficacy parameters all undergo similar scrutiny, although differences arise in determining therapeutic categories and dosing administration. Because many orphan diseases are serious or life-threatening, development is expedited (as is efficacy testing and data collection) and costs may be minimized; as a result, the reduction in time and the tax credits afforded orphan drug research make the development of drugs with orphan status appealing.

---

* The following Internet site provides a list of products currently designated as orphans by the Office of Orphan Products Development: http://www.fda.gov/orphan/designat/list.htm.

Because research time is reduced, so is the time in potential discovery and development of related compounds and alternative indications of the orphan compound. Historically, the approval time for orphan drugs has been shorter than for non-orphan drugs. Expedited approval is indicative of the FDA's awareness of the importance of orphan drugs that may be the only treatment available for a specific life-threatening disease. The NDAs for orphan drugs, also tend to be slimmer than for non-orphan drugs because typically fewer patients are studied and analyzed and therefore the review takes less time. The institution of User Fees, however, has mandated standard review times for all marketing applications.

Orphan drug development also is expedited by the Subpart E section of the Federal Food, Drug and Cosmetic Act, which provides guidelines on developing drugs for serious and life-threatening illnesses, especially where no alternative therapies exist. This section of the legislation enables the FDA to be flexible in interpreting the standards for evaluating drugs and provides detailed guidance during the development program.

Treatment Investigational New Drug (IND) status also is often used to help speed the development and marketing of orphan drugs. In 1987 the FDA created the Treatment IND in a further attempt to help make treatments for serious or life-threatening illnesses available sooner than they would be if following the normal process. Many of the Treatment INDs that have been granted are for orphan drugs, such as mecasermin (trade name Myotrophin) for treatment of amyotrophic lateral sclerosis.

Certainly, not all drugs that begin as orphans remain orphans. Zidovudine, one of the first antiviral drugs marketed specifically to treat human immunodeficiency virus (HIV) infection, is an example of an orphan drug that, because of the devastating nature of the disease it treats, experienced rapid FDA approval and a streamlined clinical trial (10). Furthermore, with the number of patients infected with HIV reaching epidemic proportions, manufacturers reaped large profits from orphan drug development. The Orphan Drug Act did not consider the effect of an epidemic such as HIV infection.

The old pharmaceutical maxim that a drug used in one population will undoubtedly be applicable for others characterizes another advantage of orphan drug development. Human growth hormone was designated for treating hypopituitary dwarfism, but now also is used to treat severe burns and osteoporosis. Erythropoietin was developed to help patients receiving dialysis, but its usage has expanded to include treating patients with anemia related to cancer or AIDS.

The utility of orphan drug trials as probes of potential applications in other fields is limitless. There is no credo preventing a drug originally developed as an orphan drug from being applied to a much larger market. This is especially advantageous because the safety and efficacy profiles have been defined by earlier trials. Prostacyclin, a potent vasodilator, platelet inhibitor, and potentially dangerous drug, was tested in neonates with the rare and often fatal syndrome of primary pulmonary hypertension (PPH). The data from the PPH studies were then applied to the problem of secondary pulmonary hypertension, which has a considerably larger market. Invasive techniques such as catheterization were not necessary in the secondary pulmonary hypertension studies because important data from catheterized patients were obtained in earlier PPH trials. The earlier PPH trials gave the company pharmacological and clinical data that enabled it to expand the application of the drug and to streamline the investigative process.

Historically, the mechanism of action and the characteristics of the orphan compound are usually well known and may already have been given to humans in some form. This decreases the likelihood of failure (and increases the likelihood of success). Digibind, an antibody product for digitalis overdose, was first discovered by scientists seeking a method to assay digitalis in human blood serologically. Its mechanism of action was well known, as was the problem and pharmacokinetics of digitalis toxicity, which affects more than 65,000 patients annually. This life-saving drug was a spin-off from basic research in which a well-defined mechanism of action was applied to a well-defined clinical problem. With a defined mechanism of action and a defined disease state, the only problem that could prevent a drug from being approved was if the drug was found to be more toxic than the disease.

Orphan drug development also gives industry scientists the opportunity to work with novel compounds and to work with a disease and drug that are probably not being studied by anyone else: the state of the art is literally defined by their work alone. Furthermore, clinical applications for orphan diseases may be a logical extension of basic research. Similarly, some extensions of orphan research have logical applications for basic clinical problems. The research group is able to obtain good information that then can be reprocessed and applied elsewhere (as discussed above). The patient always comes out ahead, because a new compound will be available to them where once there was none.

Patients suffering from orphan diseases tend to be "clean" subjects: they lack the complicated array of confounding medicinal problems typically found in other patients and tend to manifest well-defined and characterized clinical traits that are often the result of genetic syndromes. This characteristic alone is attractive to most researchers, who seek to gather data uncontaminated by extraneous human characteristics.

V. PROBLEMS IN ORPHAN DRUG DEVELOPMENT

The crucial problems in orphan drug development center on the quality of the clinical research. Often too few patients exist to demonstrate efficacy statistically. Patients are often dispersed throughout the country, and great efforts (and money) are necessary to bring them into referral centers. The paucity of patients also affects the evaluation of different dose levels and frequencies. Furthermore, study designs, especially parallel, double-blind, placebo-controlled trials, may be virtually impossible with the few patients available for study. Safety is difficult to determine definitively because of the small patient numbers, and dosing regimens are difficult to optimize because of the lack of subjects.

Some problems with orphan drug development still center on money. There is a limit to how many orphan drugs a company can afford to develop, because companies must generate profits if they are to retain sophisticated equipment and good scientists. This financial discrepancy is balanced by the realization that new applications are often developed from orphan drugs that may have wider and more profitable applications (e.g., prostacyclin and PPH and secondary pulmonary hypertension). A breakthrough in progeria, a rare disease of rapid aging, could have a profound effect on the wider market of drugs developed to treat the associated physiological responses to aging (osteoarthritis, osteoporosis, senility, etc.).

VI. CONCLUSIONS

Orphan drug development is an emotional issue that attempts to even the odds for the underdog. The success of the Orphan Drug Act has been far greater than anticipated and continues to encourage manufacturers to develop such drugs. Government incentives to stimulate research have been successful in affording those rare patients the hope many have sought for their disease. In the first 10 years after enactment of orphan drug legislation, the pharmaceutical industry produced many new orphan drugs that helped more than 2 million Americans suffering from rare diseases (11). Today, that number is more than 10 million. Some few orphan drugs may be very profitable. Whether the motivations are philanthropic, egalitarian, or profit-based, all sectors appear to have reaped rewards from orphan drug legislation, and the future should bring even greater orphan drug availability and access to therapies. David now has a much better chance of slaying Goliath.

REFERENCES

1. The Pharmaceutical Research and Manufacturers of America. Pharmaceutical Industry Profile 2000. Washington DC: 2000:42.
2. The Pharmaceutical Research and Manufacturers of America. PhRMA Policy Papers: strong patent protection is essential. Available at http://www.phrma.org/policy/federal/protect.phtml. Accessed September 20, 2000.

3. Spilker BA. The drug development and approval process. New Medicines in Development [PhRMA Web site]. Available at http://www.phrma.org/searchcures/newmeds/devapprovprocess.phtml. Accessed October 1, 2000.

4. Barash CI, Lasagna L. The Bendectin saga: "voluntary" discontinuation. J Clin Res Drug Devel 1987; 1:277–292.

5. Hearing before the Fertility and Maternal Health Drug Advisory Committee, Department of Health and Human Services, Public Health Service, FDA, vol. 1, Sept. 15, 1980; vol. 2, Sept. 16, 1980.

6. The FDA's orphan drug development program. In: Mathieu M, Evans AG, Hurden EL, eds. New Drug Development: A Regulatory Overview. 2d ed. Waltham, Massachusetts: Parexel International, 1994:264.

7. 57 Fed Reg 62076 (Dec. 29, 1992) (codified at 21 CFR Part 316).

8. Levitt JA, Kelsey JV. The orphan drug regulations and related issues. Food Drug Law J 1993; 48:525–532.

9. Rare diseases: what patients need. In: Thoene JG, Smith DC, eds. Physicians' guide to Rare Diseases. Montvale, New Jersey: Dowden, 1992:xvii–xix.

10. Myers MW. When and at what stage should a new therapy for AIDS be evaluated in a randomized clinical trial. J Clin Res Drug Devel 1988; 2(1):47–51.

11. Haffner ME. Orphan Products—ten years later and then some. Food Drug Law J 1994; 49:593–601.

ADDITIONAL READING

Haffner ME, Kelsey JV. Evaluation of orphan products by the U.S. Food and Drug Administration. Int J Technol Assess Health Care 1992; 8(4):647–657.

Henry V. 1992 Le Tourneau Award. Problems with pharmaceutical regulation in the United States. J Leg Med 1993; 14:617–639.

14

Single-Event Adverse Drug Reactions:

Tribulations in Ascribing Causality*

Nelson S. Irey[†]
Armed Forces Institute of Pathology, Washington, D.C.

I. INTRODUCTION

The analysis and evaluation of adverse drug reactions (ADRs) is a major problem in the clinical practice of medicine, the development of new drugs, controlled clinical trials, and the postmarketing surveillance period. Just as there are standards and requirements established as guidelines in the chemical, pharmacological, and toxicological phases preceding the marketing of a new drug, there are also guidelines for causality assessment of individual human cases in both the premarketing and the postmarketing phases of new drug development.

This chapter presents an algorithm that is applicable to the individual: the single-event ADR case. This methodology, relating to the use of therapeutic, diagnostic, and prophylactic-type drugs in a clinical setting, should permit the diagnostician to make one of three responses after an assessment of an ADR case: an assured *yes*, a firm *no*, or a reasoned admission of *uncertainty*.

---

* The opinions or assertions contained herein are the private views of the author and are not to be construed as official or as reflecting the views of the Department of Defense, the Department of the Army, or the Armed Forces Institute of Pathology. The author is grateful to Phyllis S. Bojnowski for her expert typographical support.
[†] Deceased.

There are three basic points to consider:

1. The drug "explosion" that has taken place in recent decades has added a new dimension to the practice of modern medicine: an iatrogenic category-the ADR.
2. The possibility of the occurrence and presence of an ADR should be a constant component of the modern physician's differential diagnosis, along with the already well-established infectious, neoplastic, metabolic, degenerative, and vascular groups of disease.
3. The clinicopathological picture presented by the ADR case is often not readily distinguishable from non-drug-induced diseases. The clinical and morphological findings of ADRs have the same limited number of final common paths that characterize these other (non-drug) human illnesses.

II. THE ALGORITHM

There are three major requirements for establishing the occurrence of an ADR:

1. The possibility and likelihood of a causal relationship between the drug and the ADR must be confirmed by establishing its *eligibility*.
2. The drug must have a *linkage* with the clinicopathological findings.
3. The *degree of certainty* of this drug linkage should be determined.

As an initial background for developing this algorithm or methodology, Fig. 1 is offered for consideration and orientation. This figure has the basic elements of a "time flow chart," which has considerable utility in evaluating ADR cases.

In this graphical representation of an ADR, the ordinate (Q) represents any of the findings of an ADR. *Specifically*, Q may be a symptom (pain, nausea, etc.), a sign, a clinical laboratory result, a radiological finding, a morphological finding, or any combination of these. Synonyms for Q include marker, disease marker, signal, indicator, parameter, detector, response, and effect.

The abscissa is the time element (T), related to both the time of drug administration and to the dating of disease marker data. Both are usually plotted on the same time flow chart in a particular case.

This graphical representation of an ADR case will be used frequently in the assessment of eligibility and linkage determinations of ADRs. The four eligibility criteria are listed in Fig. 1, and will be discussed.

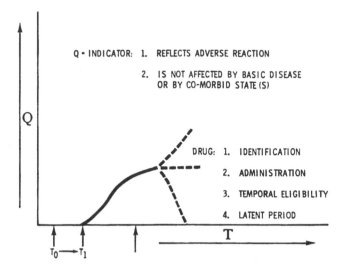

Q - INDICATOR:
1. REFLECTS ADVERSE REACTION
2. IS NOT AFFECTED BY BASIC DISEASE OR BY CO-MORBID STATE (S)

DRUG:
1. IDENTIFICATION
2. ADMINISTRATION
3. TEMPORAL ELIGIBILITY
4. LATENT PERIOD

Figure 1 An adverse drug reaction (the curve Q) is plotted against time (the abscissa T). Dashed lines show the three courses an ADR can take: increasing severity to death; leveling off to chronicity; or return to the abscissa, indicating recovery. Four criteria that must be met before the drug is eligible to be an empiric correlate of Q (the adverse drug reaction) as listed. (From Ref. 6, by permission of the publisher.)

A. Eligibility of the Drug

1. Identification of the Drug

In most cases, it is tacitly assumed that the drug ordered by the physician is the one received by the patient. This assumption is not always correct, as illustrated in the following case reported by Golbert and Patterson (1).

> *Example*: A patient complained of recurrent urticaria, with occasional wheezing, dyspnea, nausea, and vomiting. He was receiving two drugs, thyroid extract and ascorbic acid, neither being likely candidates for producing this clinical picture. As part of an assessment of this case, a laboratory analysis of the ascorbic acid revealed that it was mislabeled: it was actually benzyl penicillin.

While it is not practical or even necessary in most cases to question the "identification" of the drug, it is advisable to keep in mind the possibility of a mislabeling, particularly in a difficult case that presents unique and contradictory features. It is evident that misidentification can occur at any point along the pharmaceutical–pharmacy–physician–nurse–patient chain of events.

2. Administration of the Drug

As it is with accurate identification of a drug, so it is that its "administration" must at times be held in question. Patient compliance with the doctor's orders is an omnipresent problem in medical therapy. Complete noncompliance sometimes occurs, as in the following instance.

> *Example*: A male diabetic receiving tolbutamide developed renal dysfunction. Renal biopsy revealed interstitial granulomatous nephritis. There is precedent in the literature for an association between granulomas and sulfonylurea compounds (tolbutamide is in this group). With this possible (or even probable) relationship in mind, follow-up information disclosed that the patient had *never* taken this medication, even though prescriptions had been regularly written and given to him for more than 2 years.

3. Temporal Eligibility

The time factor in assessment of ADRs is a very important one and in some cases is of critical diagnostic importance. This is true not only in establishing "eligibility" of the drug, but also in linking the drug to the reaction. On the other hand, the time element may be equally important in denying eligibility and also may make linkage of the drug with the clinicopathological picture a most unlikely possibility.

It is quite apparent that a drug cannot be responsible for an ADR if the latter is already in progress before the drug is first administered. This dys-synchrony is illustrated in the following cases.

> *Example 1*: A 50-year-old white male with a long history of rheumatoid arthritis had a terminal illness of 5 weeks' duration that was dominated by cardiac and cerebral symptoms and signs. He had been receiving indomethacin, and a low platelet count had been one of the features of the laboratory findings during this final 5 weeks. The case was diagnosed an indomethacin-induced thrombotic thrombocytopenic purpura.
>
> At autopsy, there were thrombotic vascular lesions of the small vessels of the heart and brain that were compatible with this morphological diagnosis. However, the medication data in the patient's chart revealed that the indomethacin was not started until the beginning of the fourth week of his terminal 5-week illness. Indomethacin was therefore ineligible to have initiated his terminal illness and could not have been responsible for the thrombotic lesions found at autopsy in the heart and brain.

> *Example 2*: A jaundiced middle-aged man had been receiving prochlorperazine. A liver biopsy showed cholestasis. The drug and liver abnormality were initially through to be causally related. However, time-related chart information revealed that the jaundice was present for 3 days before this tranquilizer

was first administered. The prochlorperazine was therefore ineligible to have initiated the jaundice and cholestasis.

4. Latent Period

Latent period refers to the time interval between the initial administration of the drug and the onset of the ADR (in Fig. 1, it is the interval T_0 to T_1). The latent period is not rigidly fixed or exactly predictable, but it tends to fall within certain limits.

Characteristically, cyanide deaths occur in seconds to minutes. Most anaphylactic deaths occur within 20–30 min after contact with the lethal antigen, while jaundice associated with chlorpromazine has its onset within 3 days to 3 weeks after the beginning of therapy. The fatal pancytopenia following chloramphenicol appears in 1–3 months, while hepatic angiosarcoma related to thorium dioxide has a latent period of one to several decades. The ultimate in length of latency is one to several generations from a drug-induced mutational germ cell change to its manifestation in a conceptus.

Consideration of the latent period in an ADR is of use in an ADR assessment in one of two ways: the latent period may be too long, or it may be too short.

Example 1: An overlong latent period was noted in the case of an inadvertent overdose of meprobamate given to a 4-year-old male child, who suffered cardiorespiratory arrest 16 h later. During the intervening 16 h following the 400-mg dose there were no signs or symptoms indicating any problem. The demise of the patient was associated with a sudden cardiorespiratory arrest, with no premonitory symptoms or signs. Although meprobamate was initially blamed for this cardiorespiratory death, it was thought to be an unlikely candidate because of the prolonged latent period: this drug usually reaches a peak blood level within 2 h, and slowly declines over the next 10 h.

Further clinical information and the autopsy findings provided a more likely cause of death. There had been a number of prior episodes of non-drug-related cardiorespiratory arrests. Further, the autopsy revealed multiple congenital anomalies of the central nervous system: hypoplasia of the cerebellum and spinal cord, polymicrogyria and pachygyria, and hydrocephalus *ex vacuo*.

While the clinical history and autopsy findings showed a non-drug-related cause for this death, the prolonged latent period alone would have essentially disqualified meprobamate as the responsible agent.

Example 2: An illustration of a too-short latent period is afforded by the case of a 52-year-old woman being treated with sulfamethoxazole for a urinary tract infection, with subsequent death associated with pancytopenia. Sulfamethoxazole was initially held responsible for the blood dyscrasia.

Additional clinical and laboratory information, however, revealed that she was already described as "weak and anemic" 6 days after initiation of this therapy, and with an "abnormal" blood count (not otherwise defined). Four days later (10 days after this drug was started) the hemoglobin level was down to 6.6 g. Considering that the half-life of the red cell is 120 days, with no evidence of either hemolytic disease or blood loss, and with the assumption that she had a normal hemogram when therapy was begun (there is no evidence to the contrary), the 10-day interval between initiation of the sulfamethoxazole and the demonstrated anemia was too short to be attributed to this drug.

In summary, identification, administration, temoral eligibility, and latent period are the four criteria for establishing the eligibility of a drug to have caused an ADR. Emphasis should be placed on obtaining sufficiently detailed time-related data on drug administration and on the appearance of ADR markers. These data are a *sine qua non* in the assessment of drug eligibility.

B.   Linking the Drug with the Clinicopathological Findings

The second major task in analyzing an ADR case is to establish a connection or linkage between the drug and the clinicopathological findings (making empiric correlates of the drug and these findings).

Figure 2 is a time flow chart representing an ADR that itemizes six ways of making this linkage.

1.   Exclusion

Exclusion consists of selecting one drug from a group of drug candidates by the use of the time flow chart.

> *Example*: A 15-year-old black male with pulmonary blastomycosis was treated with a succession of five drugs over a 3-month period. During this interval, renal failure developed. A renal biopsy showed an interstitial nephritis with granulomatoid features. Cultures from this renal biopsy were negative for fungi, acid-fast bacilli, and anaerobic organism.
>
> Figure 3 plots the drugs administered, dates of administration, and the blood urea nitrogen (BUN) levels over this 3-month period. It is evident from this time flow chart that only one agent (stilbamidine) was temporally eligible to have initiated the renal dysfunction. The remaining four drugs were administered after the BUN had risen to abnormal levels and were therefore ineligible to have caused the renal dysfunction. Notably, the graph shows a return of the BUN to normal range soon after the stilbamidine was discontinued. This dechallenge response reinforces the thesis that stilbamidine caused the kidney changes.

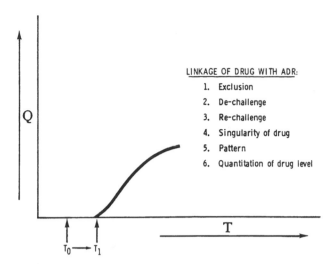

Figure 2 The six methods of linking a drug with an adverse drug reaction. (From Ref. 6, by permission of the publisher.)

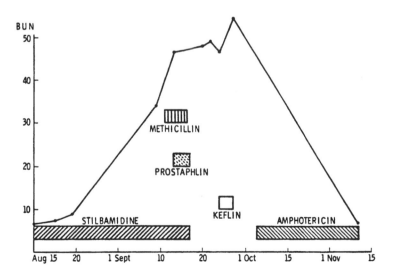

Figure 3 Time flow chart demonstrating the temporal eligibility of stilbamidine to have produced the elevation of the BUN in the case described. (From Ref. 7, by permission of the publisher.)

The exclusion method also includes instances in which drug candidates are themselves excluded from causation status because a non-drug etiology is clearly demonstrable (environmental or occupational factors, radiation injury, the underlying disease of the patient, or a co-mobrid state) that can reasonably account for the clinicopathology findings.

An illustrative case involves renal failure in which tetracycline and a thrombotic vascular lesion were candidates for having caused the renal failure.

> *Example*: A 70-year-old white male underwent repair of an atherosclerotic aneurysm of the abdominal aorta. Tetracycline was given postoperatively for 6 days. As this therapy with tetracycline was terminated, a progressive rise in the BUN began, with terminal oliguria and anuria about $2^1/2$ weeks later (Fig. 4).
>
> The drug was initially considered to be the cause of the kidney dysfunction, on the basis of temporal eligibility, latent period, and literature precedent. However, it was noted that a translumbar aortogram done 9 days before death had been reported as showing "no flow in the left kidney and a minimal or no flow in the right kidney."

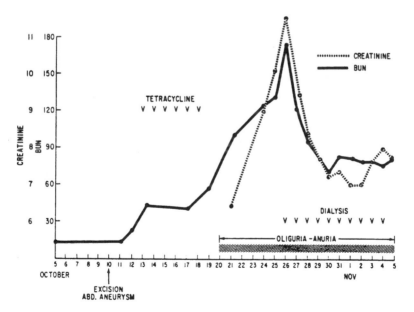

Figure 4   Time flow chart illustrating the temporal eligibility of tetracycline in relation to the subsequent renal failure (creatinine, dotted line; BUN, solid line). (From Ref. 7, by permission of the publisher.)

The reason for the vascular compromise was revealed at autopsy: both renal arteries were occluded by thrombotic masses that had propagated from a second abdominal aortic aneurysm located cephalad to the previously repaired aneurysm.

This case met the "eligibility" criteria but failed to meet the "exclusion" part of the linkage criteria. Drug causation was eliminated because of the finding of a concurrent co-morbid state (bilateral renal artery thromboses) substantiated by a special radiological procedure and by the morphologic findings at autopsy.

The value of a broadened database is illustrated in this case and is generally a requirement when attempting to analyze the frequently complex problems presented by ADR cases.

2. Dechallenge

The principle involved in the dechallenge method of linkage is that if there is a reversible effect present, then removing the cause will eliminate the effect.

Example: A 56-year-old hypertensive and diabetic white male was treated with 11 drugs for more than 5 years. About midway in this interval, he developed a progressive anemia and leukopenia.

Figure 5 presents curves on the disease markers (hemoglobin [Hgb] and white blood cells [WBC]) and time-related drug administration information on the 11 drugs with which he was being treated. The horizontal lines indicate the dates the drugs were started, duration of administration, and when they were discontinued.

Assessment was made in this case in the spring of 1977 (at the junction of the solid lines with the dashed lines on the Hgb and WBC markers). At that time, hydralazine was judged to be the most likely drug candidate, if indeed the hematological changes were drug-related. The other 10 drugs were eliminated for the following reasons: they were given for too short a time (Lasix, Pro-Banthine, and Indocin), they were temporally ineligible (quinine, Elavil, and chlorthalidone), or they were given continuously and over too long a time with no evident ADR (chlorpropamide, propranolol, hydrochlorothiazide, and Dimetapp). The one drug that was the most likely candidate, from the time flow chart, was hydralazine, which showed temporal eligibility and was given continuously during the drop in the hemogram elements.

On the basis of this graphical analysis, a presumptive diagnosis of hydralazine-induced anemia and leukopenia was made, and it was recommended that this drug be discontinued.

During the next 3 months, rises in the Hgb and WBC curves (shown in the dashed lines of the graph) were noted. The final diagnosis of a hydralazine-induced dyscrasia was based on the return toward normalcy of the hemogram and on the failure to find a non-drug-related cause for these hematological abnormalities.

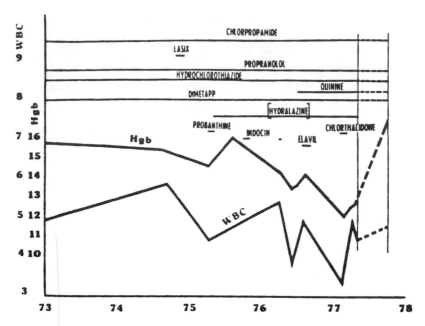

Figure 5   Time flow chart demonstrating the correction of the anemia after hydralazine was discontinued. Other drugs were eliminated because they were given for too short a time (Lasix, Pro-Banthine, and Indocin), were temporally ineligible (quinine, Elavil, and chlorthalidone), or were given continuously (chlorpropamide, propranolol, hydrochloro- thiazide, and Dimetapp). (From Ref. 8, by permission of the publisher.)

3.   Rechallenge

The principle involved in the rechallenge method of linkage of a drug to an ADR is implied in the phrase *post hoc, ergo propter hoc* (after this, therefore because of this). As applied, if a drug has been incriminated with a reaction, and the ADR disappeared when the drug was discontinued, a rechallenge with this drug followed by a return of the ADR would increase the probability that the drug and the ADR were empiric correlates.

  While intentional challenge is not often done, such a rechallenge may occur inadvertently.

  Example: A 64-year-old woman with rheumatoid arthritis, hypothyroidism, and Raynaud's disease was treated for 6 years with chlorambucil and predni- sone. She died of progressive liver failure, pancytopenia, and necrotizing bronchitis.

  Figure 6 is a time flow chart on this case. The markers of the ADR in the liver are serum glutamic oxaloautic transaminase (SGOT), lactic dehy-

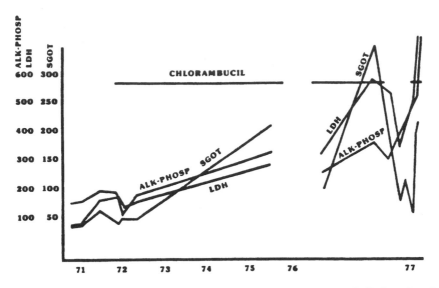

Figure 6 Time flow chart showing fluctuations in SCOT, LDH, and alkaline phosphatase during a succession of dechallenges and rechallenges with chlorambucil. (From Ref. 8, by permission of the publisher).

drogenase (LDH), and alkaline phosphatase. They show three sequences of fluctuations, each with increasing levels of these three markers during the administration of chlorambucil. During two dechallenges, these disease markers (liver function tests) dropped toward normal, but on the two rechallenges, they rose to abnormal levels.

At autopsy, the liver weighed only 800 g and was the seat of multiple foci of necrosis, moderate cholestasis, portal fibrosis, and acute and chronic triaditis.

While this case was chosen to illustrate the method of linkage by rechallenge, it also illustrates two episodes of dechallenge. Further, since there is literature precedent for an association between liver damage and chlorambucil, this case also demonstrates the fifth method of linkage (pattern) as listed in Fig. 2.

4. Singularity of the Drug

The principle involved in the singularity method of linking a drug with an ADR is based on two assumptions: Only one drug was administered, and there was no basic disease or co-morbid state that could be related to the ADR marker being used in the assessment.

Example: A 24-year-old epileptic black female had been treated with diphenylhydantoin for several years. While on a trip, she suffered a seizure and was hospitalized under the care of another physician. He prescribed this same drug in the same dosage as she had been receiving in the past.

Unbeknown to this new physician, she continued to take her usual dosage of this antiepileptic agent in addition to her "new" dosage. She thus inadvertently doubled her intake of diphenylhydantoin.

After 12 hours of this double jeopardy, she developed a complex of symptoms and signs that included fever (to 103°F), ataxia, nystagmus, confusion, hallucinations, slurred speech, and somnolence.

When it was discovered that she was receiving a double dose, the diphenylhydantoin was discontinued completely. Her symptom complex began to improve in 12 h, and 12 days later she was completely recovered. She was discharged from the hospital with no evident residuals.

The diagnosis of diphenylhydantoin-induced toxicity was made on the following basis: there was no evidence of her receiving any other medication, there was temporal eligibility and a reasonable latent period for the effects of the "overdose" to become manifest, and dechallenge was followed by recovery.

In this era of polypharmacy, it is rare to encounter a case involving only one drug, but this case had considerable evidence to support the thesis of "singularity of drug."

This method of linkage is more likely to be applicable in well-controlled preclinical trials than in the postmarketing phase of new drug development and usage.

5. Pattern

The pattern method of linking a drug with an ADR shifts the focus of attention to the clinicopathological findings in an ADR, and away from the identification of the causative drug. This shift of emphasis is necessary when detailed time-related drug and disease marker data are denied to the evaluator of the case. The site-process profile may than be used as a guideline for searching past experience and the literature for cases that have matching features. Matching features found in the literature may include associations with certain drugs or chemicals, which serve as a guideline for a focused examination of the patient's history for the causative agent.

Example: A 36-year-old white male was hospitalized after he developed jaundice. A liver biopsy revealed a generalized centrilobular zonal loss of hepatocytes (zonal necrosis), central collapse of the lobular reticulum, and prominence of Kupffer's cells containing both lipofuscin and hemosiderin.

The morphological changes seen in this liver biopsy are consistent with those produced by hepatotoxic agents, including hydrocarbons, but they are not drug- or chemical-specific. Using the "pattern" approach, the search for an etiological agent would be focused on "hepatotoxic" agents, including a variety of hydrocarbons. A retrospective search back into the history of this patient did reveal exposure to carbon tetrachloride while working in a confined and poorly ventilated room.

The sequence of assessment events included an initial determination of what morphologic changes were present in the liver; a knowledge from precedent literature of the possible etiologies of these changes; and backtracking into the history of the case, which disclosed one of the agents capable of producing these morphologic changes.

This "pattern" method may also be used in excluding drugs. If the drugs or chemicals suggested by the morphological findings are not identified or disclosed by historical or toxicological efforts, then the morphological changes appear to remain non-drug-related or non-chemical-related.

6. Quantitation of Drug Level

Assessing an ADR case by quantitation of drug level brings our focus back to the search for, and the identification of, the causative agent by quantitative and objective data based on laboratory analysis of body fluids and/or viscera. This method is applicable and essentially limited to drug overdose cases. The feasibility of this approach is based on the availability of dependable information on lethal levels from past experience. Without this comparison information, there is no judgmental significance to toxicological levels in the case at hand (2).

Quantitated levels of drugs have limitations in diagnostic value. In adverse reactions in the hypersensitivity, idiosyncratic, and pharmacogenetic categories, drugs have been administered in therapeutic (not toxic) amounts, and blood and other body fluids and tissue levels have been found to lie within therapeutic ranges. Such analyses will confirm any prior administration of the drugs, but the problem of the etiological differential diagnosis will still remain.

Example 1: A 21-year-old white male with respiratory distress was admitted to a hospital. Before he died, he stated that he was sensitive to chloroquine and that he had taken one tablet of this drug just prior to the sudden onset of his respiratory distress. He died shortly thereafter, in cardiorespiratory failure.

The subsequent autopsy revealed no anatomical cause of death. The prosector had taken samples of blood and viscera for toxicological examination. The following levels of chloroquine were reported (in mg%): blood, 6.5; kidney, 24.0; brain, 2.5; and lung, 23.0. These blood and tissue levels could not have been related to the ingestion of one 50.0-mg tablet of chloroquine. These levels were within lethal range as reported elsewhere (3).

Based on these quantitative finds, the case was placed in the toxic category (overdose). The original impression that this death was in the hypersensitivity category was discarded.

In addition to the quantitative approach, qualitative identification of a drug or chemical may be of value in appropriate instances.

Example 2: A 22-year-old woman developed (apparently *de novo*) multiple subcutaneous masses in the anterior abdominal wall. Biopsy of one of them revealed multiple cystic spaces that contained a clear viscid fluid. The lesion was a benign one and had some resemblance to a lymphangioma.

Its exact nature and etiology remained undetermined until a history was elicited of prior breast enhancement by silicone injection. Aspirated fluid from one of the cystic lesions was subjected to infrared spectrophotometry and was identified as silicone. It is presumed that gravitational migration along fascial planes moved some of the silicone from the breasts to their abdominal wall location (4).

This qualitative procedure identified *what* was there; *how* much was there was immaterial.

7. Multiple and Simultaneous Methods of Assessing ADRs

In some cases of ADRs, more than one of the six methods of drug linkage that are listed in Fig. 2 may be used in causation analysis. In fact, multiple methods in the same case strengthen either the confirmation or the rejection of an ADR and its etiology.

Example: A 55-year-old Oriental female sustained multiple and serious injuries in an auto accident. Death occurred in 7 weeks and was associated with liver failure. During this 7-week period, a number of agents and circumstances were identified that might have been responsible for her hepatic failure: she had three epidoses of hypotension, she was given blood transfusions, and she was administered halothane anesthesia twice.

Hypotension: The first episode occurred on the day of the accident and happened 21 days before the first evidence of liver disease. The latent period was too long. The other two hypotensive episodes occurred after the liver damage was already apparent. Temporal ineligibility disqualified these episodes from having initiated the liver damage. They may have had a proximate effect on the liver status, but they could not have initiated it.

Blood transfusions: The possibility that the liver failure might have been due to viral hepatitis transmitted via transfused blood was part of the differential diagnosis in this case.

It is virtually impossible on morphological grounds alone to differentiate between drug hepatotoxicity and viral hepatitis in instances of massive liver necrosis. In this case, the liver necrosis was submassive. Typically, the viral hepatitis lesion is spotty and focal while the lesion in drug-induced hepatotoxicity is universal, zonal, and centrilobular. Morphological changes in the liver in this case were centrilobular and zonal. This morphological picture was more consistent with drug hepatotoxicity than with viral hepatitis. Thus, liver damage related to the blood transfusion appeared most unlikely.

Halothane anesthesia: In this case, there were three items that favored liver damage secondary to the use of halothane:

1. Liver dysfunction (as monitored by liver function tests) was evident following the second exposure to this anesthetic (multiple exposures to halothane often precede liver damage).
2. Unexplained fever occurred on the third day after this second exposure (a part of the profile of halothane-liver damage).
3. The centrilobular and universal zonal necrosis is consistent with the findings in the liver associated with drug hepatotoxicity.

The liver damage and subsequent hepatic failure in this case was judged as probably due to the halothane anesthetic. It was possible to arrive at a reasoned choice of one of the three candidates discussed above because there were adequate, detailed, and time-related data on the therapeutic agents used, the adverse clinical circumstances, the liver function tests, and the tissue changes reflecting the liver damage. The multiple methods utilized include latent period, temporal eligibility, exclusion, and morphological/clinicopathological patterns.

8. Difficulties in Assessing ADRs

Requirements for establishing eligibility and methods of linking a drug with an illness have been presented in the preceding discussion. This algorithm should constitute a blueprint for solving many if not most of the ADR problems in this area of medical diagnostics.

However, in the hands-on practice of the assessment of ADR cases, there are at least four major difficulties that stand in the way of such high diagnostic expectations. These four obstacles include the following.

1. *Incomplete information*: Incomplete information is not unique to ADR evaluation but is common to all areas of medical practice. The lack of sufficiently detailed, time-related data on drug administration and disease markers may make it impossible to render a reasoned judgment on many ADR cases, leaving them in their original and unsatisfactory anecdotal status. Denial to the diagnostician of access to these required facts makes it impossible to make judgments on latent period and temporal eligibility; time flow charts cannot be utilized in exclusion, dechallenge, and rechallenge techniques. The diagnostic data base should also

include information on other drugs being administered, concurrent co-morbid states, and the existence of occupational and environmental hazards.

2. *Polypharmacy*: In this medical era, polypharmacy is the rule rather than the exception. Patients with complicated and prolonged illnesses may have 20–30 medications in their medical background. Cases of this sort may be of such complexity that even with ideally complete drug and disease marker information, diagnostic success may be elusive.

3. *Lack of objective means of linking the drug to the ADR*: Tests and procedures that specifically and causally connect a drug to an illness are lacking. We do not have the equivalent of the special stains and cultural methods that identify *Mycobacterium tuberculosis* with some granulomatous lesions. Our high-tech laboratory instrumentation is capable of identifying and quantifying extremely low levels of drugs and chemicals, but this type of information falls short of establishing causation.

4. *The limited number of clinicopathological reaction patterns in human disease*: There are a limited number of generic morphological reaction patterns that diseases fit into (inflammatory, congenital, neoplastic, degenerative, infiltrative, vascular, functional). In parallel, there are also a rather limited number of clinical symptoms and signs (pain, nausea, fever, lumps, etc.) that come to the attention of the practicing physician. There are a multitude of causes and a multitude of clinical conditions that funnel into these clinicopathological "final common paths." The algorithm previously described is an attempt to move from the generic to the specific in analyzing ADR causation.

Of the four difficulties cited above, only the first (incomplete information) is subject to at least some degree of improvement.

To illustrate the results that can be obtained by overcoming this first difficulty, at least in part, a study of 94 phenothiazine-related hepatic ADRs is cited (5). The bar graph on the left in Fig. 7 shows the judgment of degree of certainty as to the drug causation of the liver damage, based on initial information. The "possible" category predominated, meaning that a definitive and categorical diagnosis could not be made.

The right side of the bar graph in Fig. 7 was constructed after requesting and receiving more clinical information and additional morphological material on 95% of these 94 cases. By overcoming the handicap of inadequate information, the uncertain middle group was reduced from 43% to 13% and there were corresponding significant increases in the categorical diagnoses excluding or substantiating drug causation of the liver damage.

C. Degree of Certainty

The third major task in analyzing and assessing ADRs is determining the degree of certainty one has as to the causal relationship between the drug and the clinico-

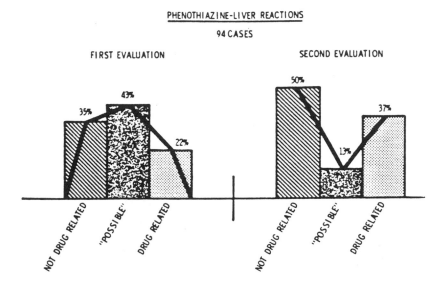

PHENOTHIAZINE-LIVER REACTIONS

94 CASES

Figure 7 Graph illustrating the value of more complete information in a study of 94 cases of phenothiazine-related hepatoses. First evaluation on left, second evaluation on right after obtaining additional information. Note inversion of curve and reduction of possible group after a more complete study. Note large overall group (50%) after second evaluation. (From Ref. 7, by permission of the publisher.)

pathological findings. Interposed between the definite *causative* and *negative* categories are three shades of certainty (probable, possible, and coincidental) that titrate between these two extremes. These degrees of certainty are defined as follows.

1. *Causative*: Cases in this class are those in which there is no doubt that a drug has caused the reaction. This category is essentially limited to drug overdose cases or those cases in which the causative agent can be objectively identified (asbestos bodies; alpha tracks of thorium dioxide, etc.).
     Parenthetically, the overdose cases with drug levels in lethal ranges should have an important negative findings: no anatomical cause of death at autopsy.
2. *Probable*: This term is equivalent to the phrase "consistent with," and cases in this category of certainty fall short of the "causative" designation because they lack an objective and quantitative laboratory finding that is the *sine qua non* of the causative category. Cases placed in this category have the following characteristics.

(a) The criteria of temporal eligibility and appropriateness of latent period have been met.
(b) The clinicopathological features are consonant with previous experience and literature precedent for the drug in question.
(c) Other causes (the basic disease, co-morbid states, and other modalities of therapy) have been eliminated from consideration.
(d) One or several means of linkage of the drug to the ADR have been utilized: exclusion, dechallenge, rechallenge, singularity of the drug, and pattern.

3. *Possible*: Cases are put in this category when the relationship between the drug and the clinicopathological findings can be neither confirmed nor denied. There are three subdivisions in this category.

(a) Cases with potential causes other than the drug in question. The clinicopathological picture could have been produced by the basic disease, a co-morbid state, or by some other modality of therapy.
(b) Cases in which some of the criteria for eligibility and linkage have been met, but some have not because of lack of adequate information. Such a case could be put in this category temporarily while awaiting more information or placed here permanently if it were evident that further data would not be forthcoming.
(c) Cases that have met all the criteria of eligibility and linkage but for which there is no known precedent literature. Such a case might be a new and emergent ADR. It could be placed in the "possible" group, awaiting the appearance of similar cases for cluster studies at a later time.

4. *Coincidental*: Cases in this category include those with a patient who was indeed exposed to the drug in question but in which assessment of the case clearly reveals only an anecdotal association.
5. *Negative*: This category applies to those cases in which the alleged drug was not or could not have been in the patient's system at the time of the ADR. This circumstance could be related either to noncompliance, mislabeling of the drug, or historical misinformation.

The statistical breakdown of 3800 cases in the Registry of Tissue Reactions to Drugs is shown in Fig. 8. Confirmation of the presence of an ADR was found in about half the cases (combining the causative and the probable categories for a consolidated "yes"); denial of the presence of a validated ADR was the judgment in about one-fifth of the cases; uncertainty as to the presence of a validated ADR was seen in one-third of the cases. This latter was the largest single group in this graph. These findings are not unexpected in view of the all-too-frequent

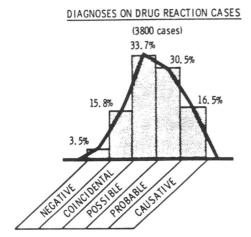

DIAGNOSES ON DRUG REACTION CASES
(3800 cases)
33.7%
30.5%
15.8%
16.5%
3.5%

NEGATIVE COINCIDENTAL POSSIBLE PROBABLE CAUSATIVE

Figure 8 Graph showing distribution of degrees of certainty as to the relationship between the drug and the alleged ADR in 3800 cases. (From Ref. 8, by permission of the
publisher.)

lack of adequate information and the resultant inadequate data base for the assessment of ADR cases.

III. CONCLUSIONS

The thrust of the foregoing development of an ADR algorithm is to outline a
methodology for assessing the relationship between a drug (or drugs) and the
clinicopathological findings of a particular illness, with emphasis on the ways
and means of evaluating the relationship between the drug and the illness. The
issue faced in this discussion on ADRs is more *how* to diagnose ADRs than *what*
to diagnose.

   This methodology should enable one to confirm, deny, or admit uncertainty
as to the role of a drug in a patient's illness, be it in the limited clinical trials of
the premarketing phase, or in the postmarketing surveillance phase of new drug
development.

REFERENCES

1.   Golbert TM, Patterson R. Recurrent anaphylaxis caused by a misidentified drug. Ann
     Intern Med 1968; 68:621–623.

2. Winek CL. Drug and Chemical Blood-Level Data 1989. Pittsburgh, PA: Fisher Scientific, 1989.
3. Kiel FW. Chloroquine suicide. JAMA 1964; 190:398–400.
4. Delage C, Shane JJ, Johnson FB. Mammary silicone granuloma: migration of silicone fluid to abdominal wall and inguinal region. Arch Dermatol. 1973; 180:104–107.
5. Ishak KG, Irey NS. Hepatic injury associated with phenothiazines, clinico-pathologic and follow-up study of 36 patients. Arch Pathol 1972; 91:283–304.
6. Irey NS. Tissue Reaction to Drugs, Teaching Monograph, American Journal of Pathology, vol. 82, no. 3, pp. 617–647, New York: Harper & Row, 1976.
7. Irey NS. Diagnostic problems in drug-induced diseases. In: Drug-Induced Diseases, vol. 4, Meyler L, Peck HM, eds. Amsterdam: Excerpta Medica, 1972:chap. 1.
8. Irey NS. When is a disease drug-induced. In: Riddell RH, ed. Pathology of Drug-Induced and Toxic Diseases. New York: Churchill Livingstone, 1982.

15

How to Deal with a Sudden, Unexpected Death in Clinical Studies

Allen Cato
Cato Research Ltd., Durham, North Carolina

Lynda Sutton
Cato Research Ltd., Durham, North Carolina

I. INTRODUCTION

Clinical trials, regardless of how well controlled and well designed, always face unavoidable potential risks and unexpected events. Perhaps the most challenging event is the unexpected death of a subject—the ultimate adverse effect (1). In spite of such events, investigational drug trials must be performed, for no alternative way exists to test new drugs safely and effectively before they are brought to the attention of the medical community. As stated in 1865 by Claude Bernard (2), a nineteenth-century physiologist:

> The principle of medical and surgical morality, therefore, consists in never performing on man an experiment which might be harmful to him to any extent, even though the results might be highly advantageous to science, i.e., to the health of others. . . . So, among the experiments that may be tried on man, those that can only harm are forbidden, those that are innocent are permissible, and those that may do good are obligatory.

II. DETERMINING CAUSE OF DEATH—STAGES OF INVESTIGATION

The possibility of a sudden, unexpected death of a patient is an event that always looms in the study monitor's mind during the course of a clinical trial. Some possible reasons for an isolated death during a clinical trial are listed below:

Natural causes
Unnatural causes (e.g., a fatal motor vehicle accident)
Disease-related causes
Study-related causes
Drug-related causes
Lack of efficacy
Unknown causes

Although the list of potential causes of a death may be long, the crucial question facing the monitor is, ''Was the death caused by the test agent?'' The future of the test agent and the clinical trial depends on the answer to that question. Important decisions must be made as quickly as possible after such a death. The results of those decisions could have a profound effect on all present and future patients and therefore must be derived through a careful, thorough investigation of the event. Because of the nature of clinical trials, the investigation is most often conducted in two stages. Each stage involves specific actions that must take place over two distinct periods.

Stage 1 of the investigation of a sudden death involves decisions that have to be made immediately—within 24 hours of the death. Investigation at the study site must begin as soon as possible to make a preliminary judgment of the relationship of the death to the test drug. A quick decision has to be made about what must be done, who will perform the investigation, and how it will be conducted. If medical monitors are not prepared to deal with an unexpected death, they may overlook important information and make faulty decisions that could jeopardize the lives of others, as well as place in question the future of the test drug. Therefore, it is important before study initiation to have a plan in place detailing how a medical monitor will address an unexpected death.

Stage 2 of the investigation involves a period of 1 week to approximately 2 months after the event. During this time, a comprehensive investigation is undertaken to arrive at a final decision regarding the relationship of the death to the test drug.

An example of the activities in these two stages can be seen in a case taken from the first Phase II study of a new anticonvulsant agent in humans in which the fifth subject died. The study was a Phase II, single-dose, increasing titration trial of six subjects. The subject was a 31-year-old woman who, at the end of a 2-week treatment period, had just been released from the hospital with no abnormal findings. Two days after discharge, the subject called the investigator, complaining of generalized aches and pains, a slight cough, and a warm feeling. She was given permission to take Darvon and was instructed to see a physician if her condition persisted. The next day she was found dead by her husband. Because this death was an isolated event, it could not be subjected to rigorous statistics. The decisions must be based on this case alone.

A. Stage 1 Investigation

Stage 1 of the investigation begins by obtaining a preliminary history of events surrounding the death. A telephone call between the medical monitor and the investigator is usually conducted before any other actions are taken. From preliminary data obtained in this telephone call, the medical monitor and the clinical team can more readily initiate the specific tasks that must begin as soon as possible. The medical monitor may then ask the investigator to request a complete autopsy, which can be very valuable in understanding the cause of death. Unless the case is deemed a medical examiner's case, however, autopsies, although often requested, are difficult to obtain because the wishes of the deceased's family must be respected. Samples of blood and cerebrospinal fluid should be obtained as soon as possible so that levels of drugs and metabolites can be measured. Cerebrospinal fluid is important to examine because some drugs cross the blood–brain barrier and some (e.g., bromide) do not. In addition, the investigator should expedite a faxed or e-mail written summary of the death to the medical monitor.

If the test agent is still in Phase I clinical trials, all dosing of the test agent at study sites should be temporarily discontinued. Even if a test agent is not known, as in a double-blind, controlled study, the blind should be broken immediately, but only for that subject. Even if the blind reveals that the medication was placebo, the investigation should proceed as though the medication were active drug. This practice will ensure that the appropriate information is collected, whether or not the patient is on placebo. It could be found later that an error in packaging or dispensing of the medication, or related factors of the study itself, including the study protocol, design, or site execution, are implicated in the death. Also at this time, analysis of the clinical trial material should begin in order to confirm the content (i.e., drug or placebo) of the clinical trial material taken by the deceased. Therefore, clinical trial material should be immediately shipped back to the sponsor or appropriate laboratory for analysis.

Having initiated the specific actions, the monitor or other qualified person should go to the study site to obtain all available additional information by thoroughly investigating all of the records, including not only the medical chart, but also nurses' notes, pharmacy records, and clinic charts. Information from the subject's history, including peculiar events such as experimental therapy that occurred before their entry, will often reveal facts that may now be relative to the death. Additional information can often be obtained by talking to relatives or friends of the subject, although these conversations are usually carried out by the investigator or the study coordinator. Table 1 summarizes Stage 1 investigations.

In our case example from the anticonvulsant Phase II study, the patient's medical records and data collection forms were intensively reviewed: the patient's compliance in taking the test drug was checked; records of concurrent medications were reviewed; and preliminary results from the autopsy, cerebrospinal fluid sample, and blood-level analyses were reviewed.

During that first 24-hour period, after all available data are obtained and scrutinized, a preliminary decision is made regarding the likelihood of the drug contributing to the death. This decision determines whether to continue with the study. Assuming the preliminary decision is made that the death is thought to be unrelated to the test drug, several actions must still be taken until a final decision is reached. If the test agent is in Phase I, the investigator can now be informed to continue dosing of patients, but not to increase dosage more than the maximum dose allowed at the time the death occurred. Also at this time, no new patients should be entered into the study. Other subjects in the study at that site should be informed of the death and given the option to discontinue. In addition, investi-

Table 1   Stage 1 Decisions to Be Made Immediately to Within 24 h of Death

1. Phone contact with investigator by medical monitor or other qualified person
    a. Obtain preliminary, general information surrounding patient's death.
    b. Discontinue temporarily all dosing at site.
    c. Break code for that patient, if a double-blind study.
    d. Request the following:
        (1) Autopsy
        (2) Blood levels for drug(s) and metabolites
        (3) Cerebrospinal fluid
    e. Initiate steps to have clinical trial material analyzed.
    f. Obtain from the investigator a written summary of the death.
2. Trip to study site by monitor or other qualified person
    a. Begin thorough investigation of all records to obtain all facts and events surrounding the death:
        (1) Review intensively all medical records and patient's data collection forms.
        (2) Check compliance, concurrent medication.
        (3) Obtain preliminary results of autopsy, cerebrospinal fluid, and blood levels.
    b. Obtain past history and information about any peculiar events or previous experimental therapy by talking to relatives.

Table 2 Stage 1 Actions to Be Taken if Preliminary Decision Indicates Death Is Probably Unrelated to the Test Drug

1. Inform investigator to continue dosing, with no increase in dose (maximum dose at time of death).
2. Enter no new patients.
3. Inform all patients at site of the death, and give the option of discontinuing.
4. Contact all other investigators (if any), informing them of preliminary results.

gators at other sites should be informed of the preliminary results of the investigation into the cause of death. Table 2 summarizes these actions.

In our anticonvulsant case example, all patients in this study were known to be taking the test agent, so the cause of death had to be determined quickly. All steps in Stage 1 of the investigation were performed, with the following results:

> Autopsy: Cause of death undetermined
> Blood levels: Normal
> Cerebrospinal fluid: Not obtained
> Compliance check: OK

Therefore, the preliminary decision was that the death was probably not drug related. Thus dosing could continue, but no new patients could be entered. The other study investigators were informed, and patients at the study site were told of the death and given the option to discontinue. Of the patients hospitalized at the site, only one chose to remain in the study.

B. Stage 2 Investigation

Stage 2 of the investigation lasts 1 week to 2 months and involves a thorough, intensive review of all information. The following actions are taken:

> Obtain and review final results of the autopsy, blood levels, and cerebrospinal fluid.
> Compile and review any available data from other study sites.
> Conduct a more intensive review of the subject's records and data collection forms.
> Review the literature for any epidemiological factors that may be relevant to the diseases or the population being studied.
> Contact outside consultants.

Table 3   Stage 2 Investigation Activities 1 Week to 2 Months After Event

1. Obtain final results of autopsy, blood levels, and cerebrospinal fluid.
2. Conduct intensive review of data (data collection forms and hospital records).
3. Contact outside consultants from pertinent branch of FDA, academia, etc.
4. Compile and review all available data from other study sites.
5. Notify the FDA (within 3 days).
6. Check literature (epidemiological data).

> Notify the Food and Drug Administration (FDA) of the death as soon as possible, but within 3 days of the incident.

Table 3 summarizes the actions to be taken at this point in Stage 2 of the investigation.

Having obtained all results, the determination can now be made as to the relationship of the death to the test drug. Assuming the final decision is that the death was not drug related, some specific actions must be taken. The investigator can now be informed to allow an increase in dosing, permit new subjects to enter the study, and continue the study according to protocol. Also, all other investigators should be notified of the results and reminded to inform their Institutional Review Boards. The FDA should be notified, and sent a complete written report of the death. This report should include all available information on the subject, including data collection forms, autopsy report, investigator's report, clinical trial material analysis report, pharmacist's report, and monitor's report (Table 4).

Table 4   Activities After Determining the Death Is Unrelated to Test Drug

1. Inform and allow investigator to increase dosing.
2. Permit new patients to be entered into study.
3. Continue the study according to protocol.
4. Contact all other investigators:
    a. Inform them of the results.
    b. Remind them to inform their Institutional Review Boards.
5. Contact the FDA:
    a. Inform them of the results.
    b. Send them a complete written report of the death. (Report should include all available information on the patient, including data collection forms, autopsy report, investigator's report, clinical trial material analysis report, pharmacist's report, and monitor's report.)

In the case under discussion, all of the Stage 2 steps described above were performed, with the following results:

Final autopsy: Cause of death undetermined
Data review: Not drug related
Consultants' review: Not drug related

The literature was reviewed and it was found that sudden, unexpected death in patients with epilepsy is not an uncommon occurrence, even in patients with an average age of 32 years at the time of death (3). The FDA was sent a full written report of the death; they concurred that it was not drug related. Therefore, the study resumed as originally planned, without harmful effects. The only negative effect of this death occurred later, when an Institutional Review Board at another site refused approval of a proposed study because of the death.

III. SUBSEQUENT EVENTS IN OUR EXAMPLE CLINICAL TRIAL

This case report of an actual death was presented as an example to demonstrate the steps required in a two-stage investigational process to determine the cause of the death. It is worthwhile to mention the subsequent deaths that occurred in this study, and the outcome of these events.

About 6 months later, another death occurred at a different site. This death was the 50th patient entered in the study. The monitor had a serious decision to make at that point. As a monitor, what would you do? Would you continue entering patients, or would you stop the study?

This patient, too, was a 31-year-old individual who died suddenly and unexpectedly in his home. Notably, however, the patient was only at baseline in the study and had not received any medication; therefore, the decision was made to continue the study. Had he already received test drug, the decision to continue would not have been as clear-cut.

Another death occurred about 3 years later, in Phase II. The patient was a 26-year-old woman in the last week of the first treatment period of 12 weeks in a multicenter, double-blind, placebo-controlled study of outpatients with epilepsy. Because this was a placebo-controlled study, after receiving a call about her sudden, unexpected death, the code was broken for her alone. She had been assigned placebo. Immediate steps were taken to confirm that the dispensed drug contained no active medication. Analytical results confirmed within a few hours that the packaged medication contained placebo, yet the same actions were taken to investigate the cause of death, to gather information for FDA reports, and to further evaluate any relationships between the death and the study site. After a thorough investigation, it was concluded that the patient was on placebo. Additionally, the cause of death was disease related and in no way implicated the test drug, concurrent drugs, or study methodology. Therefore, clinical studies at all other sites proceeded according to protocol.

In this example study of 225 patients with epilepsy, two other deaths occurred. One death occurred in a man on treatment drug in an open Phase II study. This death, however, was deemed disease related. The patient evidently had a seizure while exercising with barbells and subsequently died of asphyxiation in the accident.

Another disease related death in this study occurred when a 31-year-old man had a tonic clonic seizure. However, he was still at baseline; thus, he had never received the test drug.

Although this project progressed to Phase III in development, and in spite of the fact that many of the patients became seizure free while on the drug even though other antiepileptic medications did not control their seizures, the development of the drug was discontinued. The placebo effect was not significantly different from the drug effect.

IV. TEST-DRUG–RELATED DEATHS

Assuming that a death is possibly or probably related to a test drug is another matter. Actions must be taken to have all test drug discontinued and to recall any unused test drug. The FDA should be notified and sent a full, written report. All other investigators should be notified of the decision to discontinue.

What evidence will prove that death is drug related? It is hard to prove a drug-related fatality conclusively. Evidence that might imply a drug effect is given in Table 5.

Table 5 Evidence Needed to Prove a Death Is Related to Test Drug

1. Abnormally high blood levels of drug or metabolite.
2. A side effect appearing just before death and known to be related to the drug from animal studies or other human data studies.
3. Some defined causes of death that would be unexpected in a given patient (e.g., acute kidney failure, aplastic anemia heart attack or stroke in a young, nonhypertensive patient)

V. PLACEBO-RELATED DEATHS

The placebo in a clinical trial should not be automatically dismissed as a possible cause of a sudden and unexpected death in a clinical study. Consider the following case from a Phase II study of an antidepressant drug. The study involved 64 depressed outpatients and had a 1-week placebo lead-in with 6 weeks of double-blind, b.i.d. dosing. A 45-year-old woman missed her Week 6 visit. The study site contacted the family and discovered that the subject had died unexpectedly. Autopsy and assays were scheduled. The medical monitor reviewed all treatment and test records, including the patient's medical chart, case report forms, compliance, clinical trial material, concurrent drugs, preliminary autopsy results, and postmortem results. The patient's history was reviewed by talking with family members, and any pertinent information about unusual events and past experimental therapies was noted. In addition, the unused clinical trial material was shipped to the sponsor for analysis. The results of these investigations were as follows:

> Prior adverse experiences: None
> Concomitant medications: None
> Prior serious medical problems: No
> Blood pressure: Normal
> Serum chemistry: Normal, except slight cholesterol elevation
> Hematology: Normal, except transient eosinophil elevation
> ECG: Occasional PVCs; one instance of shortened QTc
> Preliminary autopsy report: *Cause of death undetermined*

The patient had received clinical trial material for 5 weeks. After breaking the blind for this patient, it was found she had been on placebo. Because the death was not related to the test drug, the decision was made not to interrupt dosing at the site.

The next step was to confirm that the patient was, in fact, taking placebo. The remaining clinical trial material that had been returned to the sponsor was analyzed, and the subject's body fluids were examined for drug levels. All analyses indicated placebo, so the adverse event was deemed to be serious and unexpected, but not associated with the active drug.

VI. UNEXPECTED DEATH IN A RELATED FIELD

Although a clinical program may be progressing without any significant safety issues, it is important to follow comparable compounds. "Class effects" have been observed in the past. For example, a series of antiarrythmic compounds were discovered to produce sudden unexpected death. Several companies pursuing that class of compound choose to discontinue future studies even though sudden death may not have been observed with their compound.

On the other hand, a sudden unexpected death in the same field could negatively affect a program even if the death has no relationship to the product being studied. For example, the sudden unexpected death of Jesse Gelsinger, who was enrolled in a gene transfer protocol at the University of Pennsylvania, halted the majority of gene transfer clinical trials in the United States. After an investigation by the FDA, National Institutes of Health, Congress, and the press, the death was reported to have been related to the vehicle (adenoviral vector) used to deliver the gene to the target cells. Nonetheless, all gene transfer programs, whether or not an adenoviral vector was used, were negatively affected by this unfortunate death.

VII. CONCLUSIONS

A sudden, unexpected death is a possible occurrence in any clinical drug trial. Although such an event is never easy to deal with, being prepared for the possibility of a death will help with the subsequent investigation and decisions that must be made in the aftermath. Certainly, any unexpected death has the potential of immediately ending a clinical program. Therefore, the situation must be dealt with in a systematic and efficient manner that not only will determine the connection of the test agent to the event, but that still respects the dignity of others involved in the study and the family of the deceased. Having a plan in place and understanding the class of compound being studied and the field of use that is being pursued will prove to be integral elements in the investigation.

In this chapter, we have presented various examples of deaths occurring in clinical studies. The first death occurred in a subject known to be taking the study drug, the second subject was still in baseline, and the third subject was on placebo. The basic manner of investigating all three deaths was the same and will generally apply to any unexpected death in a clinical trial. During the stages of investigation, however, the medical monitor should keep in mind the Hippocratic oath taken by physicians before entering practice. The oath states, ''I will prescribe regimens for the good of my patients, according to my judgment and ability, and never do harm to anyone. To please no one will I prescribe a deadly drug, nor give advice which may cause his death.''

REFERENCES

1. Cato A. Premarketing adverse drug experiences: data management procedures. Unexpected death occurring early in clinical trials. Drug Inf J 1987; 21(1):3–7.
2. Bernard C. An Introduction to the Study of Experimental Medicine. Greene HC (trans.). New York: Dover, 1957:101–102.
3. Terrence CF Jr, Wisotzkey HM, Perper JA. Unexpected, unexplained death in epileptic patients. Neurology 1975; 25(6):594–598.

16

Clinical Trial Material—The Fuel for Clinical Research

David F. Bernstein
Cato Research Ltd., Corona del Mar, California

I. INTRODUCTION

In the context of clinical research, the preparation of clinical trial material (CTM) satisfies the short-term objective of providing the correct, blinded drug product (including various doses of the investigational drug, matching placebos, and matching competitive products) according to a randomized medication allocation scheme for a specific clinical study. As such, investigational products and their packaging, labeling, and assembly into patient kits are customized for each clinical study.

In the context of overall drug development, the preparation of CTM contributes to the evolving scientific database that is the basis for a New Drug Application (NDA). This satisfies a long-term objective of product approval from the chemistry, manufacturing, and controls (CMC) perspective. Often, the preparation of ever-increasing amounts of a variety of investigational drug products can identify manufacturing or processing problems that can be corrected in future batches. Stability data on CTM (which is required to support the specific clinical study) can be used to identify potential commercial packages and, in selected cases, can be used as supportive stability data for registration.

Since both clinical research and CTM preparation require a lengthy, multi-year development process, the technical issues surrounding the clinical supply chain are themselves evolutionary. The greatest challenge in drug development from the CMC perspective is that CTM preparation is a miniproduction operation conducted in a research and development (R&D) environment. The principles and practices for manufacturing, packaging, and labeling that are well established for commercial products need to be modified and adapted for the specialized clinical supply environment.

In contrast to commercial products, where manufacturing processes, formulations, specifications, analytical methods, and stability profiles are well established, CTM is prepared under an evolutionary umbrella where every technical aspect of a product is under continual change. Early in Phase I, of the clinical development process, multiple strengths of investigational drug products are required to provide flexibility in dosing for ascending-dose tolerance safety studies. Later, in Phase III of clinical development, multiple strengths may be required for dose-ranging studies. Typically, formulations and manufacturing procedures to support these two types of studies are different, reflecting advancing CMC development and focusing of the desired clinical doses.

In addition, placebo products that match the active investigational product in visual and organoleptic properties must also be developed. Often, Phase III studies include a positive control drug or comparator product, which pose particular blinding challenges. Due to extremely lengthy lead times in obtaining comparator products and then in performing manipulations to blind all products, these challenges must be identified and addressed up to 15 months before the intended start of the clinical study. The formulation and manufacturing process for capsules and ampules, which may be preferentially developed for a Phase I clinical study, will need to be continually refined to accommodate scale-up and an increasing technical knowledge base. These early dosage forms may need to be modified to tablets or vials, which are preferred for expansive late clinical-phase development and commercialization.

CTM is prepared under the legal requirements of Good Manufacturing Practices (GMP) and the International Conference on Harmonization (ICH) Good Clinical Practice Consolidated Guideline (See sections 4.6 and 5.13 of ICH E6). Complete compliance with GMP is expected for the first Phase I study, except in several well-defined areas where strict compliance is impossible or impractical. In these areas, alternative practices based on Good Common Sense, Good Documentation Practices (GDP), Good Scientific Practices (GSP), and Good Housekeeping Practices must govern CTM operations. The areas where alternative compliance strategies must be devised involve the evolutionary nature of CMC drug development.

> Validation of manufacturing processes (based on three replicate batches) is not expected in early CTM operations, since replication is the exception rather than the rule. Extensive process evaluation represents a GSP as it contributes to the evolving scientific database. However, due to the safety considerations inherent in injectable products, validation of either aseptic process parameters or terminal sterilization is required for the first-in-man (FIM) study.

Validation of analytical methods can be abbreviated. However, since far-reaching decisions (e.g., release of CTM, data suggesting future development problems) are based on analytical data, a reliable analytical method that is capable of detecting the active pharmaceutical ingredient, any impurities, and any degradation products should be available for FIM studies.

Specifications are usually wide, since an insufficient number of batches have been prepared on which to base typical tight commercial specifications.

Final, approved standard operating procedures (SOPs) may not be complete. In these cases, all CTM operations can be conducted according to a thorough, written protocol that defines exactly what will be done for this clinical supply operation.

In contrast to the above examples, where flexibility is provided by the GMP requirements, sponsors need to adopt more traditional approaches to some GMP issues, including the following.

Trained scientists and technicians are required. Due to the highly specialized nature of all aspects of the preparation of CTM, commercial manufacturing technicians are rarely suitable for the customized packaging, labeling, and assembly operations.

Manufacturing facilities may be small-scale versions of GMP-compliant commercial manufacturing or facilities devoted to investigational products. In either case, attention to facility design, equipment qualification, and written procedures governing all production operations are required.

Procedures to clean equipment and techniques to demonstrate and test that residues of either the active pharmaceutical ingredients (API) or detergents used in the cleaning do not remain are required. This cleaning issue is a particular challenge when using contractors or multi-use equipment, since neither the toxicological profile of the API or impurities has been established. Even for a Phase I study, it would be inappropriate to have yesterday's drug residue in today's investigational product.

Written formulation, manufacturing process, specifications and analytical methods must be based on good science. These are the critical elements that must be included in the IND.

GMPs provide minimum requirements. There are several areas requiring controls that are more stringent than those normally used for commercial operations, including the following.

An easy-to-use change control system is necessary. Change is inevitable during the preparation of investigational drug products, and deviations to planned operations should be expected. Documentation of these deviations contributes to a continual improvement process.

Quality assurance (QA) oversight is imperative, but the company must foster an attitude that quality is each employee's responsibility. QA personnel should be cognizant of the specialized requirements inherent in the preparation of investigational products.

Due to the lookalike nature of drug products in lookalike containers with look-alike labels, written systems to eliminate any chance of mixups must be in place. This is imperative, since mixups cannot be easily detected.

II. THE GENERAL INVESTIGATIONAL SUPPLY PROCESS

The visible portion of the investigational supply process begins with the ordering of drug supplies and ends with shipment of investigational products to the clinical site. This is a sequential process that is not amenable to conducting operations in parallel with the intent of saving time. These sequential processes require a well-developed scenario, since each investigational supply project has a defined cascade of activities. This cascade of activities needs to begin with excellent communication of the overall clinical plan to clinical supply scientists and ends with post-use accountability, reconciliation, return and destruction of CTM.

The preparation of CTM is customized in response to specific clinical protocols. The specialized nature of CTM operations does not lend itself to mass production. Consequently, there is no clinical supply drug store that could immediately supply the wide variety of investigational drug products in the wide variety of packages that are typically employed in clinical research. Packaged contents (e.g., 30 capsules, 5 mL) are selected based on dosing frequencies and the frequency of patient visits to clinical sites. Label copy, label text, and label sizes are all customized and are subject to strict approval mechanisms, control and separation of labels and inventory requirements. Global multicenter studies require language-specific labeling that addresses both domestic and international regulatory requirements. Patient kits are not standard items; a 2-week, 6-week, or 3-month supply of CTM would require three different-sized patient kits.

The investigational supply process is understandably time-consuming. It would be nice if attempts to truncate time could be associated simply with increased cost; however, projections of time frames are initially aggressive, and attempts to shorten them often compromise quality. Any compromise of quality during the preparation of lookalike drug products which are associated with specific patients can, and has, compromised an entire clinical study. Since it is difficult to detect mixups in even the best situation, sponsors often ask, "Are you sure you packed my CTM correctly?" when the goals of a clinical study are not realized. Only those firms that have conducted CTM operations according to GSP and GDP will be able to answer that question.

III. DEFINING THE CLINICAL SUPPLY PROJECT

Clinical supply projects are complex; they involve numerous separate functions (manufacturing, packaging, labeling, testing), all of which usually follow different departmental priorities. When multiple contractors are involved, the concept of just-in-time clinical supplies is nice theoretically, but it is almost impossible to achieve in practice.

Clinical supply projects that have had the benefit of parallel conceptualization of the CMC program, the clinical program, and the resultant CTM program have typically been completed in realistic, attainable, yet challenging time frames. Defining any clinical supply project requires an early alert of the overall clinical program so that bulk API or manufactured drug product requirements and their lead times can be anticipated.

Since even draft or final clinical protocols often overlook many clinical supply concerns (e.g., the frequency of CTM dispensing, overages needed to account for missed clinical visits, packaging options to promote patient compliance), these issues must be explored by alternative mechanisms. An early interactive discussion among clinicians, statisticians, and clinical supply scientists can identify and address the majority of issues that are inherent and unique to each clinical study. In this way, trade-offs and options can be explored and the "best way" and best time frame can be agreed to by all. Then, as the clinical protocol is being finalized, clinical supply operations create a definition document. This protocol covers all manufacturing, packaging, labeling, assembly, testing, and distribution activities and identifies the responsibilities for and the details of each of these activities.

IV. ORDERING CLINICAL SUPPLIES

Ordering CTM should occur in two stages, bulk and specific packaged product, reflecting the lengthy lead times for manufacturing and the shorter lead times for customized packaging activities.

Bulk supplies (the number of capsules, tablets, liters of liquid for an injectable product) for the immediate clinical study, as well as the entire clinical program, need to be estimated and manufactured. These projections need to include different dosage forms for bioavailability studies, different strengths for dose–response studies, comparator products for comparisons with the innovator, and placebos.

It is understandably difficult for clinical researchers to predict with certainty their needs 6 or 12 months in advance in the specificity required by CMC development experts. However, a substantial attempt must be made to identify the maximum number of bulk supplies that could be required, since the clinical supply chain begins with the availability of the API, which itself requires 4 to 12 months in advance of CTM operations.

Once a clinical site is initiated, specific shipments can be directed to designated investigators for a specified number of potentially enrolled patients.

Obviously, due to the sequential nature of clinical supply operations and the lengthy lead times for the preparation of the API (especially for complex biotech products), projections of bulk supplies must be made early in the development process and must consider all users, including toxicology, CMC development, analytical development, as well as projected clinical requirements. Projection of specific shipments needs to be finalized at the time that the CTM definition document is created, since numerous components (e.g., containers, closures, labels, kit boxes, and shippers) need to be identified and acquired in addition to the bulk drug product.

V. MANUFACTURE OF CTM

Investigational drug products are often manufactured to supply CTM for specific clinical trials. The preparation of CTM is conducted under the umbrella of evolutionary CMC activities that are directed at developing increasingly rugged and sophisticated formulations and manufacturing processes. At some point in development, CMC activities that have focused on CTM preparation need to be redirected to supply the scientific and technical database for marketing registration documents and commercial manufacturing.

An example of this evolutionary dosage form development process would involve the development of a rudimentary, "simple" drug plus lactose hand-filled capsule suitable for Phase 1 studies. Manual capsule operations can produce 500–1000 capsules per hour. As clinical requirements become larger, it will be necessary to incorporate additional formulation ingredients (starch, lubricants) that would be amenable to a semi-automatic encapsulation machine with its output of 4000–8000 capsules per hour. The next variation suitable for expanded Phase III studies and commercialization would involve high-speed encapsulation (1000–1500 capsules per minute) and require the incorporation of additional formulation ingredients (binders, disintegrants). If all three variations of this capsule dosage form were to be developed, each would require preformulation studies to determine drug–excipient compatibility and formulation studies to determine the qualitative and quantitative amounts of all formula ingredients. Each variation would require stability programs to demonstrate that the respective clinical products were stable throughout the clinical study.

Alternatively, and depending on the degree of difficulty of formula and process development and the sales and marketing preferences between capsules and tablets, one could develop a first-generation capsule that would be used early in clinical development and supplanted by a second-generation sophisticated capsule for later studies. During the lengthy Phase III studies, the CMC pharmaceutics group would develop a tablet and offer that product to the clinical program when available. In this case, a bioequivalence trial between the capsule and tablet dosage form would ensure that the clinical data generated from the capsule dosage form would be relevant to the intended tablet commercial dosage form that is the subject of the NDA.

The evolving dosage form development process requires an appreciation of the following two key interactions between clinical and product development.

> What dose strengths will need to be developed? For Phase I ascending-dose tolerance studies, subjects could receive multiple dosage units of the no-effect dose, which would minimize the number of different formulations to be developed and, hence, the total development time.
>
> What dosage form and dose strength will be needed for the next series of clinical trials?

The second question is of critical importance due to the asynchronous nature of CMC and CTM development. This out-of-synchrony is due to the much longer time frame for dosage form development, and manufacturing, packaging, and labeling of CTM compared with clinical protocol development. Simply stated, CTM for Phase I clinical trials must be formulated and manufactured prior to the IND, and Phase III CTM must be developed and manufactured while Phase II clinical trials are being conducted. These strategic issues are unique to each clinical program and each clinical study, and efficient drug development programs will incorporate concomitant development of the overall clinical program with the overall CMC program.

In contrast to commercially approved products, solid-dosage-form CTM cannot contain a logo or other identifying trade dress in order to supply suitable drug products for blinded studies. Bulk solid-dosage-form drug products are usually manufactured based on projected clinical requirements, equipment capabilities, and availability of the API. Only the immediately identified clinical requirements and the nonclinical regulatory requirements (i.e., retained samples, test samples, stability samples) are packaged. The balance is kept in bulk drums until it is needed for future clinical or CMC studies. For injectable products, sterility concerns require that the compounded liquid is filled into ampules or vials as part of a manufacturing process. Since manufacturing operations for blinded clinical studies often involve matching placebos, these look-alike drug products must be strictly segregated, since there is no easy nondestructive technique to tell them apart.

VI. PACKAGING OF INVESTIGATIONAL SUPPLIES

The packaging of CTM is driven by the clinical protocol. Usually, to minimize waste and maximize in-trial accountability, primary packages containing the drug product are designed to accommodate a patient-visit schedule or a medication-dispensing scheme. In an attempt to streamline this customized activity, large pharmaceutical companies have attempted to standardize the bottle sizes that are available from commercial production stock and to use them for a variety of products regardless of the number of dosage units within the container. Small companies without production facilities or companies that outsource clinical packaging must treat the acquisition of packaging components (e.g., containers, closures, seals, liner, rubber stoppers) as a custom activity in response to the particular requirement of the protocol.

Primary packaging involves the selection of the container that is in contact with the medication. The packaging components should be selected on the basis of availability of adequate amounts of appropriate components, compatibility between the container closure system and the drug product, and corporate culture (ampules versus vials, glass versus plastic bottles). Secondary packaging is discussed below in Sec. VIII.

VII. LABELING

Label is defined as the information and directions printed on the immediate container; labeling refers to all other printed matter. In the United States, the only legal requirement for label information is the "Caution—for investigational use" statement (21 CFR 312.6). However, other information is usually contained on a label; some of this information is referred to in 21 CFR 201. The following are usually included on CTM labels:

Name of sponsor.
Patient number or kit reference number.
Directions for use: For outpatient studies, specific patient directions are recommended to promote patient compliance. Directions to refer to the protocol are not helpful, since CTM dispensers and the pharmacy dispensing the medication do not usually have access to the protocol.
Code number, which is a reference to the specific assembly operation. Since this number must be the same for all products in a clinical trial, traceability from an assembly operation to the specific batches of each product used must be assured.

Caution statement, or in the European Union (EU), a statement that the drug is intended for clinical trial use only.

Contents, which refers to the quantitative contents and dosage form or route of administration (30 capsules, 10 mL for IV injection).

Clinical protocol number (or IND number)

A Caution Statement to keep the drug out of reach of children (for outpatient studies only).

Storage statement (e.g., keep in refrigerator, store below 30°C [86°F]).

*Name of an investigator or clinical site reference code.

*Use by date, expiry or retest date.

Those items marked with an * are also required in the EU.

Multiple tear-off panels are used to document the manufacturing activity downstream from primary packaging (e.g., reconstitution of a powder by the clinical-site hospital pharmacist) or a dispensing operation (this panel would be placed on the case report form). A variety of suppliers of computer-generated labels or print shop labels are available, as well as several excellent systems intended for in-house label generation. As in most CTM operations, due to the specialized nature of clinical labeling, the generation of labels should be preferentially handled by those familiar with the uniqueness of CTM labeling activities rather than by a commercial printer.

Traditionally, patient numbers were preprinted on labels that were affixed to the immediate container of the various drug products according to the medication allocation randomization code. This technique preallocated CTM to the specific patients who could be enrolled at a given site. Since predicted patient enrollment often does not materialize and dropouts do occur, there is a greater potential for unused CTM. While the preprinted patient number remains the major technique to associate a specific patient with the randomized treatment, alternative techniques intended to conserve CTM are also being used.

These alternative techniques have been referred to as minimization, double randomization, or material pooling. Basically, these techniques link specific patient kits to specific patients only at the time of enrollment. Since label operations must attach specific labels to specific medication containers according to GMP documentation requirements and the randomization code, each container is labeled with a unique alphanumeric code, which itself can be randomly generated as shown in Table 1. This "kit randomization" needs to be associated with the traditional patient randomization, and this linkage is done at the time of patient enrollment. Table 1 illustrates that CTM containers for the active product are labeled with randomized reference codes 521, 364, 905, and 872, while the placebo product is similarly labeled with its unique reference codes. As the first patient is enrolled, a link is made between the patient name and Patient Number 101. The clinical site calls a central registration office that assigns the kit number to be dispensed. The central registration office may be manned or will utilize an

Table 1 Double Randomization

Patient randomization		Kit randomization	
Patient	Drug	Drug	Kit
101	A	A	521
102	P	A	364
103	P	A	905
104	A	A	872
105	P	P	244
106	P	P	385
107	A	P	191
108	A	P	774

Interactive Voice Response System. The central office will then look up the drug assignment for Patient 101 (which is active) and inform the site to dispense Kit 521. Similarly, the second patient at that site would be assigned Kit 244. Both the clinical site, and central office document that Patient 101 received Kit 521. This technique minimizes the CTM required at any clinical site, where space for CTM is often at a premium, and reduces the potential for unused CTM due to incomplete enrollment.

VIII. ASSEMBLY OF CTM INTO PATIENT KITS

Assembly of CTM into patient kits is also known as secondary packaging, since the actual drug product is not exposed to environmental conditions during this operation. The use of patient kits facilitates dispensing by the clinical site, usage by the patient, and return goods accountability by the clinical monitor.

The specific configuration of a patient kit depends on the frequency of dispensing visits during the clinical trial. Examples of the contents of patient kits are provided in Figs. 1 and 2.

Patient kits are often used even for "simple" Phase I studies involving a less than simple dispensing scheme. In a placebo-controlled, ascending-dose tolerance safety study, the no-effect dose of 10 mg was followed by dose escalation to 20, 40, 80, 160, and 240 mg. Two cohorts of nine subjects (six on active, three on placebo) would alternate doses so that each would take three doses. Since it was impractical to develop seven different formulations (the six different drug doses plus placebo), capsules containing placebo and 10 and 40 mg of drug product were developed. Each subject took six capsules; depending on the dose and the random allocation to active or placebo, the subject would need to take

Daily Medication Box

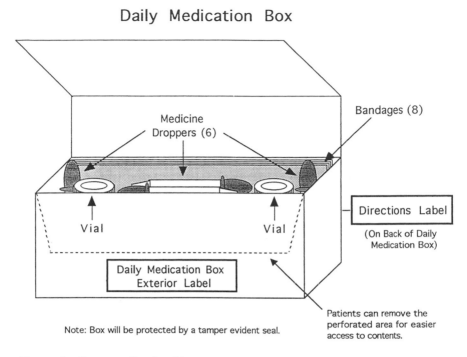

Figure 1 Contents of patient kit.

a combination of the various capsules in order to obtain the correct dose, as shown in Table 2.

Each individual patient bottle contained six capsules. Since each subject was to take three doses (e.g., the subjects in cohort A were randomized to receive 10, 40, and 160 mg, while the subjects in cohort B were randomized to receive 20, 80, and 240 mg) and one of the three doses would be placebo, it was imperative that the clinical site dispense the correct bottle in the exact sequence that would preserve the ascending dose scheme and the random, predetermined assignment to placebo. There were two options for the preparation of the subject kits.

Dose-level boxes that contained nine bottles of CTM, one bottle for each patient could be prepared. In this option, six dose-level boxes, each containing nine bottles and each bottle containing six capsules, would be required. Label information would require that the dose level and patient number be clearly highlighted. Since subjects for the initial 10-mg dose level would be enrolled over a very short time period and all nine subjects

Packaging   Diagrams

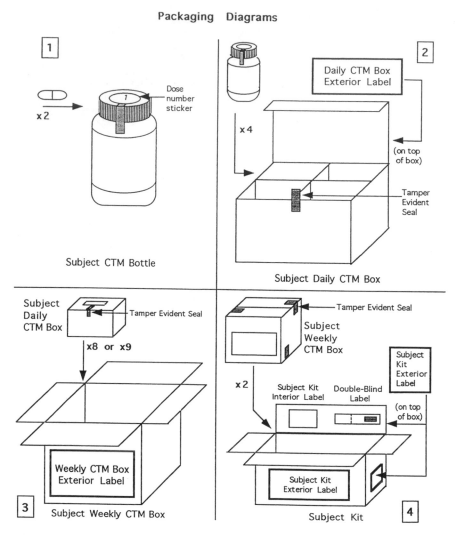

Figure 2   Contents of patient kit.

dosed on the same day, the dose-level box option facilitated the dispensing process at the clinical site.

Subject kits that contained only the three bottles of CTM required for each subject could be prepared. Eighteen subject kits, each containing three bottles and each bottle containing six capsules, would be required. This option provided greater control over specific subject CTM, but would

Table 2 CTM Configuration for a "Simple" Phase I Protocol

		Number capsules/bottles		
Dose group		Placebo	10 mg	40 mg
10	Active	5	1	—
10	Placebo	6	—	—
20	Active	4	2	—
20	Placebo	6	—	—
40	Active	5	—	1
40	Placebo	6	—	—
80	Active	4	—	2
80	Placebo	6	—	—
160	Active	2	—	4
160	Placebo	6	—	—
240	Active	—	—	6
240	Placebo	6	—	—

require that a specific bottle be located and dispensed to preserve the ascending-dose scheme. While this can be easily accommodated by using cap labels (since the caps are seen when the kit box is opened; see Fig. 2) that indicate first dose, second dose, and third dose, this scenario requires the clinical site to search for one of 18 boxes.

Since the dose-level option involved only six boxes and since all subjects would be dosed on the same day, the first option was chosen. Since this option required customized labels (the dose-level box label would indicate "Contents— nine bottles, dose level A, each containing six capsules," while the subject kit box label would indicate "Contents-three bottles, patient XXX, each containing six capsules" and a "use first, use second label"), a dialogue between clinical/ medical and clinical supply professionals encourages the "best way" to prevail. These interactive discussions help to avoid false starts and last-minute changes that can delay the initiation of clinical studies.

IX. TESTING

The release of CTM for distribution involves procedures that are similar to those required for commercial products. However, basic differences between commercial products and CTM require additional attention due to the following.

Since early CMC efforts may be minimal, the resulting formulation of an early clinical drug product may be regarded as rudimentary. Manufacturing processes have not been validated and since reasonable dose-to-dose variations and acceptance limits cannot be any less stringent, occasional batch failures can be anticipated. In one unfortunate case, a Phase III clinical study was initiated using a "rudimentary Phase I formulation" for which powder blending time and efficiency had not been studied or optimized.

While the assay value (obtained by compositing the contents of 20 capsules) was within the 95%–105% of label-claim acceptance limits, the content uniformity (obtained by the analysis of 10 individual capsules) did not pass the 85%–115% limit for this test. In this case, individual capsules contained from 65% to 155% of label claim. Since individual capsules were administered, a patient could receive a dose that was randomly $2/3$ to $1^1/2$ times what was intended. Obviously, any clinical results would not be based on a definitive dose and, hence, would be worthless.

Investigational drug products are prepared from APIs that are undergoing continuous refinement. During attempts to increase efficiency, yield, or economies of larger scale, modifications of the chemical or biotech synthesis are continual during early development. Often, unanticipated and unintended new impurities appear in the API and are incorporated into the drug product. Since toxicology studies have not been conducted on these materials, the analytical method used to test investigational drug products must be capable of detecting any new impurities. In addition, since stability data are very limited for investigational drug products, the analytical method must be equally capable of detecting degradation products. It is important to note that degradation products occur as a result of chemical change of the API or impurity over time, while impurities are organic volatile compounds or other unwanted chemicals that result directly from the API synthesis.

In contrast to the testing and issuance of a Certificate of Analysis for the entire batch of commercial products, investigational products involve a two-step release. The GMP release (known in the EU as the technical green light) may involve the release of only the portion of the batch actually packaged for a specific clinical study. This approval must be followed by a GCP release (known in the EU as the regulatory green light), where it must be evaluated whether and confirmed that the IND is current, Forms FDA 1571 and 1572 are filed and Institutional Review Board (IRB) approval has been obtained.

X. DISTRIBUTION

Once CTM is prepared into patient kits, shipment to clinical sites can be dictated by patient enrollment. For multicenter studies, initial supplies can be used to open a clinical site where resupply frequency is dependent on actual patient enrollment at any given site.

Shipment of CTM should ensure that the drug products are protected against exposure to undesirable environmental conditions. Often, early in the development process, the absolute sensitivity of a drug product to excursions outside acceptable ranges of temperature, humidity, or shear are unknown. In the cases where drug is very expensive or in very limited supply, trial shipments to a variety of dummy locations are made using placebo drug product where actual environmental conditions are measured by markers, recorders, or high-tech devices involving computer chips. These techniques are highly recommended for biologics, proteins, or topical semisolid products, where freezing or refrigerated conditions must be maintained or avoided or where freeze/thaw or refrigerated/room-temperature cycling would be detrimental to product integrity.

Shipment by the sponsor is usually accompanied by a shipment/receipt form intended to be completed by the clinical-site pharmacist or CTM study coordinator and returned to the sponsor. This form represents the point in the chain of custody of CTM which is at the interface of GMP (21 CFR 211.150) and GCP (21 CFR 312.57, 312.59, and 312.62) requirements.

XI. RETURNS

Returns of commercial products are usually associated with a recall situation caused by a drug product not meeting its stability and shelf-life specifications. In contrast, returns of CTM (or empty primary containers) are specifically required (refer to 312.59) regardless of whether it was unused, partially used, or completely used so that reconciliation and accountability can be performed. Reconciliation and accountability contribute to assessments of patient compliance, the degree of which can influence the reliability of the clinical data. A growing trend is to perform this accountability at the clinical site and then to send the CTM directly for disposal.

In the EU, because of the requirement that an expiry or use date be printed on the label, CTM that reaches the expiry date prior to the trial completion must be returned so that replacement CTM can be supplied or, if warranted, the expiry date can be extended. In the latter case, a relabeling operation (with the trial reference number and the new revised expiry date) would need to be performed.

This operation could also be performed at the clinical site. If this option is selected, the relabeling should be performed by sponsor representatives who are trained in the documentation procedures required by GMP.

XII. USE OF CTM CONTRACTORS

In recent years, there has been a growing trend for outsourcing of various portions of the investigational supply process. This need has resulted from the growth of the large number of small, emerging firms that do not have facilities or the internal expertise for manufacturing, packaging, or testing of CTM, coupled with the trend for large pharmaceutical companies to out-source portions or all of their clinical supply chain.

This trend can be seen by examining any list of contract services; there are now over 12 formulation groups that focus on the preclinical development of divergent dosage forms; over 25 analytical laboratories that can develop new analytical methods, especially those for complex proteins; 7 manufacturing organizations devoted solely to CTM (not commercial) manufacturing; and 8 contract packagers dedicated to clinical supply packaging and labeling.

Most contractors, especially those dedicated to clinical supply operations, do a good job. Their effort can be universally measured by how well the project is defined. Virtual companies that do not possess internal CMC/CTM expertise are particularly vulnerable, since simply giving a contractor a draft clinical protocol and short time frame may result in a CTM configuration being barely adequate and not meeting the overall project needs. Such firms should enlist the services of competent clinical supply consultants who can assist them in the definition process, suggesting the best approaches, and monitor contractor operations.

Since CTM operations are customized, contingency plans should be developed and changes should be anticipated because even the best definition document may not address all the realities that appear during actual production operations. This is easily done by having a person in the plant during all critical CTM activities; any deviations or unanticipated contingencies can then be addressed, and client input and approval can be obtained immediately.

XIII. CONCLUSION

The preparation of CTM under GCP, GMP, GDP, and GSP represents good business practices, since quality investigational materials need to meet both short-term (i.e., specific clinical study) and long-term (i.e., NDA) objectives. As clinical research progresses from Phase I to Phase III, early rudimentary investigational drug products are replaced by sophisticated, fully evaluated formulations and manufacturing procedures. Since changes to the formulation and manufacturing process can effect product performance and, hence, clinical efficacy, a critical concept that needs to be clearly addressed in the preparation of the NDA is the link between the investigational drug product used for clinical studies and the proposed commercial product.

The ideal scenario would require that a final formula, validated manufacturing process, final analytical test methods and specifications, and the commercial container closure system be identified and used during Phase III studies; therefore the only difference between the investigational drug product and commercial drug product is a less than 10-fold manufacturing-scale difference and specific trade dress. Since most scenarios involve multiple changes in one or more of the above aspects, product equivalence must be assured.

When CMC development has been compromised due to an early bare-bones program, poor or inadequate technology transfer, last-minute changes to marketing package configurations, or increases in manufacturing batch size beyond the 10-fold limit, this linkage becomes more challenging and difficult. In some cases, a bioequivalence study between the investigational drug product and proposed commercial product may be needed. While this requires additional time and money (estimates of 4 months and $100,000 would be reasonable), there is no guarantee that these two products will indeed be bioequivalent. Accordingly, any change in any of the CMC parameters discussed above should be evaluated according to strict scientific guidelines (e.g., Scale Up and Post Approval Change [SUPAC]). If this analysis indicates that a bioequivalence study would be prudent (regardless of whether a regulatory agency would require one), good business practices suggest that the study be conducted prior to submission of the NDA. If this approach is adopted, a side benefit would be obtaining the experience of producing a full-scale commercial batch.

Under contemporary regulatory policies, an NDA can be approved when full-scale commercial manufacturing formulas and procedures are specified in the submission even though this batch size has never been produced. Firms must complete a formal process validation exercise prior to shipment, where three replicate commercial batches must be prepared and meet predetermined specifications. In several cases, failure to validate the commercial manufacturing process has been traced to an inadequate CMC development program. In these cases, the manufacturing process must be tweaked or changed so that a commercial drug product meeting the specifications can be consistently produced. These new, changed process parameters also necessitate the demonstration of the link between the investigational drug product performance and the revised commercial product. In isolated cases, these last-minute changes to manufacturing parameters, coupled with an inadequate explanation of this link, have resulted in the clinical database being questioned and the need to repeat one or more clinical studies. These unfortunate scenarios, although rare, have occurred and could have been prevented by proactive conceptualization of the clinical program in concert with the CMC program.

17

The Role of Pharmacokinetics in Drug Development

Allen Cato III
Cato Research Ltd., San Diego, California

Richard Granneman
Abbott Laboratories, Abbott Park, Illinois

I. INTRODUCTION

Pharmacokinetics, a branch of biopharmaceutics, is a part of the pharmaceutical sciences that describes the relationship between the processes of drug absorption, distribution, metabolism (biotransformation), and excretion (ADME) to the time course of therapeutic or adverse effects of drugs (1). Efficacy is determined by the drug concentration at the site of action, which generally is correlated with the drug concentration in the blood. The ultimate goal of pharmacokinetics is to characterize the sources of variability in the concentration–time profile which may be correlated with variability in efficacy and adverse events. Pharmacokinetics can be used to guide dosage regimen selection and thereby optimize pharmacological effects and minimize toxicological effects when a drug is administered to an individual patient. Thus, while the basic pharmacokinetic properties of a drug are identified during the earliest stage of clinical drug development, the many factors affecting the pharmacokinetics in the patient population must be identified throughout the drug development process to enable proper dose selection for individuals.

Many factors within an individual are potentially capable of influencing the drug concentration at the active site. These factors include (a) demographics such as age, body weight or surface area, gender, and race; (b) genetics, particularly for drugs metabolized by the polymorphic cytochrome P450 isoforms (e.g.,

CYP2D6, CYP2C19, CYP2A6); (c) environmental factors, such as smoking, diet, and exposure to pollutants; (d) physiological and pathophysiological factors, such as pregnancy, renal or hepatic impairment, and other disease states; (e) interactions from concurrent administration of other compounds; and (f) other factors which have been shown to affect drug pharmacokinetics, such as nature and timing of meals, circadian effects, activity and posture, and adherence to the dosage regimen (compliance). Reduced efficacy or increased toxicity may result from the inability to predict the resulting systemic drug concentration–time profile.

While pharmacokinetics describes physiological disposition events and rates of a drug, it is a tool for achieving a variety of multidisciplinary research and therapeutic goals. Pharmacokinetics is an applied, hybrid scientific discipline that achieves its greatest potential when applied prospectively during the earliest stages of drug development (2). Linking the pharmacokinetics and pharmacodynamics (observable pharmacological response) of a drug in a descriptive quantitative model may provide further insight into the factors influencing drug effects. Additionally, population pharmacokinetic analysis can supplement information obtained from classical pharmacokinetic studies, particularly for special populations of patients for which few complete pharmacokinetic profiles exists.

Recent advancements in molecular biology have led to an enhanced understanding of the diversity of function and expression of the drug-metabolizing enzymes which may ultimately allow a more rational dosage selection. During the drug development process, pharmacokinetics can provide a wide range of information, from generalized ADME information to predictions based on sophisticated mathematical models, all of which help to enable the safe and effective therapeutic management of the individual patient. This chapter will first provide a description of several basic pharmacokinetic concepts. The generalized scheme of pharmacokinetic studies during drug development has changed little from the description provided by Drs. Lai, Fleck, and Caplan in the first edition (3). Also, many sources of pharmacokinetic variability and typical pharmacokinetic studies conducted to characterize the variability will be highlighted. Finally, another approach to identifying the sources of pharmacokinetic variability, population pharmacokinetic analysis, will be presented.

II. FUNDAMENTALS

The brief history of pharmacokinetics has been described in detail previously (4). The dramatic growth in the discipline of pharmacokinetics within the past 30 years may be attributed to the advent of digital computers and improved analytical instrumentation allowing the measurement of very low concentrations of drugs in biological fluids, on the order of a few picograms per milliliter (3). The processes of absorption, distribution, biotransformation, excretion, and pharmacological response are quite complex, but fortunately, fairly simplistic models may be used to describe the observed concentration–time profile of many drugs. In fact, model-independent methods are used to characterize the pharmacokinetics of many drugs, particularly during the initial stages of drug development. Development of models to accurately describe the pharmacokinetics may assist in the design of future studies (i.e., dosage regimen and sample collection times).

A. Pharmacokinetic Models and Parameter Estimates

One of the most important applications of pharmacokinetics is the ability to make predictions based on available data. To predict concentrations, a model must be developed which can apply mathematical principles to the various physiological processes involved in the pharmacokinetics of a compound. Compartmental models may be used to describe the pharmacokinetics of a compound; one-compartment, two-compartment, or other multicompartment models may be developed. The type of model is reflective of the pharmacokinetics of the drug. Some models that attempt to incorporate specific physiological processes can become quite complex, but all models are extremely simplistic depictions of the actual fate of a drug in vivo. Fortunately, models need only to be adequate for the intended use, and simple one- or two-compartment models describe the disposition of many drugs fairly accurately. The most simplistic model is often selected, particularly in the analyses of sparse "population pharmacokinetic" data from Phase II and Phase III studies.

B. Absorption Rate and Extent

Particularly for immediate release formulations, the factors that influence the rate and extent of absorption must be determined. During the preclinical phase of drug development, the basic physicochemical properties are characterized, two of which are the aqueous solubility as a function of pH and a measure of lipophilicity (e.g., the octanol–water partition coefficient, expressed as log P). For drugs with high solubility, a positive log P value, and a low rate of degradation under acidic conditions, few development difficulties would be expected for an oral formulation. If these characteristics are not met, development of an oral formulation with good bioavailability may pose significant challenges, and additional in-vitro testing such as Caco-2 cell line examination of absorptive processes may be warranted.

Routinely, promising drug candidates are screened in vivo through intravenous (IV) and oral (PO) crossover studies to determine the absolute bioavailability in animals. If the PO/IV area under the curve (AUC) ratio is high in one or more species, this provides a cautiously encouraging projection for humans. If the ratio is low but log P and solubility are high, low bioavailability could be due to poor absorption or extensive first-pass loss of the drug. Examination of the clearance after intravenous administration would provide additional insight. The well-stirred model of hepatic metabolism is a useful tool in the estimation of the extent of first-pass metabolism. According to this model, which assumes extensive hepatic metabolism and complete absorption, the degree of hepatic extraction (E) is the ratio of clearance (CL) after intravenous administration to the hepatic blood flow (Q_h):

$$E = \frac{CL}{Q_h} \tag{1}$$

If the IV blood CL of the drug is in the range of hepatic blood flow in that species (2.5 L/h in the dog to 5 L/h in the mouse), low bioavailability may be due to extensive first-pass metabolism.

For drugs with high first-pass metabolism in animals, many approaches exist for predicting the CL and first-pass metabolism in humans. These are beyond the scope of the present review, but there are several techniques which have had varying degrees of success (5). Allometric scaling (6,7), which assumes that CL is dependent on body weight taken to some fractional power, often is used to predict human CL by regressing the log CL in animals against weight and extrapolating to the average weight for a person (70 kg). Unfortunately, CL in people does not often fall on the regression line, usually deviating low, which has prompted empirical corrections based on factors such as species longevity. Other approaches involve scaling from *in-vitro* parameters, which also often require correction factors to account for disparities between animal *in-vivo* versus *in-vitro* results. In any case, interspecies scaling usually has limited use in drug discovery and development because typically few animal data are available when the initial dose in humans is chosen.

Once human data are available, the apparent extent of first-pass metabolism can be estimated with or without intravenous data. Using the foregoing assumptions for the well-stirred model, the apparent clearance after oral administration,

$$CL_{oral} = \frac{dose}{AUC} \tag{2}$$

reflects the intrinsic clearance (Cl_{int}) of the drug. The fraction of the dose surviving first-pass hepatic metabolism (f_h) may be estimated as

$$f_h = \frac{Q_h}{Q_h + Cl_{oral}} \tag{3}$$

assuming complete absorption (f_{abs}) and no metabolism within gastrointestinal cells (f_{gi}). In general, if CL_{oral} is substantially lower than hepatic blood flow (human hepatic blood flow rate $\approx$ 90 L/h, plasma $\approx$ 50 L/h), the extent of first-pass metabolism is probably low. If CL_{oral} is higher than hepatic flow, it is likely that either first-pass loss or poor absorption or both contribute to the low systemic bioavailability. Intravenous administration of the drug and mass balance data are essential to further define the pharmacokinetics of the compound.

Thus, the extent of absorption may be estimated, but substantial caveats exist. The systemic bioavailability of a drug (F) is a composite product of f_{abs}, f_{gi}, f_h, and perhaps additional factors in some cases. Certain drugs are highly metabolized by enzymes within the gastrointestinal (GI) cells, particularly the metabolizing enzyme cytochrome P450 3A (CYP3A). Estimation of f_{gi} is not easily obtained. Determination of portal blood drug concentrations in hepatic transplant patients during the anhepatic phase have shown that for some drugs f_{gi} may be as important of a determinant of bioavailability as f_h. Absorption of these drugs, many of which are CYP3A substrates, may be affected by a carrier-mediated transporter composed of an ATP-dependent exsorptive system identified as the multidrug-resistant protein P-glycoprotein (Pgp) (8,9). This transporter returns absorbed drug back to the lumen, where the drug may be reabsorbed or excreted. If reabsorbed, the increase in GI tissue residence time provides additional opportunities for metabolism, which in turn affects f_{gi}.

Traditionally, the rate of absorption is characterized by the pharmacokinetic parameters peak concentration (C_{max}) and the time elapsed to C_{max} (T_{max}). Other approaches to characterize the rate of absorption have been suggested, most of which are deficient under certain conditions. In addition to having the dimension of a rate constant (h^{-1}), C_{max}/AUC takes into account differences in the extent of absorption (10). While the apparent absorption rate constant (k_a) can be estimated through modeling, it is a composite term that reflects the rate of systemic appearance of the drug and does not allow differentiation of the potentially complex rates of dissolution (k_{diss}), transit to the absorptive site (k_t) and absorption (k_{abs}). Additionally, modeling without IV data as a reference is subject to identifiability errors for cases in which k_a is comparable in magnitude to other processes of distribution or elimination. With IV reference data, simultaneous modeling and deconvolution techniques can characterize the rate of appearance of drug, but still do not necessarily distinguish absorption from other presystemic events. With controlled-release formulations where $k_{diss} < k_{abs}$, resolution is possible. In this case, extensive regulatory guidelines exist for *in vitro* (dissolution)/*in vivo* correlations.

Sources of interpatient differences in the rate and extent of absorption often vary on a case-by-case basis. For drugs that are slowly or incompletely absorbed, fundamental questions to be considered include: (a) the effect of GI pH on drug degradation, which may be affected by antacids or antisecretory drugs, (b) the effect of complexation or precipitation, (c) the effect of drugs that alter gastrointestinal motility such as prokinetic drugs or macrolides, and (d) disease states or physiological conditions that might affect absorption or GI transit.

C. Distribution

For many drugs, distribution of the drug throughout the body is essentially instantaneous. Conceptually, the entire body is contained within this compartment (one-compartment model), and the drug is dosed into and is eliminated from a single compartment. If a drug distributes immediately throughout a central compartment which is composed of blood and highly perfused organs such as the liver, and more slowly into a peripheral compartment such as adipose tissue, the disposition profile may be described with a two-compartment or other multicompartment model. The amount of drug administered and the apparent volume within which the drug distributes (volume of distribution, V) will determine the concentration of the drug within the systemic circulation. Although the blood volume is about 5 L in a typical adult (11), the apparent volume of distribution could be much greater due to the distribution of the drug into extracellular or intracellular fluid or into body tissue. If a drug distributes into an apparent volume of about 15 L, its distribution may be limited to extracellular fluid. Volumes of distribution larger than 15 L generally indicate intracellular partitioning and reflect the ratio of unbound drug in the intracellular and extracellular compartments

$$V = 7.5 + 7.5 \cdot f_u + 27 \cdot \left(\frac{f_u}{f_{uR}} \right) \tag{4}$$

where f_u is the fraction unbound in plasma and f_{uR} is the fraction unbound in tissue (12). If binding is similar for plasma and cellular components, the distribution volume may approximate body water (42 L). If tissue binding is high, such as for many basic, lipophilic drugs, distribution volumes of 1000 L or more can result (13). The distribution of a drug into tissues may vary widely, depending on the nature of tissue, but the distribution volume is strongly affected by the tissue to plasma (T/P) ratios of muscle and fat, which together comprise approximately half of total body weight.

D. Clearance

Expressed as volume/time, CL refers to the volume of plasma from which the drug is totally removed over a specified period of time. The total CL of a drug is a combination of individual clearances by any mechanism such as biotransformation, renal excretion, or biliary excretion. Clearance is one of the most important of the pharmacokinetic parameters because it determines the AUC for a given dose, and along with the distribution volume, determines the terminal-phase half-life. In particular, clearance provides significant insight when compared to the blood or plasma flow to the eliminating organs.

For renally eliminated drugs, the net plasma renal clearance,

$$CL_R = \frac{A_e}{\text{AUC}} \tag{5}$$

where A_e is the amount excreted unchanged, is the sum of glomerular filtration (maximum of 7.5 L/h, or 125 mL/min) and tubular secretion (maximum of around 40 L/h) minus the effect of reabsorption. The glomerular renal clearance of a drug is dependent on the product of the glomerular filtration rate (GFR) and f_u, whereas tubular secretion is dependent on total renal blood flow and the intrinsic clearance of the carrier protein. Tubular reabsorption is sensitive to luminal/plasma pH gradients for ionized drugs (*e.g.*, urine alkalization enhances elimination of weak acids), and is often affected by urinary flow rates (*e.g.*, low urinary output may enhance reabsorption). Drugs with significant secretion components ($CL_R > f_u \cdot$ GFR) may display nonlinear clearance and be subject to competitive inhibitory effects mediated at the same carrier (*e.g.*, cephalosporins and probenecid). For any drug in which CL_R is a significant component of total CL, the characterization of the pharmacokinetics in subjects or patients with various degrees of renal dysfunction is essential.

For drugs that are extensively metabolized, a number of models have been developed to predict the factors affecting CL. Of these, the well-stirred model is the most basic and widely used for conceptual purposes. Briefly, the CL of unbound drug after IV administration is dependent on two factors: blood flow rate to the liver and the intrinsic clearance of the eliminating enzymes:

$$\text{CL} = \frac{Q_h \cdot f_u \cdot \text{CL}_{int}}{(Q_h + f_u \cdot \text{CL}_{int})} \tag{6}$$

where Q_h is hepatic blood (or plasma) flow, f_u is the unbound fraction, and CL_{int} is the intrinsic clearance. The Michaelis-Menten equation describes CL_{int}:

$$\text{CL}_{int} = \frac{V_{max}}{C_s + K_m} \tag{7}$$

where V_{max} is the capacity of the enzyme (or carrier) system, C_s is the systemic concentration, and K_m is the Michaelis constant.

For drugs with low intrinsic clearance in which $f_u \cdot \text{CL}_{int} < Q_h$, first-pass hepatic metabolism is low after oral administration, and interpatient differences in clearance are mainly dependent on the level of expression of the enzyme (*i.e.*, CL $\sim f_u \cdot \text{CL}_{int}$). For drugs with high intrinsic clearance in which $f_u \cdot CL_{int} \gg Q_h$, first pass metabolism is extensive, and clearance is largely affected by hepatic blood flow (*i.e.*, CL $\sim Q_h$). The interpatient variability tends to be high for drugs with high intrinsic clearance because a number of factors affecting Q_h can affect first-pass and postabsorptive metabolism. For example, changes in posture, meals, and concomitant administration of certain other drugs can produce transient changes in Q_h by 50%.

E. Biotransformation

Screening of potential new drug candidates is now a multifaceted, interdisciplinary effort. An essential aspect of screening is the initial characterization of the enzymes involved in the clearance of extensively metabolized drugs. Knowledge of the cytochrome P450 (CYP) isoforms involved in the metabolism allows initial predictions of the potential for nonlinearity, high interpatient variability, and drug–drug interactions. CYP isoform identification commonly involves (a) correlation studies in which the rate of metabolism for the drug is regressed against the rate of metabolism for standard specific probe substrates in a library of human microsomes, (b) inhibitor studies in which specific inhibitors for the various isoforms are added to incubations of the probe substrate, (c) isoform-specific antibody studies, and (d) studies of the kinetics of oxidation of the drug using microsomes from cell lines that have been transfected with high levels of a specific human CYP isoform. Given comparable pharmacological, toxicological and pharmacokinetic characteristics, a drug with metabolism by multiple isoforms, or elimination by several routes, would typically be selected over a drug that depends on a single CYP isoform or route of elimination. Similarly, drugs with dominant metabolism by one of the genetically polymorphic enzymes have a higher risk factor for continued development.

In addition to identification of the isoform(s) involved in metabolism of the drug, the interaction potential of the new drug, including its effects on cosubstrates, and the effects of known inhibitors on the new drug candidate may be determined. From a simplistic approach, drugs with high affinity (low K_m) to a specific isoform have a high potential of being inhibitors of that isoform. Drugs with low affinity are prone to large effects from other drugs that are potent inhibitors of that isoform. With two-way interaction data *in vitro* with human microsomes or cDNA expressed systems, the qualitative spectrum of drug interactions may be estimated, and occasionally the estimates of the magnitudes of effects may be similar to observed clinical effects. With appropriate *in-vitro* information, and the knowledge of the drugs likely to be used concomitantly with the new drug, a rational program of drug–drug interaction studies can be devised.

In humans, seven isoforms account for most of the identified CYP-mediated metabolism: CYP1A2, CYP2A6, CYP2C8/9/10, CYP2C19, CYP2D6, CYP2E1, and CYP3A4 (14). It has been estimated that CYP3A is involved in the metabolism of more than 50% of the CYP-metabolized drugs in current use (15). The fraction of total P450 for the isoforms has been characterized in human microsomes as 30% CYP3A, 20% CYP2C, 13% CYP1A2, 7% CYP2E1, 4% CYP2A6, 1–5% CYP2D6, and <1% CYP2A6 (16).

The most abundant and voracious isozyme, CYP3A is capable of metabolizing a wide variety of substrates, including calcium channel antagonists, triazolobenzodiazepines, and numerous natural products. Although polymorphism for

CYP3A4 has not been demonstrated, it is highly variably ($>$10-fold) expressed across individuals, and is induced by dexamethasone, rifampicin, and several anticonvulsants (17). CYP3A is also present in several tissues, most notably intestine (18).

Because CYP3A metabolizes a large number of substrates, a new drug with dominant CYP3A metabolism may exhibit competitive inhibition. *In-vitro* experiments that define the drug as a strong inhibitor or easily affected by strong inhibitors are valuable information. Strong inhibitors of CYP3A include the azole antifungals, macrolides, and calcium channel antagonists. If the drug does not appear to be a likely inhibitor of other CYP3A substrates (*i.e.*, typical steady-state concentration $\ll K_i$ or IC_{50} for a probe substrate), then formal clinical interaction studies may be unnecessary. However, *in-vitro* to *in-vivo* extrapolation is generally only semiquantitative, and at least one confirmation of *in-vitro* results typically is necessary.

For a new drug that has a high fraction of total clearance by CYP3A metabolism, interactions with other drugs that are strong inhibitors of CYP3A would be expected. The magnitude and relevance of the interaction are difficult to predict, and typically require a clinical drug–drug interaction study. For example, for a drug with 40% CYP3A metabolism and a wide therapeutic index, 50% CYP3A inhibition (*i.e.*, an AUC increase of less than 30%) is not likely to achieve clinical relevance. While formal Phase I interaction studies can be conducted with strong inhibitors, another approach that is becoming increasingly utilized is population pharmacokinetic analyses of data obtained from Phase III studies.

CYP2D6 is polymorphic, but most people have the extensive metabolizer (EM) phenotype. Approximately 8% of the Caucasian population have the poor metabolizer (PM) phenotype of CYP2D6 (19). The PM phenotype is more rare in African-Americans (20–22), Spanish (23), Turkish (24), and Saudi Arabian populations (25), with the lowest prevalence among Orientals ($\sim$1%) (26). A small fraction of the population are very rapid metabolizers, apparently because of gene amplification (27) or duplication (28). Induction of CYP2D6 activity has not been demonstrated. CYP2D6 has relatively well-defined requirements for substrates: an extended hydrophobic region and a positively charged basic nitrogen positioned from 5 to 7 Å from the site of oxidation (29,30). Quinidine, fluoxetine, norfluoxetine, and paroxetine are potent inhibitors of CYP2D6, and can confer PM status to extensive metabolizers (31–38).

For drugs that are extensively metabolized by CYP2D6, there is often high interpatient variability in the pharmacokinetics. The high variability is due in part to polymorphism of the isozyme, but other aspects, such as the overall low level of expression of this enzyme resulting in a low V_{max}, also contribute to high variability. For some substrates of CYP2D6, the binding affinity can be quite high with a low capacity, potentially resulting in nonlinear pharmacokinetics. Also, because many agonists and antagonists of biogenic amines have a basic nitrogen with oxidizable functional groups at the requisite distance, a variety of psychotropic and cardiovascular drugs are substrates of CYP2D6.

In the selection of drug candidates for development, extensive metabolism by CYP2D6 is generally viewed as a liability. Genotyping or phenotyping patients prior to treatment may be required. Accordingly, evidence of partial metabolism (>50%) by other enzymes (CYP1A2, CYP3A) or glucuronidation is adequate for advancement of a candidate to clinical status. Even if a drug candidate is partially metabolized by CYP2D6 and K_m or K_i are 0.1 µM or higher (compared to typical concentrations of less than 0.1 µM), the predictability of *in-vivo* interactions based on *in-vitro* data generally is poor. The reasons for the low predictability are not entirely clear; however, the tissue-to-plasma ratios for these drugs tend to be high (>5), and plasma concentration-to-K_i ratios (C_p/K_i) tend to underestimate the magnitude of interactions *in vivo*.

The CYP2C family comprises CYP2C8, CYP2C9, CYP2C10, and CYP2C19 (CYP2C$_{mp}$). The most information is available for CYP2C9 and CYP2C19. Phenytoin, hexibarbital, and S-warfarin are well-known substrates of CYP2C9 (39), which appears to be inducible. One of the most noteworthy substrates of the CYP2C19 isoform is S-mephenytoin, which is used for phenotyping (40). CYP2C19 also oxidizes the proton pump inhibitors (*e.g.*, omeprazole and lansoprazole), and diazepam (41–43). The enzyme is polymorphically expressed, with the PM phenotype being more prevalent in Orientals (~20%) than in Caucasians (<5%) (42). A small portion (less than 1%) of the population may be deficient in this isoform.

CYP2E1 oxidizes a limited number of small substrates (*e.g.*, acetaminophen, chlorzoxazone, and volatile anesthetics), and has been widely studied in relationship to toxic metabolites and alcoholism (44,45). CYP2E1 is inducible by ethanol, which could lead to an increase in the metabolism of drugs that are metabolized at least in part by CYP2E1 (46). In addition, isoniazid can change CYP2E1 activity (47).

CYP2A6 is best known for its role in the metabolism of coumarin, and CYP2A6 is one of several enzymes capable of converting nicotine to cotinine. Expression of the enzyme is low and genetic polymorphism has been described, with approximately 2–5% deficient alleles (48). The enzyme is inhibited by several compounds, including imidazole antifungals, methoxsalen, and pilocarpine (49).

The CYP1A family consists of CYP1A1 and CYP1A2. CYP1A1 is expressed in extrahepatic tissues, notably lung, lymphocytes, and placenta. CYP1A2 substrates are typically planar aromatics, including antipyrine (50), acetaminophen (51), tacrine (52), clozapine (53,54), theophylline (55), and caffeine (55). CYP1A2-mediated oxidation is a minor pathway in the metabolism of many other drugs, and this isoform is inhibited by fluvoxamine (56). CYP1A2 is easily inducible, and induction has been associated with carcinogen activation.

Potent inducers of this isoform are typically small planar aromatics. Most substrates with significant CYP1A2 metabolism also have relatively large differences (typically two-fold) in CL between people who smoke and those who do not. Thus, evaluation of the effect of smoking on CL is standard for any drug with substantial elimination by CYP1A2. For theophylline, interpatient differences in clearance by CYP1A2 appear to be affected by numerous factors related to diet, including protein content, caloric content, and intake of cruciferous vegetables and charbroiled meats.

Although glucuronidation by glucuronosyl transferases (GTs) is often a secondary metabolic pathway for elimination of oxidation products, there are a large number of drugs that are directly conjugated (57). The most common substrates are carboxylic acids (*e.g.*, valproic acid and nonsteroidal anti-inflammatory drugs), and hydroxy-substituted drugs such as alcohols and phenols (*e.g.*, morphine, propranolol, steroids). Tertiary amines (*e.g.*, imipramine, amitriptyline) and aromatic amines (*e.g.*, nicotine, lamotrigine) are also directly conjugated. Compared with CYP isozymes, less information is available about the substrate specificity of the human GTs, and predictions of pharmacokinetic consequences of GT metabolism based on *in-vitro* data are rarely accurate.

There are three major GT gene families, of which two—UGT1A and UGT2B—are the most frequently involved in drug elimination. Nine human GTs have been cloned, and there is considerable overlap of substrate specificity. Within the two families, three isozymes are the most frequently involved in glucuronidation: UGT1A4 (conjugation of amines), UGT1A7 (flavonoids, β-blockers, propofol), and UGT2B7 (valproate, NSAIDS, morphine). The genes are independently regulated, but several drugs that induce CYP isoforms also increase the activity of GTs. At least two inborn errors, Crigler-Najar disease and Gilbert's syndrome, result from conjugative defects. The latter is fairly common (5–12%), but the kinetic consequences for drugs that are conjugated are not well characterized.

Conjugation by GTs presents several pharmacokinetic challenges in drug development. For drugs forming glucuronides, animal data may reflect a high degree of enterohepatic recycling (ER), particularly for the rat. Unfortunately, data in animals may not be relevant to humans, and estimation of the extent of ER in humans is formidable. Often, secondary peaks in the plasma concentration-versus-time profile accompanied by recovery of unchanged parent drug in feces is indicative of ER. Pharmacokinetic modeling of ER in some cases may provide estimates of the degree of ER. Unrecognized extensive ER can result in substantial errors for prediction of the extent of first-pass metabolism based on oral clearances using the well-stirred model. In some cases, the glucuronides are unstable at physiological pH.

In addition to the extent of glucuronidation, predictions of drug interactions based on *in-vitro* or animal data are difficult for GT substrates. For example, co-administration of valproate (UGT2B7) can decrease the clearance of several compounds conjugated by the same or even different isoforms, such as lorazepam (presumptively, UGT2B7), lamotrigine (UGT1A4), and zidovudine (unknown). However, valproate has no effect on some other conjugated substrates such as acetaminophen (UGT1A6). Although competitive inhibitory effects are certainly a likely mechanism for interaction, transient depletion of UDP-glucuronic acid also is a possibility.

F. Pharmacodynamics

While pharmacokinetics describe the processes and rates of drug movement from the site of absorption into the blood, distribution into the tissues, and elimination by biotransformation or excretion, pharmacodynamics describes the drug effects once it has reached the site of action (58). Typically, pharmacodynamics are described by the parameters estimated from a mathematical model which may have a biological or empirical basis. Pharmacokinetics and pharmacodynamics are often modeled simultaneously because estimation of pharmacodynamic parameters using observations of drug effects *in vivo* requires a description of drug concentrations at the time of the effect. A commonly used pharmacodynamic model is the E_{max} (or sigmoid E_{max}) model. Concentration is the link between the pharmacokinetic model (PK), relating dose to concentration, and the pharmacodynamic model (PD), relating concentration to effect.

For drugs that cause an effect that is easily measured (*e.g.*, change in blood pressure), PK/PD modeling can provide insight to various factors influencing the effects. Once the concentration–effect relationship has been defined, pharmacokinetic changes can be used to predict the change in intensity of a specific therapeutic effect or adverse event. Predictions based on pharmacokinetic changes can help optimize experimental designs and potentially can reduce the number of studies conducted to improve the speed of drug development. In addition, the results of PK/PD modeling can help to chose an appropriate dosage form and regimen with respect to both efficacy and safety (59). Unfortunately, for many drugs (*e.g.*, anticancer drugs), PK/PD modeling is difficult at best because of the nature of the efficacy data. However, PK/PD modeling of toxicity data may be useful.

III. CLINICAL PHARMACOKINETIC STUDIES DURING DRUG DEVELOPMENT

Clinical drug development follows a sequential process, with preapproval segments Phase I–III and a postapproval segment Phase IV. The definitions of the three preapproval phases have relatively clear separations. However, the different phases refer to different types of studies rather than a specific time course of studies. For example, bioequivalence studies or drug–drug interaction studies are both Phase I studies, but they may be conducted after Phase III studies have been initiated. The generalized sequence of studies may be tailored to each new drug during development. Regulatory agencies have specific guidelines for the format and content of the clinical pharmacokinetics and bioavailability section of a New Drug Application (NDA). The pharmacokinetic section of a NDA typically contains information pertaining to the following:

Metabolism
Protein binding
Formulation
In-vitro testing methodology
Analytical methodology
Bioavailability/bioequivalence information (including food effects)
Pharmacokinetic parameter estimates
Dose proportionality
Special populations
Drug–drug interactions
PK/PD relationships
Population PK/PD analyses
Support of labeling

A. Phase I

New drugs should be studied in people as early as safety allows. The initial introduction of a new drug into subjects are the first Phase I studies. These studies are closely monitored, typically conducted in healthy adult men, and are designed to obtain information on the safety, pharmacokinetics, and pharmacological effects of the drug. In addition, the metabolic profile, adverse events associated with increasing doses, and evidence of efficacy may be obtained. The primary goal of Phase I studies is to demonstrate safety in humans while collecting sufficient pharmacokinetic and pharmacological information to permit the determination of the dosage strength and regimen for Phase II studies. Because most compounds are available for initial studies as an oral formulation, the initial pharmacokinetic profile usually includes information about the absorption phase. Additional studies, such as drug–drug interactions, assessment of bioequivalence of various formulations, or other studies involving normal subjects are included in Phase I.

Generally, the first study in humans is a rising, single-dose tolerance study. The initial dose may be based on animal pharmacology data, such as 10% of the no-effect dose. Doses are increased gradually according to a predetermined scheme, often some modification of the Fibonacci dose escalation scheme (60), until an adverse event is observed which satisfies the predetermined criteria of a maximum tolerated dose (MTD). While the primary objective is the determination of acute safety in humans, the studies are designed to collect meaningful pharmacokinetic information. Efficacy information or surrogate efficacy measurements also may be collected. However, because a multitude of clinical measurements and tests must be collected to demonstrate safety, measurements of efficacy parameters must not compromise the collection of safety and pharmacokinetic data.

Appropriate biological samples for pharmacokinetic assessment, typically blood and urine, should be collected at discrete time intervals based on extrapolations from the pharmacokinetics of the drug in animals. Depending on the assay sensitivity, the half-life and other pharmacokinetic parameters in healthy volunteers should be evaluable, particularly at the higher doses. The degree of exposure of the drug is an important factor in understanding the toxicological results of the study. Pharmacokinetic linearity (dose linearity) or nonlinearity will be an important factor in the design of future studies.

Once the initial dose has been determined, a placebo-controlled, double-blind, escalating single-dose study is initiated. Generally, healthy male volunteers are recruited, although patients sometimes are utilized (*e.g.*, in testing a potential anticancer drug which may be too toxic to be administered to healthy volunteers). These studies may include two or three cohorts of six or eight subjects receiving the active drug and two subjects receiving placebo. The groups may receive alternating dose levels which allows assessment of dose linearity, intrasubject variability of pharmacokinetics, and dose response (*i.e.*, adverse events) relationship within individual subjects.

Participants in the first study are hospitalized or institutionalized so that clinical measurements can be performed under controlled conditions and any medical emergency can be handled in the most expeditious manner. The study is placebo-controlled and double-blind so that the drug effects (*e.g.*, drug-induced ataxia) can be distinguished from the non-drug effects (*e.g.*, ataxia secondary to viral infection). The first study in humans should not be considered successfully completed until an MTD has been reached, because the relationship between a clinical event (*e.g.*, emesis) and a particular dose level observed under controlled conditions could be extremely useful information for the design of future trials. Also, the dose range and route of administration should be established in Phase I studies.

A multidose safety study typically follows completion of the first study in humans. The primary goal of the second study is to define an MTD with multidosing prior to the initiation of well-controlled efficacy testing. The study design of the multidose safety study should simulate actual clinical conditions in as many ways as possible; however, scientific and statistical validity must be maintained.

The inclusion of a placebo group is essential to allow the determination of drug-related versus non-drug-related events. The dosing schedule, including dosages, frequency, dose escalations, and dose tapering should simulate the regimen to be followed in efficacy testing.

Typically, dosing in the second study lasts for a minimum of 2 weeks. The length of the study may be increased depending on the pharmacokinetics of the drug so that both drug and metabolite concentrations reach steady state. Also, if the drug is to be used to treat a chronic condition, a study duration of 4 weeks may be appropriate. To obtain information for six dose levels with six subjects receiving active drug and two receiving placebo for each of two cohorts, a minimum of 24 subjects would be anticipated to be enrolled. Similar to the first study in humans, these subjects would be institutionalized for the duration of the study.

Also similar to the first study, obtaining pharmacokinetic data is an important objective, because these data will be used to help design dosage regimens in future efficacy trials. The new pharmacokinetic information that can be gathered includes: (a) whether the pharmacokinetic parameters obtained in the previous acute safety study accurately predicted the multidose pharmacokinetic behavior of the drug, (b) verification of pharmacokinetic linearity (*i.e.*, dose proportionality of C_{max} and AUC) observed in the acute study, (c) whether the drug is subject to autoinduction of clearance upon multidosing, and (d) the existence and accumulation of metabolites that could not be detected in the previous single-dose study. A number of experimental approaches can be utilized to gather this information, and all require frequent collection of blood and urine samples. The challenge to the clinical pharmacokineticist is to design an appropriate blood sample collection schedule to maximize the pharmacokinetic information that can be gathered without biasing the primary objective—determination of safety parameters.

B. Phase II

After the initial introduction of a new drug into humans, Phase II studies focus on efficacy while using the pharmacokinetic information obtained in Phase I studies to optimize the dosage regimen. Phase II studies are not as closely monitored as Phase I studies, and are conducted in patients. These studies are designed to obtain information on the efficacy and pharmacological effects of the drug in addition to the pharmacokinetics. Additional pharmacokinetic and pharmacological information collected in Phase II studies may help to optimization the dosage strength and regimen, and may provide additional information on the drug's safety profile (*e.g.*, determine potential drug–drug interactions).

Efficacy trials of the drug should not to be initiated until the MTD has been defined. In addition, the availability of pharmacokinetic information in healthy volunteers is key to the design of successful efficacy trials. The clinical pharmacokineticist assists in the design and execution of these trials in addition to analyzing the plasma drug concentration data upon the completion of the efficacy studies.

During the planning stage of an efficacy trial, the focus of the clinical pharmacokineticist is the dosage regimen and its relationship to efficacy measurements. Based on the mathematical model derived from the first two studies in humans, the pharmacokineticist can simulate plasma drug concentrations for various dosage regiments. The disease and/or physiological states of the test patients (*e.g.*, organ dysfunction as a function of age), concurrent medications (*e.g.*, enzyme inducers or inhibitors), and the safety data obtained earlier must be taken into consideration before arriving at an optimal regimen for inclusion in the protocol. In addition, if the targeted site of the drug is in a tissue compartment, the clinical pharmacokineticist can simulate theoretical drug levels in this compartment and recommend appropriate times for efficacy measurements.

During the execution of the study, the services of a clinical pharmacokineticist can be especially useful when serious adverse experiences occur. A clear understanding of the pharmacokinetics of the drug definitely helps in tackling overdose cases with respect to the selection of a remedy. Furthermore, plasma drug level data in combination with pharmacodynamic information sometimes may allow the distinction of whether an unusual response to the drug has a pharmacokinetic versus a pharmacodynamic basis. For drugs with narrow therapeutic margins such as antiarrhythmics, therapeutic drug monitoring by a clinical pharmacokineticist will increase the safety of the patients during efficacy trials. Therapeutic drug monitoring becomes even more important if there exists the possibility of a toxic metabolite.

Upon completion of the efficacy trial, the clinical pharmacokineticist can define a therapeutic window in terms of plasma drug levels by reviewing the correlation between plasma drug concentrations and key safety and efficacy parameters. The goal is to improve efficacy and safety of the drug by individualization of dosage regimen, based on previous plasma drug concentrations in the same patient.

1. Clinical Pharmacokinetic Studies to Evaluate Drug Formulations

For the clinical development program of an oral drug, the drug can only be evaluated in patients as a formulation containing several other excipients. A vehicle must be developed for the delivery of the drug, and hence the drug generally is formulated as a solution or an immediate-release tablet or capsule. Furthermore, the original formulation used in clinical trials often will not be selected for marketing for a variety of reasons. The justifications for developing a new formulation for marketing are many and may include the need for a more stable product (*i.e.*, a longer shelf life), minimization of production cost via streamlining the manufacturing processes, portability of the medication by patients, patient acceptance of the formulation as revealed by marketing surveys, and specially shaped tablets (*e.g.*, to identify an innovator's compound from a generic formulation).

A bioequivalence study is the key to applying data collected in clinical trials that utilized the original formulation to the new formulation. While the desirable outcome of efficacy trials is to find a statistically significant difference (*i.e.*, to find the drug superior to placebo), the desirable outcome of a bioequivalence study is the lack of difference between two formulations. If the new formulation delivers to the systemic circulation the same amount of drug as the original formulation, the new formulation should elicit the same clinical response. Bioequivalence studies generally are conducted in healthy volunteers because of the extensive sampling regimen, but there is no specific reason that patients could not be included. The studies can follow an open-label, crossover, single-dose design.

Although the data of bioequivalence studies continues to be analyzed by analysis of variance (ANOVA), confidence-interval techniques for C_{max} and $AUC_{0-\infty}$ are the primary parameters used to test for bioequivalence. In addition, failing to demonstrate a difference between formulations is not the same as demonstrating that they are the same. Bioequivalence is achieved when the confidence intervals for C_{max} and AUC are between 0.8 and 1.25, and there is at least an 80% chance of detecting a 20% difference. For most drugs, 18 to 36 subjects are adequate. Relatively simple methods to determine sample size for bioequivalence studies exist (61), but an estimate of intrasubject variability is required. Data from the first two studies in which at least two cohorts of subjects were included may be used to estimate the intrasubject variability. A four-way crossover study may be required to determine bioequivalence for highly variable drugs (62).

IV. SOURCES OF PHARMACOKINETIC VARIABILITY

In the application packages submitted to regulatory agencies, certain pharmacokinetic data are required, and serve as the foundation for product labeling. Characterization of the sources of variability in the pharmacokinetics should be detailed, which most often requires elucidation of the factors affecting interpatient differences in both CL and response (desired and undesired). Even for identical doses of a drug within a group of individuals, large differences in pharmacological response may occur. Interindividual variability in the response may be due either to differences in effect produced by a given drug concentration (pharmacodynamic variability) or differences in the drug concentration produced by a given dose (pharmacokinetic variability).

Traditionally, the pharmacodynamic variability of most drugs was assumed to be low, and variability in effect was assumed to be related to high pharmacokinetic variability, particularly for compounds with nonlinear pharmacokinetics or high first-pass metabolism. This hypothesis led to many concentration-controlled trials with dosage alterations based on Bayesian forecasting algorithms. Unfortunately, the results were generally not encouraging, often because of the high intrapatient variability which defeated the feedback controls and high interpatient variability in response to a given concentration. In fact, it is often the pharmacodynamic response that is highly variable, as demonstrated by Levy, who found in a survey of a number of drugs across several therapeutic classes that variability in EC_{50} was 10-fold or greater (63).

A major challenge to predicting interpatient variability is that drug concentration only predicts 20% or less of the variability in response. The reasons for poor predictability are numerous and often obscure. Many physiological or disease states are multifactorial, and drugs with high specificity for one enzyme or receptor may have limited effect due to differences in expression of the target receptor. In certain serious indications, such as some infections, the drug may be administered at high dosages to ensure that average concentrations greatly exceed the EC_{95} (effective concentration in 95% of the organisms). Thus, individuals with a high drug clearance are given the best opportunity for successful treatment. For the treatment of HIV infection, in which viral turnover is extraordinarily high (10^{10}/day) and mutation is frequent, even the EC_{95} goal may be inadequate, as is demonstrated by the current use of multiple drugs with different mechanisms of action to treat this disease.

Pharmacokinetic variability is often more easily characterized than pharmacodynamic variability, because pharmacokinetic variability is usually dependent on a variety of identifiable factors, including demographics, disease states, drug–drug interactions, environmental components, and genetics.

A. Demographics

1. Body Size and Composition

Several factors relating to body size and composition often affect clearance and apparent distribution volume (hence half-life) of a drug. Weight, gender, and age are often confounded because early pharmacokinetic studies during drug development generally require a narrow age range of subjects, exclude women, and stipulate that subjects have a body size within $\pm 10\%$ of their ideal body weight based on their height. Population pharmacokinetic analysis of data from Phase III studies which include women can be a powerful source of information because the number of patients studied is much greater and the ranges in body size and age are larger than in previous studies.

Body size is often correlated with drug CL because CL is often correlated with liver size, which is related to overall metabolic capacity. The relationship between CL and body weight is often nonlinear, but may be proportional to weight raised to a fractional power. With large data sets, lean body mass (LBM) or body surface area (BSA) may be better predictors of interpatient differences in clearance than weight. Typically, dosage adjustments due to body size are unnecessary except for children and for unusually small or obese adults. Because body surface area may be a more accurate indicator of organ size and function (*i.e.*, cardiac output, glomerular filtration rate, and hepatic metabolic ability), estimates of the dosages for children may be based on the recommended adult dose, corrected for body surface area differences.

The volume of both total body water and extracellular fluid in adults with average body size is directly proportional to body weight. Thus, there is a relationship between the apparent volume of distribution and body weight, particularly for drugs with low protein or tissue binding. If both clearance and distribution volume are directly dependent on weight, then half-life would be independent of body size. However, this relationship also may be nonlinear, and log(CL) is often more highly correlated with weight than untransformed CL. For drugs that have greater distribution into adipose than muscle, differences in the amount of adipose tissue may affect the distribution volume. If the tissue/plasma ratio for muscle is greater than that for fat, men may have a larger distribution volume per unit weight than women, and women may have higher maximum concentration values but shorter half-lives for equal clearances.

2. Gender

Although gender-dependent differences in the pharmacokinetics of many drugs have been demonstrated, these differences are often minor. The recent review by Harris et al. provides comprehensive details (64). Apparent gender differences in clearance are usually not as pronounced when corrected for weight or BSA differences. However, for some drugs, relatively small mean differences in plasma concentrations can mask large differences for some individuals, thus understating the individual effect on efficacy or toxicity. There is no *a-priori* basis for the assumption that pharmacological effects would be the same in men and women.

The sources of nonanthropometric differences due to gender are diverse, ranging from absorptive effects attributed to differences in gastric secretion and gastrointestinal motility (65,66) to effects of estrogen on metabolic activity (67–70). In addition, the inhibitory effect of ethinylestradiol on CYP3A and CYP1A2 activity (17) demonstrate the potential importance of obtaining information about the effects of menopause and the use of oral contraceptives for population pharmacokinetic analysis. Thus, while early Phase I and sometimes Phase II studies typically have been conducted with young healthy men, women are being included in studies sooner for drugs intended for use in both men and women.

3. Race

The effects of race on pharmacokinetics and pharmacodynamics should be assessed for new drugs, particularly for those that are metabolized by the polymorphic CYP isoforms. Differences in clearance may be associated with race. Population pharmacokinetic analysis may be the best method to study the effects of race, assuming a database of a large number of patients of various races exists, allowing comparison among groups other than Caucasian and African-American. Particularly now that new drugs may be developed globally, differences between Caucasians and other races should be evaluated. For example, the frequency of CYP2D6 deactivating mutations is greatest in Caucasians, whereas Orientals have a higher fraction of CYP2C19 PMs compared to other races. Other than genetic effects, unexpected apparent interracial differences may be a secondary result from lifestyle and diet.

4. Age

In the past, new drugs were studied almost exclusively in adults due to safety concerns. Today, there is increased emphasis by regulatory agencies on the collection of pharmacokinetic information for children and elderly populations. Again, due to safety concerns, it is vitally important to combine the pharmacokinetic information obtained for adults with the knowledge of the potential age-dependent changes in the pharmacokinetics of individual drugs to chose an effective and safe dosage for children and elderly. Age-dependent changes in pharmacokinetics may be the most complex source of variability. The functioning of many different organs may change with age. Also, protein binding, percent lean body mass, volume of extracellular fluid, and other characteristics of individuals may change with age.

In general, renal function is lower in neonates and the elderly compared with young adults. Similarly, hepatic function typically is lowest in newborns, improves with age (most efficient in children and young adults), and declines during aging (71). In addition, phase I reactions (*e.g.*, oxidation) generally occur at a slower rate in newborn as compared to adults; cytochrome P450, NADPH, and cytochrome c reductase activities are approximately one-half the adult values (72).

Unfortunately, the heterogeneity of the CYP system precludes the use of total CYP enzyme content as a meaningful predictor of the rate at which an individual substrate is metabolized. Both the absolute amount and the relative proportion of different isozymes may be age-dependent. The fact that enzymatic activities involving various substrates are influenced by gestational age to different extents and follow different maturational patterns (73) may be due to age-dependent changes in isozymes as opposed to total CYP content.

Although information in humans regarding age-dependent changes in specific isozymes is limited, the CYP3A subfamily changes substantially as a function of gestational age. The predominant prenatal isoform is CYP3A7. In the perinatal period, expression of this isoform declines with concurrent appearance of CYP3A4. The overall metabolic capacity increases in the early neonatal period, although longitudinal data are lacking to characterize the time course and variability thereof. CYP3A7 constructs (*e.g.*, lymphoblastoid microsomal preparations) are not currently commercially available to allow determination of the catalytic spectrum and affinity of CYP3A7 relative to CYP3A4. Age-dependent metabolism *in vivo* is complicated further by the fact that the rate of biotransformation is affected not only by enzyme activity but also by factors such as hepatic blood flow and the degree of protein binding (74). In addition, age-dependent changes in endogenous compounds such as free fatty acids (75) and dietary differences may affect metabolism.

As an example of age-dependent change in pharmacokinetics, the mean half-life of diazepam varies from 55 ± 35 h in premature newborns to 31 ± 2 h in full-term newborns, 10 ± 2 h in infants, 17 ± 3 h in children, and 24 ± 12 h in young adults (76). However, because diazepam is metabolized by both CYP2C19 and CYP3A, extrapolations from these data should be guarded, particularly since half-lives reflect both intrinsic clearance and distributional differences. Phenobarbital shows similar changes, with a serum half-life ranging from 234 ± 43 h in premature newborns to 146 ± 23 h in full-term newborns, 58 ± 7 h in infants, 37–73 h in children (data from separate studies), and 132 ± 18 h in adults (76,77). The CYP isoforms involved in the metabolism of phenobarbital are unknown, and transintestinal elimination appears to contribute substantially to the overall clearance.

Another example of age-dependent change in the rate of metabolism is the change in clearance of phenytoin. Larger dosage on a body-weight basis for pediatric patients compared with that for adults are required for phenytion (78). *In vivo* estimates of the Michaelis-Menten parameters have shown that while V_{max} is not influenced by age, K_m values in children less than 15 years of age are 43% less than those of older patients (79). A similar increased rate of metabolism in childhood compared with both neonatal and adult rates requiring dosage adjustments also has been described for carbamazepine and ethosuximide (74). However, these apparent differences may be an artifact originating with the assumption that clearance is directly proportional to total body weight.

Clearly, changes in the rate of metabolism of some compounds may be altered during development. Oxidative metabolism of several drugs has been shown to decline (*e.g.*, antipyrine, quinidine, nortriptyline, and verapamil) or remain relatively constant (*e.g.*, acetanilide, digitoxin, midazolam, prazosin, warfarin) during aging (80–82). A reduced rate of oxidative metabolism during aging has been reported for various anticonvulsants, including benzodiazepines, diazepam, chlordiazepoxide, desmethyldiazepam, desalkylflurazepam, alprazolam, and clobazam (83). Providing further evidence that hepatic enzymatic activity may be not only age-dependent but also isozyme-dependent, enzyme induction has been shown to decrease (80,82) or remain relatively constant with age (81). In general, the rate of biotransformation (*i.e.*, oxidative metabolism) increases during development, reaching peak rates that may be higher than those observed in mature adults, then declines during aging.

Age-dependent changes in protein binding may affect the pharmacokinetics of a drug. In elderly patients with hypoalbuminemia, systemic phenytoin clearance may be accelerated due to the lower degree of plasma protein binding, which facilitates hepatic uptake (84). In contrast, reduction in the intrinsic clearance of valproate in the elderly may result in higher unbound serum valproate concentrations in the elderly compared to young subjects given equivalent doses. However, the total concentrations of valproate in serum may not differ in the two groups because of the concurrent reduction in valproate binding to serum proteins in the elderly (74).

While similarities in the age-dependent changes in the rate of metabolism by phase I and phase II reactions exists, phase II reactions (*e.g.*, conjugation, such as glucuronidation) are generally more compound-specific. Many phase II reactions occur at a slower rate in newborn humans (particularly premature neonates) compared with adults (74,78). During development, the enzyme systems responsible for conjugation mature at different rates—more slowly for glucuronide conjugation compared with other pathways such as sulfate conjugation. Development of the glucuronidation capacity varies depending on the substrate being investigated because of the heterogeneity of the GTs (83). However, adult values of glucuronidation activity usually are reached within 3 years of age (74).

Information on the rate of phase II reactions in the elderly human is limited. Aging, however, seems to affect the rate of glucuronidation much less than the rate of oxidation. The elimination of compounds that are primarily glucuronidated (*e.g.*, oxazepam, lorazepam, and temazepam) is not much different in the elderly compared with the young adult (80,81). High compound specificity and extensive variability in age-dependent changes in the rate of glucuronidation make it difficult to predict age-dependent changes in the rate of conjugation of a new drug.

The significance of these observations is that clearance in neonates and children or clearance in the elderly are not always prospectively predictable based on adult values. A pharmacokinetic study must be conducted to characterize age-related differences if the drug is to be used in these populations. The traditional approach to detect age-related pharmacokinetic differences is to conduct a single-dose pharmacokinetic study with tight inclusion and exclusion criteria in age groups. Often, specific studies are not conducted, and data from Phase I and II studies are compared after categorizing by young and old. Because a large number of patients over a range of ages are enrolled in Phase III efficacy studies, population pharmacokinetic analysis may be a more efficient tool to study the effect of age on pharmacokinetics.

Both approaches have their respective merits, and the selection of a particular approach will depend on the drug being developed and the overall strategy. Obviously, the success of the hypothesis-testing approach depends on the accuracy in predicting specific problems that might or might not occur in geriatric patients, whereas the success of the pharmacokinetic screen usually depends on the sample size of each subgroup, since statistical power is needed to support any meaningful statement for the package insert.

For pediatric patients, defining age-related differences in pharmacokinetics is more problematic than for elderly patients. While similar reasoning can be evoked in the design of clinical studies with pharmacokinetic components in pediatric patients, ethical concerns should carry more weight, because minors legally cannot give written informed consent for themselves. Thus, pharmacokinetic studies in healthy pediatric volunteers are unusual, but studies in pediatric patients can provide invaluable pharmacokinetic information.

5. Disease States

The two standard approaches to evaluating the effects of disease states on the pharmacokinetics of a new drug are controlled Phase I evaluations, and Phase II–III population pharmacokinetic approaches. The latter has the benefit of greater heterogeneity as well as reflecting actual usage in the target population. Drug disposition may be altered in many disease states, particularly renal or hepatic diseases for drugs that are primarily eliminated by those routes.

Dysfunction of the major organs of drug elimination may lead to reduced drug clearance and increased $t_{1/2}$. If clearance is reduced with no change in the volume of distribution, the dose may be similar to that of a healthy person, but the interval between doses may be increased to provide similar systemic exposure while preventing accumulation of the drug to toxic concentrations. Thus, the pharmacokinetics of new drugs often are determined in patients with renal or hepatic impairment. The design of these studies is dependent on the sources of clearance and routes of elimination of the drug.

The typical study conducted to assess the effects of renal impairment on the pharmacokinetics of the drug includes subjects with end-stage renal disease who require hemodialysis, subjects with various levels of renal function, and subjects with normal renal function. Because subjects who require hemodialysis have virtually no renal function, interpatient variability should be relatively low and meaningful information can be obtained from a few (4–6) subjects. Information on the ability of hemodialysis to remove the drug from the subjects also can be obtained from end-stage renal failure subjects, and may prove beneficial in the management of overdoses.

End-stage renal-failure subjects represent the worst possible case of renal dysfunction, and it can be assumed that all other subjects with renal impairment will fall between the subjects with normal renal function and those with end-stage disease. Depending on the therapeutic index of the drug, the duration of therapy, and the magnitude of the difference between subjects with normal renal function and those with end-stage renal disease, data from the subjects with end-stage renal disease may be adequate to describe the effects of renal function on the pharmacokinetics of the drug.

For most drugs with renal-dependent elimination, it is necessary to study the pharmacokinetics of the drug in subjects with various degrees of renal function. Because of the large potential for intersubject variability, it is necessary to study a greater number of subjects than in the previously mentioned study; however, it is often easier to obtain these subjects than it is to obtain subjects with total renal failure. When the relationship between renal function and clearance of the drug is known, dosing nomograms or guidelines can be established to ensure safe usage of the drug in patients with renal disease.

One of the major problems in studying subjects with mild to moderate renal failure is in determining accurately the level of renal function. Creatinine is produced by muscle tissue at a fairly constant rate, and is filtered by the glomerulus but neither secreted nor reabsorbed in the renal tubule. Thus, creatinine clearance is a reflection of the glomerular filtration rate. To determine creatinine clearance accurately, it is necessary to collect all urine formed over a given time interval (usually 24h) to determine the amount of creatinine excreted during the interval. It also is necessary to determine the serum creatinine concentration at some time point during the interval. Creatinine clearance is defined as the ratio of the amount of creatinine in the urine to the concentration of creatinine in the serum adjusted for the time of the urine collection and the units of measurement so that the result can be expressed as milliliters per minute.

Methods of estimating creatinine clearance based on the patient's age, weight, height, gender, and serum creatinine concentration (85–88) have been developed because timed urine collections are difficult to obtain. Implicit in all of these methods of estimation of creatinine clearance is that the rate of creatinine formation is a function only of muscle mass, and that muscle mass can be determined from the more readily measured variables of age, weight, height, and gender. It has been demonstrated that these methods of estimation of creatinine clearance tend to be inaccurate when the patient's actual weight differs significantly from his or her ideal weight. Thus, the usefulness of creatinine clearance as an indicator of renal function is only as good as the assessment of creatinine clearance.

In contrast to renal dysfunction, it remains difficult to apply the results of a well-controlled pharmacokinetic study in patients with liver dysfunction to design dosage regimens without collecting some efficacy and safety information in the same subpopulation. Although there is a wealth of information about the influence of hepatic disease and impairment on drug disposition (89), hepatic diseases (including cirrhosis, acute viral hepatitis, chronic active hepatitis, fibrosis, tumor, and fatty liver) are heterogeneous. Regardless of the etiology, they can affect other vital organs and, hence, affect both the pharmacokinetics and pharmacodynamics of a drug. In addition, biotransformation of foreign compounds by the liver is an extremely complex process—one that can be impacted by both changes in physiological variables such as hepatic blood flow and cardiac output and biochemical variables such as effect of liver disease on the activity of different CYP enzymes and other proteins produced in the liver. An additional complication is that the correlation between common blood chemistry tests such as serum bilirubin concentration and pharmacokinetics of model drugs such as antipyrine is sporadic at best, often depending on the stage of the disease.

The effect of hepatic disease or impairment is not consistent and can have highly variable, sometimes opposite, effects on the plasma concentrations of the drug and its active metabolites. As a result, the efficacy and safety of a drug which is subjected to extensive metabolism in this subgroup of patients should be evaluated in a specific clinical trial. Pharmacokinetic studies can serve the useful functions of explaining the outcomes of these trials. It is also advisable to match the age, weight, height, and gender of the subjects with hepatic impairment to those with normal hepatic function. For example, in a study to determine the effect of hepatic impairment on azimilide pharmacokinetics, subjects with normal hepatic function were demographically matched to subjects with mild or subjects with moderate hepatic impairment (90). The two groups of subjects with normal hepatic function had substantially different mean pharmacokinetic parameter values (AUC and C_{max} differences of 40% and 60%, respectively), but mean pharmacokinetic parameter values were similar to their respective demographically matched group of subjects with hepatic impairment.

B. Drug Interactions

In many disease states, the use of polytherapy is quite common, and the risk of drug–drug interactions is high, both from pharmacokinetic and pharmacodynamic perspectives. The likelihood of drug interactions and semiquantitative estimates of magnitude may be predicted from *in-vitro* data (17). The potential for interactions needs to be evaluated from two perspectives: (a) the potential that the new drug may affect the kinetics of other drugs, and (b) the potential that other drugs may affect the kinetics of the new drug. The former generally depends on the ability of the new drug to affect various enzyme- and carrier-mediated clearance processes. Most notably, this concerns the CYP isoforms, but could also involve conjugative enzymes and transporters such as Pgp. Drugs may be an effective inhibitor without being a substrate of the CYP isoform, as is the case for quinidine's inhibition of CYP2D6.

The potential for significant drug–drug interactions caused by other drugs requires knowledge of the components of clearance for the new drug, and the likelihood that known inhibitors will be co-administered. For drugs with multiple pathways and a broad therapeutic index, the need for formal interaction studies may be limited. Population pharmacokinetic analyses of data obtained from Phase III studies may help to discover and quantify drug interactions due to classes of drugs often associated with inhibition (*e.g.*, macrolides, systemic antifungals, calcium channel antagonists, fluoxetine, and paroxetine) or induction (*e.g.*, anticonvulsants and rifampin).

Pharmacokinetic drug–drug interactions can be classified into two main categories: interactions that take place at the absorption site (including incompatibility of two dosage forms, effect on gastrointestinal tract motility, or chelation) and those that occur after the drug has been absorbed (including enzyme induction, enzyme inhibition, and displacement from binding sites). Pharmacokinetic drug–drug interaction studies generally have two key purposes: confirmation of the phenomenon and demonstration of the extent and time course of the interaction. Such information is essential in developing dosage recommendations for use by clinicians.

Although drug–food interactions have been documented for many drugs, from a clinical drug development perspective it still is not possible to predict with certainty whether food will significantly affect the bioavailability of the drug. Furthermore, if there is an interaction with food, the next question naturally is whether food interacts with the drug substance or with the formulation. Thus, a drug–food interaction study should be conducted. A three-way single-dose study of the solid dosage form administered after fasting, the solid dosage form administered with food, and an oral solution administered with food can determine whether the food effect, if there is one, is on the drug substance itself or on the formulation. For drugs with a narrow therapeutic margin, a food effect on the order of 15–20% decrease or increase may be considered clinically significant and must be noted in the package insert. A food effect on the order of 50% may seriously jeopardize the continual development of the drug if the margin of safety between therapeutic and toxic doses is between 1.5 and 2.0.

C. Environmental Components

Another factor contributing to intersubject pharmacokinetic variability is the environment, in particular, alcohol, tobacco, and diet. The effects of alcohol are complicated because alcohol may either inhibit or induce drug metabolism. Tobacco smoke tends to have a general induction effect on hepatic isozymes, particularly CYP1A1 and CYP1A2, and can lead to increased clearance. Thus, subjects who regularly consume relatively large amounts of alcohol and subjects who smoke are usually excluded from pharmacokinetic studies during the early phases of drug development. However, the effects of alcohol consumption and smoking on the pharmacokinetics of the drug often are evaluated at some time during development, particularly for drugs metabolized by CYP2E1, CYP1A1, or CYP1A2.

Dietary factors have been shown to have various effects on drug metabolism, ranging from induction to inhibition, and knowledge of the principle processes of elimination can direct the research in this area. Recently, foods such as grapefruit juice (91–93) and watercress (94) have been shown to substantially decrease clearance by interacting with CYP3A4 (95) or CYP2E1 (96), respectively. Dietary-induced inhibition of CYP activity may cause increased drug concentrations in plasma resulting from not only decreased hepatic metabolism but also decreased intestinal metabolism and a higher bioavailability. Compounds with extensive first-pass metabolism that are metabolized by CYP3A are apparently the most affected by dietary factors compared with drugs metabolized by other isozymes. Dietary effects on drugs metabolized by CYP1A2 may be similar to those of caffeine and theophylline, which have well-defined effects associated with diet protein content, cruciferous vegetables, and charbroiled meats. Although foods that may alter CYP activity are often avoided and all meals are standardized and identical between regimens of pharmacokinetic studies, dietary effects of various food classes on the pharmacokinetics of the drug should be addressed at some stage.

D. Genetics

Genetic factors may have the most substantial impact on intersubject variability of the hepatic CYP mono-oxygenases (97). The ability to predict the rate of drug metabolism in individuals depends on the ability to gauge the activity of the CYP enzymes in various human subpopulations. Special attention may be required for drugs in which a polymorphic enzyme such as CYP2D6 or CYP2C19 is responsible for a large fraction of total clearance. In these cases, the magnitude of difference in clearance between PMs and EMs of probe substrates or genotyped individuals should be assessed. Inevitably, the question will arise as to whether PM status confers greater efficacy or increased rates of adverse events under fixed-dosage study designs.

The current technology allows genotyping for CYP mutations at a reasonable cost. Proponents of genotyping claim that knowledge of genotype predicts clearance which would allow prospective dosage adjustment for better control over therapy. While this may be true for the "average" patient (*i.e.*, population mean), the success for an individual patient is dependent on the product of the percentages of variance in clearance that is predicted by genotype and in efficacy (or adverse events) that is predicted by concentration. If the two percentages are 50% and 20%, the overall predictability of 10% is not likely to have a large impact on clinical practice. For example, if the percentages are higher, success becomes more likely, but broad utilization, including the education of physicians and pharmacists, may take some time to develop.

While much attention has been focused on CYP2D6 and CYP2C19, other CYP isoforms are polymorphically expressed, including CYP2A6 and CYP2C9. Polymorphisms are described for other enzymes as well, including N-acetyl trans-ferases (NAT-1 and NAT-2) (98,99) and thiopurine methyltransferase (TPMT) (100). Differences in these isoforms can be clinically relevant. For example, indi-viduals with low erythrocyte expression of TPMT have greater azathioprine-associated neutropenia and are more susceptible to the toxic effects of the 6-mercaptopurine metabolite.

E. Other Sources of Pharmacokinetic Variability

1. Circadian Effects

A number of physiological processes have circadian rhythms or diurnal fluctua-tions, and in some cases efficacy can be enhanced and adverse effects minimized with proper selection of dosing times (101). In addition, circadian rhythms may affect the pharmacokinetics of the drug. For drugs that are administered two or more times daily, absorption after an evening meal often is delayed and more protracted compared with an isocaloric morning meal (102). Absorption of poorly soluble drugs may be related to the presence of bile acid, and biliary secretion is variable throughout the day (103).

2. Activity and Posture

Because both activity and posture can affect GI transit, they are standardized in bioequivalence studies. More important, drugs with high extraction ratios are greatly affected by hepatic blood flow, and their clearance may fluctuate through-out the day as a function of changes in cardiac output and portal blood flow associated with changes in activity and posture.

3. Dose Regimen Adherence

While adherence is generally guaranteed under the rigid controls of Phase I stud-ies, adherence is not guaranteed under Phase III trials. Assessment of adherence is an important element in evaluating efficacy and in population pharmacokinetic analyses. A useful review of adherence monitoring has recently been published (104). Electronic devices with time- and date-stamping microcircuitry is perhaps the best current method to objectively assess adherence. Coformulation of the drug with small amounts of a chemical with slow metabolism used as a marker may complement the electronic method, which does not ensure that vial opening is followed by ingestion of the drug.

Techniques used to monitor adherence have shown surprisingly low levels of adherence, which tends to be lower with drugs that have to be administered several times daily. According to a survey of several studies, 1 of 3 patients adheres more than 40% but less than 80% of the time, and another 1 of 6 patients adheres less than 40% of the time (104). In addition, patients may follow a certain administration regimen meticulously, but fail to follow the guidelines of the study. For example, in a study in which patients apply a topical medication for a type of skin cancer, control lesions should not to be treated. It would be difficult for patients who attain efficacy for the treated lesions to avoid applying the medication to the control lesions. Similarly, it can sometimes be impossible to prevent a patient from determining whether their drug is active or placebo. For example, it may be quite easy to determine the difference between a drug that is formulated as a solution and the placebo which is the vehicle with identical taste and appearance. If the drug has low solubility in water, the vehicle alone may be miscible with water, but addition of the drug formulation to water may produce a precipitate indicative of the presence of the drug.

4. Enterohepatic Recirculation

ER is a recurrent cycle in which compounds are excreted by the liver as components of bile into the intestine, reabsorbed from the gastrointestinal tract into the systemic circulation, and reexcreted after reuptake by the hepatic cells. For some drugs and compounds such as bile acids, no change in the structure of the compound occurs during recirculation. For drugs such as valproate, the glucuronide metabolite is excreted in the bile, and the parent drug is regenerated by hydrolysis of the glucuronide by β-glucuronidase before being reabsorbed. The process of ER would be expected to increase the time during which the compound is present in the systemic circulation and possibly increase the duration of effects. For compounds that are toxic or are metabolized within hepatocytes to toxic metabolites, enhanced toxicity could result from efficient ER.

Glucuronidation is one of several critical steps in the process, and a suitable functional group (*i.e.*, phenols, alcohols, and carboxylic acids) must be present in order for glucuronidation to occur. As an example, glucuronidation of valproate occurs at the carboxylic acid group. Other compounds eliminated in the bile as glucuronides that undergo ER include morphine, DDT, diphenylacetic acid, mefamanic acid, and the nonsteroidal anti-inflammatory drug carprofen (105).

Changes in the extent of ER (*e.g.*, age-related changes in glucuronidation) may lead to changes in the duration of effect or degree of toxicity of the compound. Perhaps the most widely recognized example of a perturbation in ER leading to potentially serious consequences is the interaction between oral contraceptives and antibiotics. Reduction in the ER of oral contraceptives by antibiotic-induced reduction in hydrolysis of the glucuronide could lead to inadequate blood concentrations of the oral contraceptive resulting in ovulation and the potential to become pregnant.

V. POPULATION ANALYSIS

Population analyses allows characterization of pharmacokinetics of a drug using data collected in treated patients, without extensive plasma sampling from any single individual. Usually, Phase III pivotal and long-term studies can be the source of substantial information about the factors affecting drug clearance. Typically a relatively large number of patients is studied, with several concentrations at various times postdose for each patient. When properly planned and with sufficient controls and data collection, the additional sample collection and analyses can usually be cost-effective. For example, a 300-patient study with an average of four samples per patient will generate 1200 samples, requiring the expenditure of approximately $48,000 to $60,000 for analytical costs. For each pharmacokinetic question answered by the analysis (effect of age, renal function, gender, race, concurrent disease, or drug interactions), the need for certain Phase I studies, costing in excess of $100,000 each, may be averted.

From these data, estimates of the population central values as well as factors affecting inter- and intra-subject variability are obtained. Several computer programs are available for analyses of population pharmacokinetic data. NONMEM, the nonlinear mixed effects modeling program introduced by Sheiner and co-workers (106–108), is the most widely used program. Other computer population analysis programs (P-Pharm and NPEM) are available.

While these analyses hold substantial promise, there are several restrictions. First, adequate simple models must be available from preceding traditional pharmacokinetic studies. Second, the dosage history of the drug (timing of the sampled dose, and several preceding doses) and concomitant medications is crucial to the success of the analyses. Success is more likely when the population analysis is prospectively planned. This ensures that critical information is collected in the case report forms. If absorption rate or extent is dependent on meals, the timing of meals relative to dosing may be important for certain drugs. In general, drugs with short half-lives and frequent dosing present difficulties because of adherence issues and the likelihood of diurnal effects in absorption.

The important pharmacokinetic issues are entirely different for a renally eliminated drug versus a CYP3A substrate, versus a CYP2D6 substrate. If the major component of clearance is due to one of the genetically polymorphic enzymes, this will be critical in the modeling of the interpatient variability, which may be bimodal or a mixture of distributions, and which may be racially dependent. For these cases, genotyping or phenotyping patients may be necessary. In some cases the metabolite-to-parent concentration ratio may serve as an internal phenotype, thus correlating with overall clearance. Complete information about concomitant drug use (and underlying rationale), including over-the-counter preparations, may be quite beneficial in identifying causes for outlying data, as would objective measures of adherence.

The sampling times chosen depend on the issues to be addressed. Often, random sampling across a dosing interval taken at several of the visits during the duration of the study will provide information about the basic parameters (*e.g.*, k_a, CL/F, and V/F) as well as addressing issues of time dependence of both the pharmacokinetics and pharmacodynamics. It has been our experience in open, long-term safety trials, that if only interdose "minima" are specified by the protocol, samples are collected over a wide variety of times postdose, and estimation of k_a is difficult. For this reason, partitioning the dosing interval into segments, with equal randomization of sample collection times for the segments, may improve the final analysis . Another approach that has been used is to have more extensive sampling at selected clinical sites to serve as a foundation data set, with more sparse sampling from the other study sites.

The standard analysis involves preparation of the data set, followed by an initial analysis with a basic pharmacokinetic model. At this stage, the Bayesian post-hoc estimates of clearance and the residual errors for each sample for the individuals are obtained and are subjected to stepwise multiple regression with the various covariates. Because scores of exploratory covariates may be tested, standard statistical approaches are more efficient than population analysis programs. Significant factors (after accounting for multiplicity of testing and repeated observations) are then examined through the population analysis modeling. Special attention is directed to extremely outlying data, often prompting additional inquiries. Once a final model is constructed, the individual clearances can be used to explore relationships between concentration and effect, including logistic regression of adverse events against concentration. Although population analyses require additional expense and more rigid experimental control, the traditionally underutilized data from these trials can provide a wealth of information in the understanding of the drug's pharmacokinetics and effects.

REFERENCES

1. Gibaldi M, Levy G. Pharmacokinetics in clinical practice I. Concepts. JAMA 1976; 235:1864.

2. Kaplan SA. Pharmacokinetics research: more than a simple disposition profile of a new chemical entity. TIBS 1983; 8:372.

3. Lai AA, Fleck RJ, Caplan NB. Clinical pharmacokinetics and the pharmacist's role in drug development and evaluation. In: Cato AE, ed. New Drug Development: Trials and Tribulations. New York: Marcel Dekker, 1989.

4. Wagner JG. History of pharmacokinetics. Pharmacol Ther 1981; 12:537.

5. Lin J. Species similarities and differences in pharmacokinetics. Drug Metab Dispos 1995; 23:1008.

6. Chappell WR, Mordenti J. Extrapolation of toxicological and pharmacological data from animals to humans. In: Testa B, ed. Advances in Drug Research. London: Academic Press, 1991:1.

7. Boxenbaum H, D'Souza RW. Interspecies pharmacokinetic scaling, biological design and neoteny. In: Testa B, ed. Advances in Drug Research. London: Academic Press, 1990:139.

8. .Hunter J, Jepson MA, Tsuruo T, Simmons NL, Hirst BH. Functional expression of P-glycoprotein in apical membranes of human intestinal Caco-2 cells. Kinetics of vinblastine secretion and interaction with modulators. J Biol Chem 1993; 268: 14991.

9. Thiebaut F, Tsuruo T, Hamada H, Gottesman MM, Pastan I, Willingham MC. Cellular localization of the multidrug-resistance gene product P- glycoprotein in normal human tissues. Proc Natl Acad Sci USA 1987; 84:7735.

10. Endrenyi L, Fritsch S, Yan W. Cmax/AUC is a clearer measure than Cmax for absorption rates in investigations of bioequivalence. Int J Clin Pharmacol Ther Toxicol 1991; 29:394.

11. Walker RH, ed. American Association of Blood Banks Technical Manual. 11th ed. Bethesda, MD: American Association of Blood Banks, 1993.

12. Øie S, Tozer TN. Effect of altered plasma protein binding on apparent volume of distribution. J Pharm Sci 1979; 68:1203.

13. Yata N, Toyoda T, Murakami T, Nishiura A, Higashi Y. Phosphatidylserine as a determinant for the tissue distribution of weakly basic drugs. Pharm Res 1990; 10: 1019.

14. Gonzalez FJ. The molecular biology of cytochrome P450s. Pharmacol Rev 1989; 40:243.

15. Benet LZ, Kroetz DL, Sheiner LB. Pharmacokinetics: the dynamics of drug absorption, distribution, and elimination. In: Hardman JG, Limbird LE, Molinoff PB, eds. Goodman and Gillmans the Pharmacological Basis of Therapeutics. 9th ed. New York: McGraw-Hill, 1996:3.

16. Shimada T, Yamazaki H, Mimura M, Inui Y, Guengerich P. Interindividual variations in human liver cytrochrome P-450 enzymes involved in the oxidation of drugs, carcinogens, and toxic chemicals: studies with liver microsomes of 30 Japanese and 30 Caucasians. Pharmacol Exp Ther 1984; 270:414.

17. Bertz RJ, Granneman GR. Use of in vitro and in vivo data to estimate the likelihood of metabolic pharmacokinetic interactions. Clin Pharmacokinet 1997; 32:210.

18. Kolars JC, Awni WM, Merion RM, Watkins PB. First-pass metabolism of cyclosporin by the gut. Lancet 1991; 338:1488.

19. Eichelbaum M, Gross AS. The genetic polymorphism of debrisoquine/sparteine metabolism—clinical aspects. Pharmacol Ther 1990; 46:377.

20. Relling MV, Cherrie J, Schell MJ, Petros WP, Meyer WH, Evans WE. Lower prevalence of the debrisoquin oxidative metabolizer phenotype in American black versus white subjects. Clin Pharmacol Ther 1991; 50:308.

21. Evans WE, Relling MV, Rahman A, McLeod HL, Scott EP, Ling J.-S. Genetic basis for a lower prevalence of deficient CYP2D6 oxidative drug metabolism phenotypes in Black Americans. J Clin Invest 1993; 91:2150.

22. Marinac JS, Foxworth JW, Willsie SK. Dextromethorphan polymorphic hepatic oxidation (CYP2D6) in healthy Black American adult subjects. Ther Drug Monitor 1995; 17:120.

23. Agúndez JAG, Martinez C, Ledesma MC, Ladona MG, Ladero JM, Benítez J. Genetic basis for differences in debrisoquin polymorphism between a Spanish and other white populations. Clin Pharmacol Ther 1994; 55:412.

24. Bozkurt A, Basci NE, Isimer A, Sayal A, Kayaalp SO. Polymorphic debrisoquin metabolism in a Turkish population. Clin Pharmacol Ther. 1994; 55:399

25. Islam SI, Idle JR, Smith RL. The polymorphic 4-hydroxylation of debrisoquin in a Saudi arab population. Xenobiotica 1980; 10:819

26. Bertilsson L, Lou Y.-Q. Du Y.-L., et al. Pronounced differences between native Chinese and Swedish populations in the polymorphic hydroxylations of debrisoquin and S-mephenytoin. Clin Pharmacol Ther 1992; 51:388.

27. Johansson I, Lundqvist E, Bertilsson L, Dahl ML, Sjöqvist F, Ingelman-Sundberg M. Inherited amplification of an active gene in the cytochrome P450 CYP2D locus as a cause of ultrarapid metabolism of debrisoquine. Proc Natl Acad Sci USA 1993; 90:11825.

28. Agúndez JAG, Ledesma MC, Ladero JM, Benítez J. Prevalence of CYP2D6 gene duplication and its repercussion on the oxidative phenotype in a white population. Clin Pharmacol Ther 1995; 57:265.

29. Smith DA, Jones BC. Speculations on the substrate structure-activity relationship (SSAR) of cytochrome P450 enzymes. Biochem Pharmacol 1992; 44:2089.

30. Strobl GR, von Kruedener S, Stöckigt J, Guenerich FP, Wolff T. Development of a pharmacophore for inhibition of human liver cytochrome P-450 2D6: molecular modeling and inhibition studies. J Med Chem 1993; 36:1136.

31. von Moltke LL, Greenblatt DJ, Cotreau-Bibbo MM, Duan SX, Harmatz JS, Shader RI. Inhibition of desipramine hydroxylation by serotonin-reuptake inhibitor antidepressants and by quinidine and ketoconazole: a model system to predict drug intractions in vivo. J Pharmacol Exp Ther 1994; 268:1278.

32. Otton SV, Wu D, Joffe RT, Cheung SW, Sellers EM. Inhibition by fluoxetine of cytochrome P450 2D6 activity. Clin Pharmacol Ther 1993; 53:401.

33. Brøsen K, Hansen JG, Nielsen KK, Sindrup SH, Gram LF. Inhibition by paroxetine of desipramine metabolism in extensive but not in poor metabolizers of sparteine. Eur J Clin Pharmacol 1993; 44:349.

34. von Moltke LL, Greenblatt DJ, Court MH, Duan SX, Harmatz JS, Shader RI. Inhibition of alprazolam and desipramine hydroxylation in vitro by paroxetine and fluvoxamine: comparison with other selective serotonin reuptake inhibitor antidepressants. J Clin Psychopharmacol 1995; 15:125.

35. Inaba T, Jurima M, Mahon WA, Kalow W. In vitro inhibition studies of two iso-zymes of human liver cytochrome P450: mephentoin P-hydroxylase and sparteine monoxygenase. Drug Metab Dispos 1985; 13:443.
36. Brinn R, Borsen K, Gram LF, Haghfelt T, Otton V. Sparteine oxidation is practically abolished in quinidine-treated patients. Br J Clin Pharmacol 1986; 22:194.
37. Brøsen K, Gram LF, Haghfelt T, Bertilsson L. Extensive metabolizers of debriso-quine become poor metabolizers during quinidine treatment. Pharmacol Toxicol 1987; 60:312.
38. Zhou H.-H., Anthony LB, Roden DM, Wood AJJ. Quinidine reduces clearance of (+)-propranolol more than (−)-propranolol through marked reduction in 4-hydroxylation. Clin Pharmacol Ther 1990; 47:686.
39. Rettie AE, Korzewaka KR, Kunze KL, et al. Hydroxylation of warfarin by human cDNA-expressed cytochrome P-450: a role for P-450-2C9 in the etiology of (S)-warfarin-drug interactions. Chem Res Toxicol 1992; 5:54.
40. de Morais SM, Wilkinson GR, Blaisdell J, Nakamura K, Meyer UA, Goldstein JA. The major genetic defect responsible for the polymorphism of S-mephenytoin metabolism in humans. J Biol Chem 1994; 269:15419.
41. Andersson T, Regardh CG, Dahl-Puustinen ML, Bertilsson L. Slow omeprazole metabolizers are also poor S-mephenytoin hydroxylators. Ther Drug Monit 1990; 12:415.
42. Andersson T, Regardh CG, Lou YC, Zhang Y, Dahl ML, Bertilsson L. Polymorphic hydroxylation of S-mephenytoin and omeprazole metabolism in Caucasian and Chinese subjects. Pharmacogenetics 1992; 2:25.
43. Caraco Y, Tateishi T, Wood AJ. Interethnic difference in omeprazole's inhibition of diazepam metabolism. Clin Pharmacol Ther 1995; 58:62.
44. Koop DR. Oxidative and reductive metabolism by cytochrome P450 2E1. FASEB J 1992; 6:724.
45. Peter R, Bocker R, Beaune PH, Iwasaki M, FP Guengerich, Yang CS. Hydroxylation of chlorzoxazone as a specific probe for human liver cytochrome P-450IIE1 [published erratum appears in Chem Res Toxicol 1991 May–Jun; 4(3):389]. Chem Res Toxicol 1990; 3:566.
46. Klotz U, Ammon E. Clinical and toxicological consequences of the inductive potential of ethanol. Eur J Clin Pharmacol 1998; 54:7.
47. O'Shea D, Kim RB, Wilkinson GR. Modulation of CYP2E1 activity by isoniazid in rapid and slow N-acetylators. Br J Clin Pharmacol 1997; 43:99.
48. Daly AK, Cholerton S, Gregory W, Idle JR. Metabolic polymorphisms. Pharmacol Ther 1993; 57:129.
49. Kinonen T, Pasanen M, Gynther J, et al. Competitive inhibition of coumarin 7-hydroxylation by pilocarpine and its interaction with mouse CYP 2A5 and human CYP 2A6. Br J Pharmacol 1995; 116:2625.
50. Dahlqvist R, Bertilsson L, Birkett DJ, M. Eichelbaum, Sawe J, F. Sjoqvist. Theophylline metabolism in relation to antipyrine, debrisoquine, and sparteine metabolism. Clin Pharmacol Ther 1984; 35:815.
51. Patten CJ, Thomas PE, Guy RL, et al. Cytochrome P450 enzymes involved in acetaminophen activation by rat and human liver microsomes and their kinetics. Chem Res Toxicol 1993; 6:511.

52. Woolf TF, Pool WF, Kukan M, Bezek S, Kunze K, Trager WF. Characterization of tacrine metabolism and bioactivation using heterologous expression systems and inhbition studies: evidence for CYP1A2 involvment. 5th North American Meeting, ISSX. Tuscon, AZ, 1993:139.
53. Bertilsson L, Carrillo JA, Dahl ML, et al. Clozapine disposition covaries with CYP1A2 activity determined by a caffeine test. Br J Clin Pharmacol 1994; 38:471.
54. Pirmohamed M, Williams D, Madden S, Templeton E, Park BK. Metabolism and bioactivation of clozapine by human liver in vitro. J Pharmacol Exp Ther 1995; 272:984.
55. Gu L, Gonzalez FJ, Kalow W, Tang BK. Biotransformation of caffeine, paraxanthine, theobromine and theophylline by cDNA-expressed human CYP1A2 and CYP2E1. Pharmacogenetics 1992; 2:73.
56. Wagner W, Vause EW. Fluvoxamine. A review of global drug-drug interaction data. Clin Pharmacokinet 1995; 29:26.
57. Burchell B, Brierley CH, Clarke DJ. Cloning and expression of human UDP-glucuronosyl transferase genes. In: Pacifici GM, Fracchia GN, eds. Advances in Drug Metabolism. Brussels, Luxembourg: European Commision, 1995:609.
58. Holford NH, Sheiner LB. Kinetics of pharmacologic response. Pharmacol. Ther 1982; 16:143.
59. Kroboth PD, Schmith VD, Smith RB. Pharmacodynamic modelling application to new drug development Clin. Pharmacokinet 1991; 20:91.
60. L. Edler. Statistical requirements of Phase I studies. Onkologie 1990; 13:90.
61. Machin D, Campbell MJ, Fayers PM, Pinol APY. Sample size tables for clinical studies. (2d ed.) London: Blackwell Science, 1997.
62. Schall R, Williams RL. Towards a practical strategy for assessing individual bioequivalence. Food and Drug Administration Individual Bioequivalence Working Group. J Pharmacokinet Biopharm 1996; 24:133.
63. Fullerton T, Forrest A, Levy G. Pharmacodynamic analysis of sparse data from concentration- and effect-controlled clinical trials guided by a pilot study. An investigation by simulations. J Pharm Sci 1996; 85:600.
64. Harris RZ, Benet LZ, Schwartz JB. Gender effects in pharmacokinetics and pharmacodynamics. Drugs 1995; 50:222.
65. Wald A, Van Thiel DH, Hoechstetter L, et al. Gastrointestinal transit: the effect of the menstrual cycle. Gastroenterology 1981; 80:1497.
66. Datz FL, Christian PE, Moore J. Gender-related differences in gastric emptying. J Nuclear Med 1987; 28:1204.
67. Abernethy DR, Greenblatt DJ, Divoll M, Arendt R, Ochs HR, Shader RI. Impairment of diazepam metabolism by low-dose estrogen-containing oral-contraceptive steroids. N Engl J Med 1982; 306:791.
68. Hunt CM, Westerkam WR, Stave GM. Effect of age and gender on the activity of human hepatic CYP3A. Biochem Pharmacol 1992; 44:275.
69. Somani SM, Khurana RC. Mechanism of estrogen-imipramine interaction. JAMA 1973; 223:560.
70. Walle T, Walle UK, Cowart TD, Conradi EC. Pathway-selective sex differences in the metabolic clearance of propranolol in human subjects. Clin Pharmacol Ther 1989; 46:257.

71. M. Gibaldi. Biopharmaceutics and Clinical Pharmacokinetics. (3d ed.) Philadelphia: Lea & Febiger, 1984.

72. Aranda JV, Louridas AT, Vitullo BB, Thom P, Aldridge A, Haber R. Metabolism of theophylline to caffeine in human fetal liver. Science 1979; 206:1319.

73. Morselli PL, R. Franco-Morselli, L. Bossi. Clinical pharmacokinetics in newborns and infants. Age-related differences and therapeutic implications. Clin Pharmacokinet 1980; 5:485.

74. E. Perucca. Drug metabolism in pregnancy, infancy and childhood. Pharmacol Ther 1987; 34:129.

75. Slattum P, Cato AE, Pollack GM, Brouwer KLR. Age-related changes in valproic acid (VPA) binding to rat serum proteins *in vitro*. Pharm Res 1993; 10:S392.

76. Morselli PL. Psychotropic drugs. In: Morselli PL, ed. Drug Disposition during Development. New York: Spectrum, 1977:431.

77. Dodson WE. Antiepileptic drugs utilization in pediatric patients. Epilepsia 25(Suppl. 2):S132 (1984).

78. Assael BM. Pharmacokinetics and drug distribution during postnatal development. Pharmacol Ther 1982; 18:159.

79. Grasela TH, Sheiner LB, Rambeck B, et al. Steady-state pharmacokinetics of phenytoin from routinely collected patient data. Clin Pharmacokinet 1983; 8:355.

80. Schmucker DL. Aging and drug disposition: An update. Pharmacol Rev 1985; 37:133.

81. Loi C.-M., Vestal RE. Drug metabolism in the elderly. Pharmacol Ther 1988; 36:131.

82. Greenblatt DJ, Sellers EM, Shader RI. Drug disposition in old age. N Engl J Med 1983; 306:1081.

83. E. Perucca. Biotransformation. In: Levy R, Mattson R, Meldrum B, Penry JK, Dreifuss FE, eds. Antiepileptic Drugs. 3d ed. New York: Raven, 1989:23.

84. Hayes MJL, Langman MJS, Short AH. Changes in drug metabolism with increasing age. II. Phenytoin clearance and protein binding. Br J Clin Pharmacol 1975; 2:73.

85. Cockcroft DW, Gault MH. Prediction of creatinine clearance from serum creatinine. Nephron 1976; 16:31.

86. Jelliffe RW. Estimation of creatinine clearance when urine cannot be collected. Lancet 1971; 1:975.

87. Jelliffe RW, Jelliffe SM. A computer program for estimation of creatinine clearance from unstable serum creatinine levels, age, sex, and weight. Math. Biosci 1972; 14:17.

88. K. Siersbaek-Nielsen, Hansen JM, Kampmann J, Kristensen M. Rapid evaluation of creatinine clearance. Lancet 1971; 1:1133.

89. Williams RL, Mamelok RD. Hepatic disease and drug pharmacokinetics. Clin Pharmacokinet 1980; 5:528.

90. Corey AE, Agnew JR, Comer PF, et al. Effect of hepatic impairment on azimilide pharmacokinetics following single dose oral administration. American Association of Pharmaceutical Scientists Annual Meeting. San Francisco, 1998:S464.

91. Proppe DG, Hoch OD, McLean AJ, Visser KE. Influence of chronic ingestion of grapefruit juice on steady-state blood concentrations of cyclosporin A in renal transplant patients with stable graft function. Br J Clin Pharmacol 1995; 39:337.

92. Honig PK, Wortham DC, Lazarev A, LR Cantilena. Grapefruit juice alters the systemic bioavailability and cardiac repolarization of terfenadine in poor metabolizers of terfenadine. J Clin Pharmacol 1996; 36:345.

93. Miniscalo A, Lundahl J, CG Regårdh, Edgar B, U. G. Eriksson. Inhibition of dihydropyridine metabolism in rat and human liver microsomes by flavonoids found in grapefruit juice. J Pharmacol Exp Ther 1992; 261:1195.

94. Kim RB, Wilkinson GR. Watercress inhibits human CYP2E1 activity *in vivo* as measured by chlorzoxazone 6-hydroxylation. Clin Pharmacol Ther 1996; 59:170.

95. Lilja JJ, Kivisto KT, Neuvonen PJ. Grapefruit juice-simvastatin interaction: effect on serum concentrations of simvastatin, simvastatin acid, and HMG-CoA reductase inhibitors [in process citation]. Clin Pharmacol Ther 1988; 64:477.

96. Leclercq I, Desager JP, Y. Horsmans. Inhibition of chlorzoxazone metabolism, a clinical probe for CYP2E1, by a single ingestion of watercress. Clin Pharmacol Ther 1998; 64:144.

97. Guengerich FP. Human cytochrome P-450 enzymes. Life Sci 1992; 50:1471.

98. Hickman D, Sim E. N-acetyltransferase polymorphism. Comparison of phenotype and genotype in humans. Biochem Pharmacol 1991; 42:1007.

99. Hickman D, Risch A, Camilleri JP, Sim E. Genotyping human polymorphic arylamine N-acetyltransferase: identification of new slow allotypic variants. Pharmacogenetics 1992; 2:217.

100. Lennard L, Van Loon JA, Weinshilboum RM. Pharmacogenetics of acute azathioprine toxicity: relationship to thiopurine methyltransferase genetic polymorphism. Clin Pharmacol Ther 1989; 46:149.

101. Ritschel WA, H. Forusz. Chronopharmacology: a review of drugs studied. Meth Find Exp Clin Pharmacol 1994; 16:57.

102. Goo RH, Moore JG, Greenberg E, Alazraki NP. Circadian variation in gastric emptying of meals in humans. Gastroenterology 1987; 93:515.

103. GP van Berge Henegouwen, Hofmann AF. Nocturnal gallbladder storage and emptying in gallstone patients and healthy subjects. Gastroenterology 1978; 75:879.

104. J. Urquhart. Role of patient compliance in clinical pharmacokinetics. A review of recent research. Clin Pharmacokinet 1994; 27:202.

105. Renwick AG. Gut bacteria and the enterohepatic circulation of foreign compounds. In: Hill MJ, ed. Microbial Metabolism in the Digestive Tract. Boca Raton; FL: Press CRC, 1986.

106. Sheiner LB, Beal SL. Evaluation of methods for estimating population pharmacokinetic parameters. III. Monoexponential model: routine clinical pharmacokinetic data. J Pharmacokinet Biopharm 1983; 11:303.

107. Sheiner BL, Beal SL. Evaluation of methods for estimating population pharmacokinetic parameters. II. Biexponential model and experimental pharmacokinetic data. J Pharmacokinet Biopharm 1981; 9:635.

108. Sheiner LB, Beal SL. Evaluation of methods for estimating population pharmacokinetics parameters. I. Michaelis-Menten model: routine clinical pharmacokinetic data. J Pharmacokinet Biopharm 1980; 8:553.

18
Building an NDA/BLA

Diana E. Fordyce
Cato Research Ltd., Durham, North Carolina

Angela Cahill
Bethesda, Maryland

I. INTRODUCTION

This chapter provides an overview of the process used in submitting New Drug Applications (NDAs) and Biologics License Applications (BLAs) to the U.S. Food and Drug Administration (FDA) and provides methods for organizing information in the marketing application.

A. What Is an NDA/BLA?

A marketing application, as defined in Title 21 of the Code of Federal Regulations (hereinafter referred to as 21 CFR) § 312.3(b), is an application for a new drug submitted under section 505(b) of the act or a biologics license application for a biological product under the Public Health Service Act. The ultimate goal of clinical development of a new medicinal product is to obtain regulatory agency authorization to sell and market the product. In the United States, the Food and Drug Administration must approve the marketing application (*i.e.*, the NDA or BLA) before the new medicine can be marketed.

The marketing application is meant to provide evidence that the product is both safe and effective when used under specified conditions and manufactured appropriately and, therefore, provides all the information that supports each statement in the proposed labeling for the product. Whether paper or electronic, from the United States or of international origin, the marketing application consists of many pages of documentation that support one to two pages of product labeling (*i.e.*, the Package Insert or the foreign Summary of Product Characteristics, and labels on the containers) that the general public and physicians read and use.

B. Roadmaps for an NDA/BLA—Begin with the End in Mind

A fundamental rule of constructing and executing the product development plan is to "begin with the end in mind" (FDA. CDER. ODE IV Pilot. Targeted Product Information). Two documents—the proposed product labeling and the comprehensive table of contents for the NDA/BLA—should be used as "roadmaps" for the development plan and should be updated as a continuum to ensure compliance with appropriate regulations and guidelines and to solicit FDA feedback. When used jointly, these two documents can facilitate the expeditious completion of NDA/BLA information.

The advent of initiatives such as the FDA Modernization Act of 1997 and the International Conference on Harmonisation (ICH) initiatives for the global dossier or Common Technical Document (CTD, ICH guidance document M4), scheduled to be completed and implemented by 2002 or 2003, may change the information format and content standards. In addition, there are the electronic submission standards to consider. It is therefore important to choose a technique for compiling information that can be flexible and adaptable to incorporation of completed modules of technical information (nonclinical reports, nonclinical summary tables, etc.). The information compiled must be appropriate for current regulations (*i.e.*, for U.S. NDAs and BLAs and for foreign Marketing Authorization Applications) and for future applications (*i.e.*, for the CTD). Many software developers for the pharmaceutical industry are now tapping into the potential to sell a variety of systems to help sponsors organize marketing applications.

II. CONTENTS AND REQUIREMENTS—ANALYSIS OF FORM FDA 356H

Form FDA 356h (*Application to Market a New Drug, Biologic, or an Antibiotic Drug for Human Use*) is used for the NDA, the BLA, and the Abbreviated New Drug Application (ANDA). Regulations for these applications can be found in 21 CFR Part 314 for NDAs and abbreviated applications and in Part 601 for BLAs. Form FDA 356h can provide valuable insight into content and requirements of the applications, and give strategic considerations for the product. Form FDA 356h is provided with an instruction sheet entitled "Instructions for Filling Out Form FDA 356h." Components of the form are described in detail in the following sections.

A. Product Information—Naming, Indication, and Review Classification Considerations

The product description information should be determined early in the development process, to avoid possible confusion and costly changes to documentation.

Establishing product name conventions may require early consultation with United States Pharmacopeia (USP) or United States Adopted Names (USAN) and the FDA Nomenclature Standards Committee (*Washington Drug Letter, 1997*). Because the trade name may change at the time of FDA approval, the trade name should be used only in the proposed labeling, and the established or generic name should be used on all other NDA and BLA documentation.

The application number for drugs, but not for biologics, can be obtained before submission. The application number is then part of the FDA's Orange Book, or *Approved Drug Products with Therapeutic Equivalence Evaluations* (the List) guide to obtaining information regarding the application. The Orange Book also includes the application number, the generic and trade names, the strengths, the applicant (holder of the application), patent number and expiration date, exclusivity code (including orphan drug) and expiration date, and equivalence evaluation information.

The indication is the part of the proposed product labeling that is used to guide expedient product development. Determination of the proposed indication(s) early in development will ensure adherence to appropriate treatment-related regulations and guidelines, and it provides a way of determining if the product has any existing comparator treatments. The existence and review of comparator treatments can be used early in the development program to determine the regulatory and marketing strategies involved. For example, clinical trials may involve comparator controls and the proposed labeling claims may indicate no difference, equivalence, or superiority. In addition, the product and the proposed indication may have been the subject of a recent marketing application that was submitted, reportedly close to receiving approval, or approved. The product may have an active patent and terms of exclusivity that should be considered in the regulatory and marketing strategy considerations (exclusivity considerations are discussed in the next section of this chapter).

The "uniform" terms provided in the Orange Book are helpful indicators of appropriate listing of dosage forms and routes of administration. The dosage form, strengths, and route of administration may affect the classification* of the

---

* FDA classification policy [Center for Drug Evaluation and Research (CDER); http://www.fda.gov/cder/da/da.htm#notes] includes:

Type 1: New molecular entity
Type 2: New derivative
Type 3: New formulation (new dosage form or new formulation of an active ingredient already on the market)
Type 4: New combination
Type 5: New manufacturer, already marketed
Type 6: New use
Type 7: Drug already legally marketed, but without an approved NDA

A product can be assigned more than one type.

product, which in turn may affect regulatory or marketing strategy considerations such as the application type, associated development program, and exclusivity considerations. As an example, if XY is a fixed combination drug product being considered for clinical product development, consider the scenarios described below.

1. If X and Y are currently sold separately for the same indication

    in the same formulation, then combination XY may be considered a New Combination and must follow the regulations (21 CFR § 300.50) for these types of products, which stipulate specific types of clinical trials. The application may be considered a 505(b)(1)-type or 505(b)(2)-type NDA application depending on the amount of, and right to reference, information from the original application(s).

    in a different formulation, then combination XY may be considered both a New Combination and a New Formulation, which may require clinical trials for the new combination (21 CFR § 300.50) and the new formulation. The application may be considered a 505(b)(1)-type or 505(b)(2)-type NDA application depending on the amount of, and right to reference, information from the original application(s).

2. If X and Y are already sold as a fixed combination XY for the same indication

    in the same formulation, then combination XY may be considered suitable for an ANDA (*i.e.*, a generic product), which stipulates bioequivalence trials (21 CFR Part 320).

    in a different formulation, then combination XY may be considered a New Formulation, which may require clinical trials to demonstrate a comparison with the existing formulation. The application may be considered a 505(b)(1)-type or 505(b)(2)-type NDA or efficacy supplement application depending on the product and on the amount

---

Efficacy supplement codes: SE1 (a new indication or significant modification of an existing indication, including removal of a major limitation to use, such as second line status); SE2 (a new dosage regimen, including an increase or decrease in daily dosage, or a change in frequency of administration); SE3 (a new route of administration); SE4 (a comparative efficacy claim, including comparative pharmacokinetic claim); SE5 (a change in sections other than the "Indications and Usage" section that would significantly alter the patient population to be treated, such as addition of pediatric use and/or dosing information or geriatric use and/or dosing information); SE6 (an Rx-to-OTC switch); SE7 (supplement–accelerated approval); SE8 (efficacy supplement with clinical data to support labeling claim).

The classification policy also includes status identifiers such as P (priority review), S (standard review), orphan (V), E [Subpart E at Investigational New Drug Application (IND) stage; Subpart H at NDA stage for drugs or equivalent to Subpart E at license application stage for biologics].

of, and right to reference, information from the original application(s). Alternatively, a formulation may differ only in inactives that are permissible within ANDA regulations. In addition, if an applicant is seeking approval for a different dosage form for an already-approved combination product, an ANDA suitability petition could be submitted to request permission to file an ANDA for a new dosage form (21 CFR § 314.93). If the petition is approved, an ANDA may be submitted. The ANDA applicant would have to conduct and meet the appropriate bioequivalence/bioavailability requirements for approval.

Clearly, in this example, careful consideration of the product characteristics and associated classification with appropriate FDA consultation, consideration of the applicant's patent and exclusivity terms, and the ability to conduct an appropriate development program are critical early in the development process.

B. Marketing Application Types—NDA [505(b)(1), 505(b)(2)], ANDA, BLA—Regulatory, Strategic, and Exclusivity Considerations

The application types (NDA, BLA, ANDA) are provided on Form FDA 356h with the appropriate regulatory reference.

The type of NDA is specified according to the section of the Federal Food, Drug, and Cosmetic Act in which it is described [*i.e.*, 505(b)(1), 505(b)(2)]. The types of applications differ in terms of content (codified in 21 CFR Part 314 Subparts B and C) and possible terms of exclusivity (codified in 21 CFR § 314.108). The submission and effective approval of ANDAs or 505(b)(2) applications for similar conditions of approval is affected by the terms of exclusivity. Exclusivity does not prevent the submission or approval of a full NDA. Exclusivity provisions begin on the effective date of approval, which refers to the date of final approval and not to the date of tentative approval. Exclusivity considerations should be considered in concert with patent term information. Briefly, the types of NDAs are described as follows:

505(b)(1)
> The 505(b)(1) is characterized as a "full NDA."
> The required content is codified in 21 CFR § 314.50; all information is required.
> Up to 5 years' exclusivity (as codified in 21 CFR § 314.108) may be received for a new chemical entity.

505(b)(2)
> The 505(b)(2) is characterized as an NDA for a drug that represents a modification (such as a new formulation or new indication) from

a listed drug* (21 CFR § 314.54) in which one or more of the investigations relied upon by the applicant "were not conducted by or for the applicant and for which the applicant has not obtained a right of reference† or use" from the original applicant [21 CFR § 314.3(b)]. Drug products with a rate or extent of absorption that exceeds or is otherwise different from the 505(j) ANDA standards for bioequivalence compared to a listed drug may be submitted as a 505(b)(2). [Therefore, a product that is more bioavailable such that a lower dose is equivalent to the existing dose of a listed drug may be submitted as a 505(b)(2) application.] A 505(b)(2) cannot be submitted for products that could be considered an ANDA [21 CFR § 314.101(d)(9)] or for inability to qualify as an ANDA within acceptable bioequivalence criteria (*i.e*, if the product's only difference from the listed drug is that its extent of absorption is less or the rate is unintentionally less than the listed drug; 21 CFR § 314.54).

The required content is codified in 21 CFR §§ 314.3(b) and 314.54; all information is required as detailed in 21 CFR § 314.50 (including appropriate patent information and certification) with the exception that nonclinical and clinical data are required as needed to appropriately support the modification(s) from the listed drug.

Up to 3 years' exclusivity [as codified in 21 CFR §§ 314.50(j)(4) and 314.108] may be received if the clinical investigations (other than bioavailability or bioequivalence) are:

> New (*i.e.*, the results of the clinical investigation(s) have not been relied on by the FDA to demonstrate substantial evidence of effectiveness of a previously approved drug product); and
>
> Essential to approval [*i.e.*, certification that the applicant has thoroughly searched the scientific literature and, to the best of the applicant's knowledge, the list of published studies and publicly available reports of clinical investigations is

---

* In accordance with the definition provided in 21 CFR § 314.3(b), *listed drug* status is "evidenced by the drug product's identification as a drug with an effective approval in the current edition of FDA's 'Approved Drug Products with Therapeutic Equivalence Evaluations' (the List) or any supplement thereto, as a drug with an effective approval. A drug product is deemed to be a listed drug on the date of effective approval of the application or abbreviated application for that drug product."

† In accordance with the definition provided in 21 CFR § 314.3(b), *right of reference or use* refers to the "authority to rely upon, and otherwise use, an investigation for the purpose of obtaining approval of an application, including the ability to make available the underlying raw data from the investigation for FDA audit, if necessary."

complete and accurate and does not provide sufficient basis for the approval of the conditions for which the applicant is seeking without reference to the new clinical investigation(s). It should be noted that the FDA decides whether a study is essential to approval at the time of approval of the application and, therefore, scientific literature available after the time of submission and during the review process of the application is considered (*Abbreviated New Drug Application Regulations: Patent and Exclusivity Provisions, Final Rule, Federal Register, Vol. 59, No. 190, October 3, 1994*)]; and

Conducted or sponsored by the applicant [*i.e.*, the applicant was named in the Form FDA 1571 for the Investigational New Drug Application (IND) under which the new clinical investigation(s) that is essential to approval of the application was conducted] and supported by the applicant (*e.g.*, certification that the applicant provided 50% or more of the cost of conducting the study).

Interestingly, the 505(b)(2) is often described as a regulatory bridge between an ANDA and a full NDA because the 505(b)(2) provides a mechanism through which an applicant that is not the original listed drug applicant (innovator) of a product can gain approval for certain changes to that product. The 505(b)(2) is similar to a 505(b)(1) efficacy supplement except that the 505(b)(2) is typically sponsored by an applicant other than the original listed drug applicant, the investigations that are relied upon from the original listed drug application were not conducted by or for the applicant, and there is not a right to reference or use. If the drug product is an active ingredient that has been previously approved (*e.g.*, in a different formulation) under another applicant and no longer under patent or exclusivity provisions, it may be helpful to consider not duplicating some nonclinical and clinical work and filing a 505(b)(2)-type application. Appropriate bridging studies and investigations would have to be conducted to support the modification(s) from the listed drug. This strategy may shorten development time for innovative products of an existing listed drug. Up to 3 years of exclusivity possible [compared with 5 years of exclusivity possible for a 505(b)(1)-type application]. This type of application is described further and in detail in review articles such as *US Regulatory Reporter, Guide to 505(b)(2) Submissions* (1995) and the *Draft Guidance for Industry: Applications Covered by Section 505(b)(2)* (1999). Pursuing a 505(b)(2) application should be discussed with the FDA early in development of the product.

Abbreviated applications (ANDAs) are categorized and the content codified in 21 CFR § 314.94. A suitability petition to submit an ANDA may be approved for a drug product that is different from a listed drug; the product can be a new dosage form, new strength, or new route, or a change in a combination product of one of the active ingredients to a different one that is listed and in the same class (21 CFR § 314.93). A suitability petition for an ANDA will not be approved if safety and effectiveness investigations (information derived from animal or clinical studies or literature beyond limited confirmatory testing) is required.

Supplemental applications are categorized and the content is codified in 21 CFR § 314.70 for new drug applications (often referred to as SNDAs) and in 21 CFR § 314.97 for abbreviated applications.

The exclusivity provisions for drug products (up to 5 years for NDAs, 3 years for supplemental NDAs, and 0.5 years for ANDAs), according to Title I of the Drug Price Competition and Patent Term Restoration Act (Hatch-Waxman Act or 1984 Amendments), currently do not apply to biological products, but are under consideration by the FDA [*The Pink Sheet, Waxman/Hatch Should Be Expanded to Cover Biologics (1998)*].

It is also important to note that 7 years of exclusivity is possible, effective the date of FDA approval of a marketing application, for a product and indication that are the subject of orphan designation (codified in 21 CFR § 316.31).

The type of application also requires different user fees (see Item 18 of Form FDA 356h). A provision of the FDA Modernization Act of 1997 (Sections 101 to 107) is the re-authorization of the Prescription Drug User Fee Act (PDUFA) of 1992, which permits the collection of user fees from prescription drug manufacturers to augment FDA resources for the review of human drug applications. Full NDAs are subject to the full fee. Under the reauthorization provisions of the Modernization Act (PDUFA II), orphan drugs and supplements for pediatric use are exempt from a user fee.

Cross-references to related applications [License Applications, INDs, NDAs, and device applications] and drug or biologic master files (DMF or BMF) should be listed. The document type, number, holder, product, and other relevant information should be provided.

Master files may be useful to cross-reference because they may provide information about the following such that the information can be updated in only one document rather than several applications:

Manufacturing site, facilities, operating procedures, personnel (Type I)

Drug substance, drug substance intermediate, and material used in their preparation, or drug product (Type II)

Packaging material (Type III)

Excipient, colorant, flavor, essence, or material used in their preparation (Type IV)

FDA accepted reference information (Type V)

The holder of the master files can authorize an applicant to reference master file information. It should be noted, however, that the master file information is not approved or disapproved by the FDA and will be reviewed only in conjunction with the marketing application. Important information regarding master files is located in the *Guideline for Drug Master Files* and in 21 CFR § 314.420.

C. Prescription and Over-the-Counter Status—Labeling

The applicant is required to state the proposed marketing status as prescription (Rx) or over-the-counter (OTC). Labeling requirements are codified in 21 CFR § 201 Subpart B for Rx and Subpart C for OTC. A marketing application would be required for a product that deviates from the applicable OTC monograph* (21 CFR § 330.11). OTC monographs specific for some types of products are provided in 21 CFR Parts 331–358 and discussed in MAPP 6020.5. The use of the labeling requirements as a tool for development and regulatory or marketing strategy considerations is described later in this chapter.

D. Index—Comprehensive Table of Contents

The checklist for the items provided in Form FDA 356h should be used to indicate which types of information are contained within a particular submission. The Form FDA 356h instruction sheet entitled *"Instructions For Filling Out Form FDA 356h"* indicates that the numbering system is not intended to specify a particular order of inclusion of the sections in the submission, but recommends that the Index be the first section and that the Index clearly provide the location of the sections. For the purposes of ensuring easy navigation within the NDA/BLA, the numbering system in the checklist is most often used for numbering the items (*e.g.*, Item 8 is the Clinical Data section even if Item 7 is not applicable for the product; Item 10 is the Statistical section even if Item 9 is not applicable as in the case of an original submission).

It is important to note that although Item 1 is entitled *"Index,"* it is described in the regulations [21 CFR § 314.50(b)] as "a comprehensive index by volume and page numbers," which indicates that a comprehensive index is actually a comprehensive table of contents.

E. Compiling the NDA

Form FDA 356h requires that the volumes submitted be identified (referring to the archival copy of the submission) and that it is identified whether the applica-

---

* Monographs establish conditions under which OTC drugs are generally recognized as safe and effective and are not misbranded.

tion is paper, electronic, or both. Because the electronic guidelines for submission of an NDA/BLA are in the initial stages of implementation, it is important to confer with the appropriate FDA reviewing division for what is an acceptable format for electronic media.

1. Paper Copies

The paper review copies contain copies of Form FDA 356h, cover letter, letters of authorization/certification items, comprehensive table of contents (index), summary section, and particular technical sections. The review copies are distributed to the individual reviewers at the FDA, thus permitting concurrent reviews to occur. The field copy, required for drug products as of 1993, is a copy of the Chemistry review copy, and certified as such, that is sent to the applicant's "home" FDA district office and used for preapproval inspections. The archival copy is the FDA's official copy (it includes the case report forms and tabulations) and serves as a resource for reviewers.

The *Guideline on Formatting, Assembling, and Submitting the New Drug and Antibiotic Applications (1987)* includes a tabular summary for the compilation of the archival and review copies of the new drug application. It should be noted and accounted for, however, that the tabular summary in this guidance is not consistent with the updated Form FDA 356h.

2. Electronic Copies

The FDA plans to move to a paperless regulatory process by the year 2002. As part of this goal, CDER and CBER have issued guidance documents for the electronic submission of NDAs [*Guidance for Industry: Providing Regulatory Submissions in Electronic Format—NDAs (1999)*] and BLAs [*Guidance for Industry: Providing Regulatory Submissions to CBER in Electronic Format—Biologics Marketing Applications (1999)*]. A general guidance document provides a comprehensive review of the history of electronic submission guidances and procedures [*Guidance for Industry: Providing Regulatory Submissions in Electronic Format—General Considerations (1999)*]. The advent of the electronic submission should offer advantages to the FDA, the applicant, and the environment. An average archival submission is approximately 100–150 volumes (each volume is 2 in. thick), with review copies of technical information adding many more volumes to this count. The applicant has to coordinate this enormous effort with the paper copy; the FDA has to coordinate the distribution, review, and storage of the paper copy.

The guidance documents for electronic submissions provide detailed specifications and information on format. Key factors in submitting the electronic document are as follows.

The document should be hypertext linked and bookmarked to ensure appropriate and efficient navigation. Bookmarks and hypertext links should be provided to each item cited in the table of contents including tables, figures, publications/references, and appendixes. Full text indexes and document information fields are provided for technical items to find documents or search for text within documents.

The document must be submitted in Portable Document Format (PDF). PDF has been accepted as a standard for providing documents in electronic format by ICH.

A folder-naming system as provided in the guidances.

If both a paper and an electronic submission are used, the specifications for the paper and the electronic copy should be discussed and confirmed with the reviewing division at the pre-NDA/BLA meeting.

F. Certification

Form FDA 356h includes a certification statement that must be signed by the applicant's representative agent or authorized official. The statement specifies that there are no false statements in the application and that the applicant will adhere to requirements for compliance with regulations for safety updates, GMPs, labeling, prescription advertising, supplements, and annual reports.

III. CONSTRUCTING THE NDA/BLA—MODULES OF INFORMATION

Constructing the NDA/BLA should be thought of as a continuum throughout the development process. Commonly, documentation obtained during development is put together on an as-needed basis, with format and content dependent on the preference of the sponsor at that time. The NDA/BLA may not be compiled until the end of Phase 3, with considerable effort needed to compile the information in a similar format. For example, sponsors have been known to conduct five or more studies with five or more data collection and reporting standards (because of differences in contract research organizations or internal differences). That sponsor would be required to embark on the time-consuming and costly effort to rework key study information into a consistent format to logically display safety, pharmacokinetic, and efficacy information. Some pieces of information that are commonly compiled in the last months of development that should be compiled as a continuum throughout development are the package insert, data set integration, report synopses, primary quantitative tabular summaries of re-

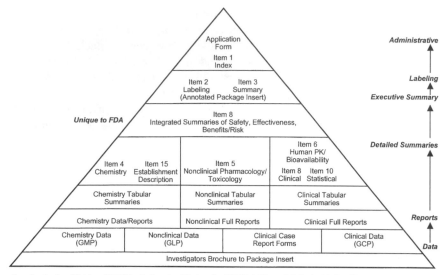

Reproduced and modified from Establishing the Format and Content of an NDA/BLA (Chapter 9, D. Fordyce) in Expediting Drugs and Biologics Development--A strategic Approach (2nd edition; S. Linberg, Editor) With permission from Parexel®.

GCP = Good Clinical Practice; GLP = Good Laboratory Practice; GMP = Good Manufacturing Practice; PK = pharmacokinetic.

Figure 1   Construction of the NDA/BLA.

sults, overall tabular summaries of clinical studies and nonclinical studies, and chemistry documentation.

Although each application presents unique considerations, our experience indicates that submission of a marketing application will be delayed significantly if the applicable information is not incorporated immediately after completion into a report, summary tables, and the proposed labeling. For an average marketing application, several months delay is often the difference between obtaining exclusivity provisions or a marketing advantage or both over a competitor's product. In addition, sponsors must deal with decisions very late in development that can greatly affect the speed at which a marketing application is compiled and possibly reviewed. Examples of some of these decisions are whether to provide a uniform format for study numbering, report synopses, tabular summaries of safety and effectiveness, patient narratives (and corresponding case report forms), and location of statements of compliance to GCPs, GLPs, or transfer of sponsor obligations.

The pyramid concept for construction of the NDA/BLA can aid in developing a sense for the building block components and organization of a marketing application. As shown in Fig. 1, the proposed labeling is developed at the IND stage (*i.e.*, the Investigator's Brochure progresses to the Package Insert). The data from each technical discipline (chemistry, nonclinical, and clinical), collected according to the appropriate regulatory requirements as appropriate (GMP, GLP, GCP, respectively), are then compiled into individual reports, overview tabular summaries, and the respective "Items" of the NDA/BLA. Unique to U.S. marketing applications, the integrated summaries of clinical information, with relevant nonclinical and chemistry information, are then developed. This information is then provided as cross-references (annotation) to support the statements in the proposed labeling.

The NDA/BLA project team assigned to the product should be very familiar with all components of the NDA/BLA. The NDA team normally includes representatives from regulatory, project management, clinical, biopharmaceutics, biostatistics, pharmacology/toxicology, and chemistry. The team should have one person or group responsible for coordination and assembly of the NDA. The team should discuss content issues, data presentation, and target dates. In addition, the team should be aware that the NDA is a document that supports each statement of the labeling. Our experience indicates that the team can ensure efficient project execution and change control with the use of status reports and meetings that review and track target completion dates of sections of the NDA/BLA working table of contents and related tasks (*i.e.*, Gantt charts).

The following sections in this chapter provide modules that can be started early in development and updated as a continuum for the most expeditious completion of clinical information for the marketing application.

A. Package Insert Annotation

The regulations require annotations to the summary and technical sections [21 CFR 314.50(c) and (d)] and the guidelines suggest annotation to the volume and page number [*Guideline for the Format and Content of the Summary for the New Drug and Antibiotic Applications (1987)*]. Annotations can be tracked throughout development by providing the study report number or comments in the annotation section that supports the proposed labeling statements.

This concept of using the proposed product labeling as a way of tracking information and updating the proposed labeling throughout product development is the subject of an FDA pilot program with CDER's Office of Drug Evaluation IV and is referred to as the Targeted Product Information document [*The Pink Sheet, "Targeted Product Information" Pilot Uses Labeling Goals at IND Stage (1999)*]. The Targeted Product Information document (or TPI) is described by the Web site (http://http://www.fda.gov/cder/tpi/default.htm) as an evolving version of the proposed labeling that can be used by the sponsor to: (a) guide the design, conduct, and analysis of clinical trials; (b) facilitate communication with the FDA; and (c) promote a shared understanding of the sponsor's drug development program. The TPI is essentially a proposed package insert with the supporting study identification information (*i.e.*, preliminary annotation). The TPI is expected by the FDA to provide a greater amount of information than the General Investigational Plan submitted with the IND and can: (a) be updated with the Annual Report to the IND (the Annual Report regulations indicate the requirement for the general investigational plan for the coming year), (b) be used at milestone meetings, and (c) enable communication about such critical subjects as the number of adequate and well-controlled studies required to support an indication and patient population.

B. Summary of Comparator Products

A summary of the product and comparator products existing for the treatment of the proposed indication(s) can be developed early in the development program and updated throughout development. This table can be in the form of a side-by-side comparison of the package inserts for the products. The information can correspond to the preliminary annotation of the package insert to support components of the clinical development plan that are ongoing. This type of table can be used as a multipurpose tool for (a) ensuring appropriate considerations and marketing strategy for the proposed labeling, and for (b) inserting into the integrated benefits/risk section of Item 8 of the NDA/BLA.

C. Summary of Studies

A summary table of studies for each technical discipline (i.e., nonclinical, clinical, and chemistry) should be created to summarize the studies and data. This summary is then supported and cross-referenced to the full study reports.

Using the summary table of clinical studies as an example, this table provides an overview of all the clinical studies, portions of which are then provided in the Clinical Pharmacology, Controlled, Uncontrolled, and Other studies sections according to the guideline for Item 8 of the NDA/BLA [*Guideline for the Format and Content of the Clinical and Statistical Sections of New Drug Applications (1988)*]. When updated as a continuum throughout the development of the product, this table can be used to present an overview of study information in the end-of-Phase 2 and pre-NDA/BLA meetings with the FDA, in addition to the final form appearing in the NDA/BLA. Information that this table should include is the following.

> 1. Identifier, title, and site(s) where the study was performed. The study identifier system should be clear to the reviewer. Status of the study such as the start and completion dates, GCP status (a statement of which is required), and the study category. It is important to note what

date was used as a cutoff date for incorporation of study information into the marketing application. Typically, the cutoff date is 3–6 months before submission of the marketing application. Studies that are ongoing at the time of submission would be listed as ongoing, but critical information up to the cutoff date such as deaths, discontinuations because of adverse experiences, serious adverse experiences, and exposure should be submitted from ongoing studies. The study category is used to identify the categories the study represents [*i.e.*, clinical pharmacology, pharmacokinetic or pharmacodynamic, and any appropriate subcategories; controlled studies in the indication(s) of the application and any appropriate subcategories; uncontrolled studies in the indications(s) of the application; and studies in indications other than those that are the subject of the application]. If there are many studies or if the categorization of the studies is complex (for example, if the studies are subcategorized into United States and foreign or sponsored by the applicant and not sponsored by the applicant), it may be appropriate to precede the table with a summary or flowchart of the categories of studies with the corresponding study identifiers.

2. Subsequent columns contain the critical information regarding the study for a succinct review of the methods used (*i.e.*, study design, control type, dose/route, regimen) and the results [*i.e.*, columns for summary data for demographics and breakdown of subpopulations (total number of subjects enrolled/completed; and total number of subjects by race, gender, and age group or provide mean age and age range); pharmacokinetics; safety; and effectiveness].

3. Cross-referencing information to the rest of the application for where such items as the full protocol, report, publication(s), raw data, case report forms, and case report tabulations (or listings) can be located. In addition, the study is cross-referenced to previous submissions to the regulatory agency (*e.g.*, the study would be cross-referenced to the IND serial number if it was previously submitted in the IND).

D. Summary of Regulatory Interactions

The guideline for Item 8 (Background/Overview) of the NDA/BLA [*Guideline for the Format and Content of Clinical and Statistical Sections of New Drug Applications (1988)*] suggests that regulatory interactions regarding major issues and agreements should be referenced. This type of tabular summary of regulatory interactions or regulatory database output may be useful to track regulatory history and ensure that FDA requests and joint sponsor–FDA agreements have been satisfied throughout the development program. Submissions of nonclinical and clinical reports and chemistry information are also recorded. Reports that have not been previously submitted to the FDA at the time of the NDA/BLA submission are to be identified in the table of contents of the submission.

This type of table can be organized into clinical, nonclinical, and chemistry technical disciplines and provided with the corresponding NDA/BLA items to facilitate review of the information. The table can also be used as an attachment to the cover letter of the application to document significant instructions or decisions with the FDA that affect the information contained in the NDA/BLA.

E. Summary of Literature-Search Strategies

The guideline for Item 8 of the NDA/BLA [*Guideline for the Format and Content of Clinical and Statistical Sections of New Drug Applications (1988)*] indicates that literature should be summarized as part of the controlled, uncontrolled, and other studies with a description of the search strategy used to assess the world literature. In addition, regulatory requirements to demonstrate that clinical investigations are "essential" for claims of exclusivity indicate that the applicant provide a "list of all published studies or publicly available reports of clinical investigations known to the applicant through a literature search that are relevant to the conditions for which the applicant is seeking approval." Also, a "certification that the applicant has thoroughly searched the scientific literature" [21 CFR § 314.50(j)(4)(ii)] must be provided. Similar to the ongoing studies, it is important to note the cutoff date for incorporation of literature search information into the marketing application.

This type of table can be organized into clinical, nonclinical, and chemistry sections and can be provided with the associated items of the marketing application to facilitate review of the information.

IV. FDA REVIEW OF THE NDA/BLA

The completed application is reviewed within the initial 60 days to determine if it is fileable or if it will be a refusal-to-file (RTF) application. Usually, a "45-day meeting" is held within the reviewing division at the FDA to determine if the application is acceptable for filing. In accordance with 21 CFR § 314.101, the FDA may refuse to file an application or abbreviated antibiotic application or may not consider an abbreviated new drug application received for any of the following reasons:

> Does not contain a completed application form (*i.e.*, Form FDA 356h)
> Is not submitted in the form or does not contain the information required

of an NDA (in accordance with 21 CFR § 314.50) or ANDA (in accordance with 21 CFR § 314.94)

Does not include a complete environmental assessment (in accordance with 21 CFR § 25.40) or provide information for categorical exclusion (in accordance with 21 CFR §§ 25.30, 25.31)

Does not contain an accurate and complete English translation of each part of the application that is not in English

Omission of statements of compliance with the requirements set forth in 21 CFR Part 58 (*i.e.*, GLP) or 21 CFR Parts 50 and 56 (*i.e.*, GCP)

Once accepted for filing, the FDA "review clock" then starts and the multi-disciplinary review process begins. Safety updates are submitted by the applicant, or a waiver requested, during the review process. The FDA "review clock," according to 21 CFR § 314.101, is 180 days; review times, however, have historically always been longer. PDUFA was enacted (originally in 1992 and reauthorized in 1997) to permit collection of prescription drug applicant submission fees to provide payment for additional reviewing staff at the FDA such that review times can be more expeditious. Review time goals are now 10–12 months for standard review and 4–6 months for priority review [*PDUFA II Five-Year Plan (1998)*]. The FDA may have questions that require responses throughout the review period. If the response to the request or of additional submitted information is substantial, the information may be considered an amendment to the application, and the review clock may be extended or restarted.

"Rolling reviews" or "rolling applications" are attractive to applicants because they represent a way in which to start the review process earlier and potentially may allow for an earlier approval date. In accordance with 21 CFR § 314.50(d)(1)(iv), the Chemistry section of an application can be submitted 90–120 days in advance of the remainder of the application, and review is dependent on resources. The FDA Modernization Act of 1997 "Fast Track" initiative (Section 112) for drugs intended to treat a serious or life-threatening conditions with an unmet medical need allows for submission of components of the application before the complete application, but stipulates that the application needs to provide a schedule for submission of sections that would make the application complete. In this case, the review clock would begin once the application is complete.

V. PRESUBMISSION AND POSTSUBMISSION PROCESSES

The marketing application requires maintenance not only before submission, but also after submission, during the review process, and after approval. Some of the presubmission and postsubmission processes that effect the NDA/BLA content are outlined below.

A. Pre-NDA/BLA Meetings

Pre-NDA/BLA meetings (*i.e.*, end-of-Phase 2 and Pre-NDA/BLA meetings) are important meetings to exchange information with the FDA regarding the product's development and resulting data and to indicate intentions for format and content of the NDA/BLA. The FDA Guidance documents entitled *Formal Meetings with Sponsors and Applicants for PDUFA Products (2000)* identifies procedures applicable to requesting and holding meetings, and it outlines recommended content for premeeting information packages.

Consistent with the FDA's 2000 guidance, a table of contents for the pre-NDA/BLA meeting information package may comprise the following*

1. Background/overview, including[†]
     Product name and application number (if available)
     Chemical name and structure
     Proposed indication(s), including scientific rationale, development plan, and regulatory information (include references to previous regulatory interactions and resolution of action items)[‡]
     Dosage form, route, regimen (frequency and duration)
     General purpose of the meeting and objectives or outcomes expected from the meeting, including the general nature of questions to be asked, how the meeting fits in with the development plan, and a brief discussion of the specifics of the NDA/BLA and the completed/planned studies/data
     Agenda
2. Specific questions[†]
3. Proposed labeling and intended use[‡]
4. Proposed NDA/BLA table of contents[‡]
5. Clinical data summary
6. Nonclinical data summary
7. Chemistry data summary

---

* Reproduced from D. Fordyce, "Establishing the Format and Content of an NDA/BLA" in S. Linberg (ed.), *Expediting Drugs and Biologics Development—A Strategic Approach*, 2nd ed., with permission from Parexel®.

[†] This information will be included in the request for the meeting and should be updated in the premeeting information package.

[‡] Although this information is not specifically cited in the aforementioned guidance document, it is appropriate to include this information to obtain FDA feedback on the structure of critical elements of labeling and the plan for organization and submission of the application (*e.g.*, plans to submit abbreviated reports versus electronic reports) and recommended in division-specific pre-NDA meeting guidance. Regulatory information should include a summary of previous meetings, agreements, and requests for information and subsequent responses, and should reference components of the submission that address any outstanding issues.

The premeeting information package should be as concise as possible. It should be fully paginated, with a table of contents and appropriate tabs, cross-references, indexes, and appendixes. The FDA's 2000 guidance indicates that the specific questions should frame much of the meeting content and, therefore, the specific questions should be as precise and comprehensive as possible.

B. Safety Update

In accordance with 21 CFR § 314.50(d)(5)(vi)(b) and 21 CFR § 601.2, safety updates are required 4 months (120 days) after filing the application, after receiving an approvable letter, and at other times as requested by the FDA. The safety updates are required to be submitted in the form of the integrated summary of safety information. In addition, case report forms for all patients who died during a clinical study* or who discontinued because of an adverse experience are required. According to the *Guideline for Format and Content of the Clinical and Statistical Sections of an Application*, if the total exposure has changed substantially, generally increased by 25% or more, the overall analysis of both new and old data is required. Because a substantial increase in exposure could greatly effect the conclusions of the application, it is appropriate to consider data cutoff/lock dates such that the information is inclusive up to several months before the submission.

VI. NEW DEVELOPMENTS—FDAMA AND THE COMMON TECHNICAL DOCUMENT

A. FDA Modernization Act (FDAMA of 1997)

A comprehensive summary of the FDA Modernization Act of 1997 can be found in several sources, including the F-D-C Reports summary prepared by Hyman, Phelps & McNamara, P.C. (1997). This legislation improves the regulation of drugs by streamlining the review process with several key initiatives. The FDAMA initiative regarding the reauthorization of PDUFA (PDUFA II) and user fees (Sections 101–107) to provide resources for application reviews was discussed briefly earlier in this chapter. Additional selected initiatives aimed at streamlining the review process are summarized as follows:

---

* Generally, this includes information 4 weeks after a study is completed, or otherwise discontinuing drug, or more if the product has a long half-life or has known late occurring effects [*Draft Guidance—Reviewer Guidance Document for Conducting a Clinical Safety Review of a New Product Application and Preparing a Report on the Review* (1996)].

Fast Track Status for drugs intended to treat serious and life-threatening conditions with an unmet medical need (Section 112): This initiative essentially codifies the FDA's accelerated approval regulations for drugs and biologics (21 CFR 314 Subpart H and 21 CFR 601 Subpart E). This information is described in detail in the *Guidance for Industry—Fast Track Drug Development Programs—Designation, Development, and Application Review* (1998).

Clinical Investigations (Section 115): This initiative allows for approval based on substantial evidence of effectiveness from one adequate and well-controlled trial and confirmatory evidence. This information was previously outlined in the *Draft Guidance for Industry—Providing Clinical Evidence of Effectiveness for Human Drug and Biological Products* (1998).

Data Requirements for Drugs and Biologics (Section 118): This initiative allows for submission of abbreviated reports for studies that are not intended to contribute to the evaluation of effectiveness or support information included in the labeling. This information is detailed in the *Draft Guidance for Industry—Submission of Abbreviated Reports and Synopses in Support of a Marketing Application* (1999).

Content and Review of Applications (Section 119): This initiative provides a requirement for the FDA, upon written request, to meet with the sponsor of an IND or applicant of and NDA or ANDA to establish the clinical trial design to form the basis of effectiveness claims and provide minutes of these agreements. This information is described, in part, in the *PDUFA II Five-Year Plan* (1998) and the *Guidance for Industry—Formal Meetings with Sponsors and Applicants for PDUFA Products* (2000).

B. International Harmonisation—Common Technical Document

The ICH initiative for the global dossier or Common Technical Document (CTD) [ICH guidance document *M4: Common Technical Document*, divided into quality (M4Q), safety (M4S), and efficacy (M4E) components], scheduled to be completed and implemented by 2002 or 2003, may change the information format and content standards of the marketing application. The CTD is based on identical modules of technical information that can be accepted worldwide.

The techniques chosen for compiling information, therefore, should be flexible and adaptable to incorporation of completed modules of technical information (*i.e.*, nonclinical reports, nonclinical summaries/summary tables; clinical reports, and clinical summaries/summary tables). The information compiled must be appropriate for current regulations (*i.e.*, for U.S. NDAs/BLAs and for foreign Marketing Authorization Applications) and for the future (*i.e.*, for the CTD).

ACKNOWLEDGMENTS

Special thanks to Gordon Johnson of Lachman Consultants and the Former Deputy Director of the Office of Generic Drugs at the FDA for his input and expertise regarding 505(b)(2) NDA applications.

REFERENCES

http://www.fda.gov/cder/regulatory/applications/NDA.htm

http://www.fda.gov/cder/da/da.htm#notes

Approved Drug Products with Therapeutic Equivalence Evaluations. 21st edition. "Orange Book." U.S. Department of Health and Human Services, Public Health Service, FDA, CDER, Office of Information Technology, Division of Data Management and Services, 2001 (http://www.fda.gov/cder/ob/default.htm).

Federal Register. Abbreviated New Drug Application Regulations: Patent and Exclusivity Provisions, Vol. 59, No. 190, October 3, 1994.

Federal Register. Biological Products Regulated Under Section 351 of the Public Health Services Act; Implementation of the Biologics License; Elimination of Establishment License and Product License, Proposed Rule, Vol. 63, No. 147, July 31, 1998.

Form FDA 356h, Application to Market a New Drug, Biologic, or Antibiotic Drug for Human Use. http://www.fda.gov/opacom/morechoices/fdaforms/cder html; http://www.fda.gov/opacom/morechoices/fdaforms/cber html; http://forms.psc.gov/forms/FDA/fda.html.

PDUFA II Five-Year Plan, 01 July 1998. http://www.fda.gov/oc/pdufa2/1998plan.html.

FDA. CDER. ODE IV Pilot. Targeted Product Information. http://www.fda.gov/cder/tpi/default.htm.

F-D-C Reports. *The Pink Sheet, FDA "Targeted Product Information" Pilot Uses Labeling Goals at IND Stage, Vol. 61, Issue 11, March 15,1999.*

F-D-C Reports. *The Pink Sheet, Waxman/Hatch Should be Expanded to Cover Biologics, Vol 60, Issue 46, November 16, 1998.*

Food and Drug Modernization Act of 1997. Summary Prepared by Hyman, Phelps, and McNamara, F-D-C Reports, Inc. Summary Prepared by the Biotechnology Industry Organization. http://www.biocentury.com/fdamod.html (by subscription only.)

Fordyce, D. *Establishing the Format and Content of the NDA/BLA*. In: S. Lindberg (ed.), *Expediting Drug and Biologics Development—A Strategic Approach, 2nd ed., chap. 9. Parexel®, 1999.*

U.S. Regulatory Reporter. Guide to 505(b)(2) Submissions. Vol. 11, No. 11, May 1995.

Washington Drug Letter. FDA to Issue "How-To" Guide for Naming Drugs. August 18, 1997.

Regulations

Title 21 Code of Federal Regulations § 201. Labeling.

Title 21 Code of Federal Regulations § 314. Applications for FDA Approval to Market a New Drug or an Antibiotic Drug.

Title 21 Code of Federal Regulations §§ 600 and 601. Biological Products: General; Licensing.

Title 21 Code of Federal Regulations § 320. Bioavailability and Bioequivalence Requirements.

Title 21 Code of Federal Regulations § 330. Over-the-Counter (OTC) Human Drugs Which Are Generally Recognized as Safe and Effective and Not Misbranded.

Guidelines

Selected FDA Guidelines (http://www.fda.gov/cder/guidance/index.htm;http://www.fda.gov/cber/guidelines.htm)

Guidance for Industry: Applications Covered by Section 505(b)(2), October 1999.

Guideline for Drug Master Files: September 1, 1989.

Guidance for Industry: Fast Track Drug Development Programs—Designation, Development, and Application Review, September 1998.

Formal Meetings with Sponsors and Applicants for PDUFA Products, February 2000.

Guideline [for Item 3]—Format and Content of the Summary for New Drug and Antibiotic Applications; February 1, 1987.

Guideline [for Item 4]—Format and Content of the Chemistry, Manufacturing and Controls Section of an Application, February 1, 1987.

Guideline [for Item 5]—Format and Content of the Nonclinical Pharmacology/Toxicology Section of an Application, February 1, 1987.

Guideline [for Item 6]—Format and Content of the Human Pharmacokinetics and Bioavailability Section of an Application, February 1, 1987.

Guideline [for Item 7]—Format and Content of the Microbiology Section of an Application, February 1, 1987.

Guideline [for Items 8 and 10]—Format and Content of the Clinical and Statistical Sections of New Drug Applications, July 1, 1988.

Guideline on Formatting, Assembling and Submitting New Drug and Antibiotic Applications, February 1, 1987.

Guidance for Industry: Organization of an ANDA, February 1999.

Guidance for Industry: Providing Electronic Regulatory Submissions in Electronic Format—General Considerations (IT 2), January 1999.

Guidance for Industry: Providing Regulatory Submissions in Electronic Format—NDAs (IT 3), January, 1999.

Guidance for Industry: Providing Regulatory Submissions to CBER in Electronic Format—Biologics Marketing Applications, November 1999.

Providing Clinical Evidence of Effectiveness for Human Drug and Biological Products, March 13, 1997.

(Draft Guidance—) Reviewer Guidance Document for Conducting a Clinical Safety Review of a New Product Application and Preparing a Report on the Review, November 1996.

Guidance for Industry: Submission of Abbreviated Reports and Synopses in Support of a Marketing Application, August, 1999.

Selected ICH Guidelines (http://www.ifpma.org/ich5.html)

ICH M4: Common Technical Document
ICH E3: Structure and Content of Clinical Study Reports, 1996.

19
International Planning of Drug Clinical Trials

David L. Horwitz
LifeScan (a Johnson & Johnson Company), Milpitas, California

I. INTRODUCTION

Today's fast-paced pharmaceutical development virtually requires that the international registration of a drug be part of the initial development plan. This requires consideration of both nonclinical and clinical requirements in every country where the drug has commercial value. If only one country's requirements are considered, valuable time is lost making up deficiencies when registration is desired in other countries. Fortunately, efforts at international harmonization have led to increasing uniformity of regulations. However, the harmonization process remains incomplete, and even when uniform regulations have been accepted the implementation of those regulations is subject to considerable local interpretation.

International clinical trial programs are desirable for several reasons (Table 1). However, implementation of an international trial program introduces several degrees of complexity that are not seen in single-country trials (Table 2). This chapter will discuss when an international clinical drug trial should be considered, explore the difficulties associated with such trials, and suggest how some of the difficulties may be resolved. In the chapter, the words "international" and "multinational" will be used interchangeably. Some authors and speakers use "international" to indicate two or more countries and "multinational" when three or more countries are involved, but the distinction is not necessary in this context.

Table 1 Reasons for International Clinical Trial Programs

Increased patient population
Explore population/genetic differences
Varying medical practice standards
Develop local base of support and expertise
Potential cost savings by use of low-cost countries

II. WHEN TO CONSIDER MULTINATIONAL TRIALS

A. Patient Population

There are various reasons to consider implementing a clinical trial program in multiple countries. The most important are summarized in Table 1. The sponsor of a clinical trial must consider the reasons that are most applicable to a particular situation. As discussed below, addition of each new country to a trial increases the complexity and incremental expense. Therefore, identification of the relevant reasons for international expansion of a trial is critical to justify the inconvenience and cost that is introduced.

In many drug trials, patient recruitment is the slowest part of the trial. Therefore, increasing the base of available patients may be the best way to speed up a trial. However, it does not always work out this way. Sometimes, adding more centers in the same country is much easier, faster, and less expensive. Typically, the centers participating in a multicenter trial will not all be equally productive, and if a study has been properly planned those centers that are likely to produce the most subjects are identified early in the planning process and entered into the trial. Hence, addition of new centers will usually mean addition of pro-

Table 2 Difficulties with Multinational Clinical Trials

Cultural differences
   Patients
   Investigators
Language differences
Regulatory differences
Communication logistics
Differences in clinical practice standards
Transportation of clinical trial drug supply and blood and tis-
    sue samples

gressively less productive centers, until there is a point of diminishing returns where the patients added by a center are not worth the additional time and money it takes to add the center. This is clearly a good time to consider international expansion of a trial if it has not already been considered for other reasons.

B. Population and Genetic Differences

Both clinicians and regulatory bodies are becoming increasingly aware of "pharmacogenetic" differences in the way populations respond to drugs. These may result from differences in drug metabolism or frequency of concomitant genetically related conditions. The disease being treated may itself be manifest differently in different populations. For instance, chronic hepatitis B seems to show a different natural history in Chinese populations than in Western or even other Asian populations. This may affect the drug's safety or effectiveness in a given diseased population. Some countries, notably Japan, insist on clinical trial data in their own population. Others do not have as rigid a requirement, but are nevertheless uncomfortable approving a drug until there has been at least some local confirmation of safety and efficacy. The sponsor must consider when it is most advantageous to get such data as part of a multinational preapproval pivotal trial, and when regional studies can be deferred to be done as smaller single-country trials after completion of the pivotal trial program.

Some guidance in these issues is provided by the International Conference on Harmonization (1). The ICH suggests that a drug's sensitivity to ethnic factors may be predicted on the basis of a number of factors, including linearity of pharmacokinetics, steepness of dose–response curve, and mode of metabolism. Potential for drug–drug, drug–diet, and drug–disease interaction are also important. Studies involving drugs with the greatest sensitivity to ethnic factors are the least transportable from region to region. This is even more reason for carefully determining whether such data are best obtained as part of the pivotal trial program or later, perhaps as a bridging study between populations.

C. Differences in Medical Practice

Some drugs may show a greater effect in one system of health care delivery than in another (for instance, as part of a "high-tech," multifaceted approach to treatment as opposed to single-agent therapy). The reasons for the differences may be difficult to elucidate. Some cultures appear to follow a doctor's instructions better than others, and hence there is a real difference in compliance with taking the study medication. Use of alcohol, tobacco, or other recreational drugs may differ from one society to another, and this can have effects on immune competence as well as overall health. Inhaled drugs, for instance, may simply behave differently in populations that have a large proportion of smokers. Availability of nursing staff or other health educators will vary, and this can affect both compliance and reporting of adverse events. Drugs for chronic injection may require daily office or hospital visits for the injection in some settings, while others may teach self-injection. Availability of advanced diagnostic equipment may make it easier to detect both changes in the studied disease and adverse drug events. Some populations may take large amounts of folk remedies, or even have a diet with a high content of pharmaceutically active food ingredients, and these do not show up on lists of concomitant medications. To some extent, it is desirable to eliminate as many of these variables as possible in the pivotal trials, so that any effects seen are limited to the investigational drug. However, even the best-designed protocol is unlikely to cover every contingency. And ultimately, of course, it is desirable to know how a drug will function in the "real world," when therapy is not controlled by a protocol. A well-designed multinational protocol will control, through entry criteria and restrictions in treatment options, those variable that can be controlled, but will give information that will be valid for a number of attainable practice settings.

D. Developing Local Support and Expertise

Once a drug has been approved in a country, the sponsor will want to establish a commercial market for the drug as quickly as possible. A recognized way of doing this is by having local thought leaders who can present the benefits (and risks) of the drug and educate other physicians in its proper use. Inclusion of these thought leaders among trial investigators will assure that they are already knowledgeable about the drug even before it is approved for marketing and, if the trial has been successful, that they are a supporters of the drug. Also, if they have been involved from the start of trial planning, it is likely that the trial will have addressed any specific national concerns that may arise in their country. On the other hand, thought leader support can be developed in other ways, such as smaller trials done following the pivotal trial, perhaps while the dossier is being reviewed. Also, many of the recognized thought leaders are at points in their careers where they spend the majority of their time in research and teaching, and have a relatively small clinical practice so they are not likely to be able to contribute many subjects to the trial. Thus, inclusion of an investigator primarily to obtain local support must be balanced against the logistical difficulties introduced each time a country is added to a trial, and is recommended only if there are other valid reasons for including a particular investigator.

E. Potential Cost Savings

It is indisputable that the conduct of clinical trials, like health care itself, can have very different costs in different parts of the world. It may be tempting to select a site primarily because it is "cheap." However, if the data quality of a site is questionable, the entire trial is at risk and then any cost savings disappear. Cost considerations are discussed in more detail below, in the section on choosing countries for clinical trials. Most important, cost should be considered a factor in deciding on a multinational trial only when use of low-cost sites will not compromise the integrity of the trial.

III. GOOD CLINICAL PRACTICE CONSIDERATIONS

For a trial to be truly international, every country should be doing the same trial in the same way. Otherwise, it is just a series of parallel single-country trials. Doing the trial in the same way in each country implies more than just having the same protocol. Trial monitoring, case report forms, and information flow should all be uniform, so the data are easily merged. The proper way of conducting a clinical trial for the purpose of obtaining drug registration is generally called Good Clinical Practice, or GCP. The initial emphasis of GCP regulations was to assure the ethical conduct of a trial, but the concept has gradually expanded to include issues of scientific conduct and data integrity. Guidelines for Good Clinical Practice specify obligations of the investigator, sponsor, and Institutional Review Board (IRB).

Ten years ago, there was sufficient diversity in GCP standards that it was useful to have publications comparing various systems (2). At the present time, considerable harmonization has been achieved (3). The ICH guidelines should guide the conduct of all international trials. For the most part they do not conflict with any national laws, but at times conflict is avoided by making the ICH guideline somewhat nonspecific and deferring to national regulatory requirements for further definition. This is especially true in the areas defining institutional review boards and informed consent. In the more technical areas such as protocol development, study monitoring, quality assurance, accountability of clinical trial drug supply, and documentation, it should be possible to use similar procedures in all countries participating in a trial. The format of the Investigators Brochure is defined somewhat differently by the ICH (3) and by the U.S. Food and Drug Administration (FDA) [21 CFR §312.23(a)(5)]. However, in the author's experience it has not been difficult to prepare an Investigators Brochure that successfully meets the requirements of both formats.

As noted, the portions of the GCP guidelines that control the ethical conduct of the study, namely, those relating to the IRB and to informed consent, are likely to be most problematic. The need to do studies in an ethical manner is not in question. However, due to legitimate cultural differences there is not uniform agreement on, for instance, the proper composition of an IRB, how much needs to be disclosed to consider a consent as "informed," and the situations in which written, as opposed to oral, consent is needed. Cultural differences arise between the assumption that the individual physician is the best-qualified person to look after a patient's interests and the assumption that the patient himself bears the ultimate responsibility. It is not easy even to approach these questions outside one's individual cultural biases. Difficulties arise when a sponsor wishes to use clinical data from one country to support approval in another country. If the sponsor is not able to document that the study was done according to the ethical precepts of the country *receiving* the data, the data may not be acceptable even though it was obtained following all of the rules of the country where it was produced. These principles arose at a time when it was felt that some sponsors of clinical trials were exploiting the population of a foreign country to conduct a study that would not be allowed in their own nation. Such practice is certainly not common today, but its regulatory legacy can continue to affect us. Planners of international clinical trials must ascertain before beginning a trial if any trial site will not meet internationally accepted GCP standards and either decide not to use that site or acknowledge the possibility that data from that site may not be internationally acceptable.

IV. CULTURAL CONSIDERATIONS

The previous section considered some cultural considerations that can affect the informed-consent process from a regulatory standpoint. Other factors to be considered are regional practices on what the physician traditionally tells the patient. For instance, in some countries, especially in Asia, physicians often do not tell patients that they have cancer. While the family is informed, both the family and the physician are expected to "protect" the patient from knowing the diagnosis. How, then, can such a patient give an informed consent to participate in a trial of a new therapy for cancer? Like many such questions, there is no answer that can be separated from one's personal ethical background. A local IRB may be very comfortable dealing with this issue, but a foreign regulatory authority may find the consent process to be unacceptable. While there is not a solution to this problem, it is critical that the sponsor understand in advance that such a situation exists, so that an intelligent decision can be made on the feasibility of a multinational trial in this circumstance.

Cultural considerations may also affect experimental design. In some countries, the concept of a placebo control is simply not acceptable. The norm is to treat everyone, and so the control must be an alternative treatment or a lower dose of the study drug. In other situations, an oral or topical placebo may be acceptable, but an injectable or suppository placebo may not be because it is felt that such intrusion without potential therapeutic benefit is not ethically acceptable. The sponsor's only alternatives may be to omit such locations from the clinical trial or using an altered protocol at those sites, with the resulting reduction in data that can be pooled.

In other environments, compensation of the patient becomes an issue. At one end of the spectrum, it may be felt that offering the patient access to potentially effective new therapies is sufficient compensation. At the other extreme, patients receive cash payments for their time, inconvenience, and possible risk taken. In between may be monetary payments limited to out-of-pocket expenses such as bus fare or parking. Access to free treatment may not be an incentive to patients who live in countries where a national health service would provide treatment in any case. Patients who learn that they have been randomized to a placebo group may resent the fact that they have seemingly received nothing for their efforts. In some settings, the investigator may be able to argue successfully that the patient has, through his or her participation, contributed to our knowledge of a disease from which the patient personally suffers. However, in some cultures the physician will also feel that placebo patients require special compensation. A commonly suggested solution is a crossover design assuring that all subjects are eventually treated. However, such a design may not be optimal for the scientific questions being studied, and conflicts between sponsor and investigator over experimental design may ensue.

The most difficult cultural issue to deal with is investigator compensation. While many would like to deny that it is an issue, the fact is that such concerns exist and, if not addressed, may undermine the best-planned trials. Many investigators participate in a trial predominantly for intellectual stimulation, for the opportunity of publication, or because their institutions urge them to seek grant support to defray a portion of salary. Modern economic realities are such that direct support of investigators is expected in some regions. This is discussed later, in the paragraph on choosing countries under the section on trial costs. A sponsor must be aware that in some cultures the need for such direct payments is not overtly brought up by the investigator and must be volunteered by the sponsor. As long as such payments are reasonable compensation for the time required to recruit and examine patients, to complete documentation, and to meet periodically with the monitor or the sponsor, such payments are fully acceptable. Sponsors are advised to determine, at the onset, whether payments will go directly to the investigator or to the host institution, and the currency of the payment. Payment tied to the outcome of the study, or payment in shares of the sponsor's stock, is almost never acceptable and will raise serious questions with regulatory authorities. It may be advisable to withhold some portion of the payment until all completed case report forms have been received; this should be specified in advance in an investigator agreement. Ownership of the data and publication rights should also be specified in advance. Many institutions will not permit an agreement that allows the sponsor to determine whether the data can be published depending on the results of the study, but it is usually acceptable to have an agreement that allows the sponsor to defer publication pending establishment of intellectual property rights. If a publication is anticipated, it is best to have agreement before the trial over who the authors will be and their order of appearance and to what national or international journals any manuscripts might be submitted.

V. LANGUAGE CONSIDERATIONS

For those of us who live in English-speaking countries, it is fortunate that English is the primary language of science. It is generally not difficult, in any country, to find a qualified investigator who is sufficiently fluent in English to permit written and verbal communications. Therefore, protocol development and investigators meetings rarely present a problem. A bigger problem can be reaching investigators through secretaries who do not speak English, or dealing with study staff, such as clinical coordinators, who have less language skills. These factors should be considered when deciding whether an international trial will be feasible.

Even though trial planning can be done in English, some documentation may need to be translated to conduct a trial. Protocols may have to be in the local language for submission to health authorities or ethics committees. Written informed-consent forms must always be in the local language. In some countries with more than one official language, or with local dialects that are not mutually understandable, some documents may need to be prepared in several languages.

Case report forms can present a real challenge (Table 3). Can English be read by those completing the forms, by those auditing the data, and by those doing data entry? Are multilingual forms necessary, or must versions be prepared in multiple languages? Even if English is used, will it be American or British spelling (hemoglobin or haemoglobin)? If abbreviations are used, are they com-

Table 3 Choosing a Language for Case Report Forms

What language is used by those completing the form?
What language is used by those monitoring the trial and
  auditing the data?
What language is used by those doing data entry?
Are there specific formats for proper names that must be
  considered. Is the family name first, last, or in the
  middle?
Are nonstandard abbreviations being used?
Are units of measurement the same in all countries?

monly used in a similar way at all sites (does the hematology laboratory do a Complete Blood Count, CBC, or a Full Blood Count, FBC)? Do all sites use SI units (many in the United States do not, but other countries generally do)? Do we instruct the investigator to mark a box with a "check" or with a "tic"? An example may be the easiest way to give the instruction.

Names can be a special problem. Patient names are often omitted from case report forms to protect confidentiality, but investigators' names and names of others completing the form are necessary. If we provide specific spaces to enter the name, we may without thinking ask for first name, middle initial, last name. It is important to be aware that the family name may come last, as it often does in names of Northern European origin, but may also come first, as in names of Chinese origin. In Spanish names, the name in the middle is of key importance. Some options are to label spaces on the form for "family name" and "given name," or to have only a single space for the entire name and use the technique often seen on customs forms of asking the person completing the form to underline the family name. Proper name completion is especially important to avoid errors at the time of data entry. With regard to patient names, use of study numbers eliminates most problems (investigator numbers can also be used to avoid confusion). However, some forms also ask for patient initials as a double check on identity. In countries with nonphonetic writing, the concept of initials does not always apply, so special provision must be made in these cases.

VI. MONITORING THE INTERNATIONAL CLINICAL TRIAL

GCP standards require that clinical trials done for registration purposes be adequately monitored. Monitoring is done to assure that the rights and well-being of human subjects are protected; that the reported trial data are accurate, complete, and verifiable from source documents; and that the conduct of the trial is in compliance with the currently approved protocol, with GCP, and with the applicable regulatory requirements. Generally, this monitoring is accomplished by periodic visits to each clinical trial site by an appropriately trained monitor.

The monitor is often the primary contact between the investigator and the sponsor, and so must play the difficult role of being both a public relations spokesperson for the sponsor and also an authoritative "police" figure when necessary. To do this well requires a person with exceptional interpersonal skills. In an international trial, it is critical that the monitor be culturally sensitive to the customs of each country visited. Especially in the early stages of a trial, errors are sometimes made in following the protocol or, more commonly, in completing case report forms. The monitor is obligated to point out these errors and see that they are corrected. However, in some cultures, acknowledging that one has made an error results in "loss of face," and many are unwilling to do it. If an error was made by a senior investigator, junior members of his or her staff may be unwilling to point out the error and may want to cover it up rather than correct it. A culturally sensitive monitor should know when it is inadvisable to say, "this is wrong," and will instead say, "let me show you how the sponsor needs to have this done to meet U.S. requirements." The stigma associated with making a mistake is so strong in some cultures that the author has seen study coordinators copy entire sets of case report forms rather than acknowledge an error through the practice, which is taken for granted in the United States, of simply drawing a line through the error, initialing and dating it, and writing in the correct information.

In addition to cultural sensitivity, adequate language skills are needed by the international monitor. As noted previously, site study coordinators may not be fluent in English. Primary source documents are usually in the local language. An ability to speak the local language is often necessary simply to find one's way to the proper location for reviewing the documents, and for requesting any needed documentation. Therefore, to conduct an international trial properly, a sponsor should carefully determine whether adequate monitoring can be done before accepting a site into the study.

VII. STRATEGIES FOR DATA COLLECTION

Data collection in all trials is being increasingly automated. Through the use of direct electronic data entry at the site, electronic transmission by modem or Internet connection, or through faxed transmission of data on paper, collection of data from multiple sites has become almost trivial. However, as the transmission process becomes simpler, the efforts needed to assure the accuracy of the data transmitted become more complex. For instance, if direct electronic entry of data is done at each site, the computer screens used to enter the data must be designed with the same attention to differences in language and specific use of terms and abbreviations that was noted above when case report forms were discussed. Because predesigning computer screens is often more complex than redesigning paper case report forms, this is sometimes more difficult to do. If data are transmitted to a data processing center directly by the investigator, rather than being collected on site by the study monitor, the data "clean-up" at the end of the study is likely to take longer and, because it is done farther in time from the actual creation of the data, may be more difficult to do—especially if investigators, co-investigators, or their staff have changed or if source documents have been misplaced. Most automated data analysis systems now being used to process clinical trial data routinely generate a "query" when results appear to be missing or inconsistent, or fall outside predetermined ranges. These queries often must be brought to the investigators' attention for resolution, and they frequently lack the cultural sensitivity discussed above under monitoring.

If case report forms have been prepared in multiple languages and are being sent to a central center for data entry and processing, some simple steps can help minimize data entry errors. Apart from the language differences, the layout of the case report forms should be similar so the data entry technician can enter data by location on the form rather than by the label of the item. As an extra safeguard, it is useful to have a small number identifying each data field on the form, and this number should be uniform across all language variants of the form. This is especially important in long columns or rows of items, so the data technician can use the field number rather than the foreign language label to confirm that the proper data field is being entered into each location in the database.

VIII. CHOOSING THE COUNTRIES FOR AN INTERNATIONAL DRUG TRIAL

Many factors must be considered when considering the countries to participate in a multinational trial (Table 4). Certainly, the considerations that apply to a single-country multicenter trial also apply here. Specifically, all centers should be able to produce data of equally high quality. One center or one country should not dominate the trial, but there should be enough subjects in various sites in the involved countries so that center-to-center and country-to-country comparisons can be made. The trial may not need to be statistically powered to detect intercountry differences (it is advisable to explore this question with regulatory authorities before starting the trial), but it should be clear that there are no major inconsistencies between centers or between countries. If the results of a trial are driven largely by unusually good results from only one site or only one country, health authority reviewers are likely to be skeptical of the overall findings.

The preceding discussion has pointed out many of the problems that may occur in international trials, and has repeated suggested factors that may lead a sponsor to decide that a particular country or individual site may not be suitable

Table 4 Choosing Countries for Multinational Clinical Trials

High prevalence of condition being studied
Appropriate patients accessible through health care system
Suitable Infrastructure
    Knowledgeable investigators
    Acceptable laboratory facilities
    Available Institutional Review Boards
    Timely regulatory review when required
Reasonable cost of conducting trial

for a specific trial. Having eliminated such sites, there will usually be many sites that remain potential trial centers. The following factors may help in this further selection.

A. Disease Prevalence

If one is expanding a trial internationally primarily to enhance patient recruitment, knowledge of the demographics of the clinical condition in question is critical. While no one is likely to go to northern Europe to study malaria, or central Africa to study cystic fibrosis, the decisions are usually more subtle than this. Often, market research will have already been done to determine the largest markets for the disease, and these will frequently (but not always) be the best places to go for clinical trials. They will also be the countries where the needs of local populations, local thought leaders, and local regulatory bodies must also be considered, and so turn out to be the logical nations to consider first.

B. Subject Accessibility

A good country for a clinical trial must not only have a reasonably high prevalence of the condition being studied; the patient population must be accessible for study. Countries with a strong national health care system may have centralized registries of patients, allowing those with a given diagnosis to be readily found. Countries with large tertiary referral centers, often associated with universities, will be helpful if the disease is one which is often referred to such centers. On the other hand, if the condition is generally managed by primary care providers, the sponsor must either find investigators with a very large practice or be able to attract patients to study centers. The local cultural climate regarding physician referral of patients, patient self-referral for a study, and patient advertising to recruit subjects must be carefully evaluated to see if adequate trial enrollment will be possible. It is unwise to assume that patient recruitment techniques that have proven successful in one's own country will be equally successful in another country. Indeed, they may prove to be illegal or ethically unacceptable to the local medical community.

C. Investigator Qualifications

In addition to a suitable patient population, a good country for a clinical trial must have a good investigator population. If the trial will be used for multinational registrations, it is imperative that the investigator have a thorough understanding of the principles of a randomized, controlled clinical trial. Investigators who are unwilling to properly randomize patients or to follow a protocol rigorously will weaken the entire clinical program. Fortunately, it is now becoming fairly easy to find investigators who have trained in internationally recognized centers and who have participated in a controlled trial at an earlier phase of their career. However, it is not rare to encounter a physician who may have considerable prestige nationally or internationally, and who may indeed be an excellent clinician and teacher, but who is not prepared to accept the limitations on free choice imposed by a defined protocol. These individuals are often most valuable when used in a consulting capacity or on a review committee, but may not be suitable trialists.

D. Laboratory Support

Laboratory measurements are frequently primary end points in drug clinical trials. Therefore, the availability of acceptable laboratories is critical. It is often desirable to use a single reference laboratory for all measurements in a multicenter clinical trial, and this is generally accomplished by having each center ship its samples to the reference lab or by using a service (often provided by commercial reference laboratories) that picks up the samples from each site. When multiple countries are involved, the logistics quickly become complex. If multiple labs are used, each must be audited for compliance with acceptable laboratory practices, an acceptable quality assurance program, and timeliness of reporting. While some laboratory proficiency testing programs are available internationally, not all labs use them. Records may be kept in different languages, and different reporting units may be used. A common requirement for clinical trials is that each center must have a certified laboratory, but not all countries have national certifying bodies, and the standards of certification may be variable. Thus, particular scrutiny is needed when multiple laboratories are to be used in a trial intended for multinational drug registration.

Other types of complexities arise if it is decided to use a common reference laboratory. The sponsor will almost always have to arrange for shipping of samples, as few, if any, commercial reference laboratories provide this service on an international basis. Because of public health concerns, there is considerable restriction on movement of medical samples that consist of body fluids. Some countries require export approval from the Ministry of Health; others require import approval. Packaging of samples must be done in ways that protect both the sample and the carrier from accidental breakage. If samples must be sent at controlled temperatures, delays in customs must be anticipated. Many air carriers will not accept any shipments in Dry Ice on a passenger flight. Shipping costs and the cost of customs brokers can add considerable expense to a trial. All of these factors must be considered early in the trial planning, and a trial site (and country) should be selected only after it is confirmed that provision can be made for adequate handling of laboratory specimens.

International standards are being developed for clinical laboratory testing (ISO TC 212). As these are implemented, comparison of laboratories and choice of a reference laboratory will be simplified. And in situations where multiple laboratories are used in a trial, comparisons between labs will be potentially far easier.

E. IRB Reviews

Regulatory requirements vary from country to country, and must also be considered in the trial process. Some countries require government approval for any trial on a new drug [similar to the U.S. Investigational New Drug (IND) application]. In other countries, there is no formal government review and the government will defer to the expertise of an institutional ethics committee. Virtually all countries require that human studies be approved by an institutional review board (IRB) or an ethics committee and, even if it is not required, the sponsor will generally want such a review to be completed to assure that the trial will be accepted internationally. Thus, in selecting trial sites the sponsor must inquire about the availability of an IRB, how frequently it meets, and the timeliness of its reviews. In some centers, an IRB may meet frequently and complete review of all protocols submitted to it, and a review can be guaranteed within a specified time period. In other jurisdictions, the IRB may meet only occasionally, meetings may not be held during holiday periods (which may last a month in some countries), and the IRB will review only a fixed number of applications at each meeting, resulting in a backlog if the protocols submitted exceed this number. All of this needs to be determined in advance.

F. Government Regulation

When formal government review is required, the length of the process must be considered. Some countries, like the United States, follow a relatively rapid procedure and allow a trial to begin 30 days after an application is received unless the government acts to delay the start. In other countries, formal approval is required before beginning. In some, the application to the government cannot be made until after IRB approval is obtained, and the delays can be considerable. In addition, for approval to begin the trial, permission must be obtained to export the drug from the country of manufacture, and import it into the trial countries. Export rules vary from country to country. In the United States, they have recently been simplified, particularly for shipments to the more developed countries. Importation, on the other hand, can be quite complex and may require multiple approvals from several government jurisdictions. Generally, an in-country resource is needed to manage the process, and sponsors without an international presence will usually require considerable consultation with experienced local advisors to carry out the process successfully.

G. Trial Cost

Finally, the cost of the trial must be considered. Sometimes, the perceived ability to reduce the cost of a trial is a primary reason for doing a trial in a specific country. Sometimes the costs reduction is very real. Particularly when a study involves hospitalization, hospital costs may be substantially less in some parts of the world. Differences in stipends to investigators may also be quite different, due to regional differences in cost of living. On the other hand, additional costs are incurred, as noted above, due to shipping of drug supply, lab samples, and case report forms. Also, cultural differences may make it difficult to settle on what the true study budget really is. In the United States, for instance, there is usually a research agreement that specifies a fixed budget that includes out-of-pocket costs (such as local lab tests) and the portion of the investigator's salary that will be provided, as well as any institutional overhead. In other parts of the world, less is committed to writing and it is assumed that the sponsor will provide investigators with travel to international meetings and other incidental costs of research. It can be very difficult, especially if one is not familiar with the local language and does not understand the culture, to gain an understanding of this. The first clue that one is not meeting the expected obligations may not come until it is noticed that an investigator who appeared to be enthusiastic is spending less time recruiting patients and may be devoting himself more to other trials. It is critical that these issues be explored prior to beginning the trial. With good communication, many potential misunderstandings may be avoided. Once again, consultation with someone who is familiar with local customs, and who may know what investigators have received in other clinical trials, may be instrumental in establishing a proper relationship with the investigator.

IX. ORGANIZATION AND IMPLEMENTATION OF INTERNATIONAL PROGRAMS

This chapter has limited its scope to those considerations that, in the author's experience, are important in assuring that an international clinical trial will go forward with the greatest possible efficiency. Many other matters may come up in the development of international trials that are similar to those seen in single-country trials. Many of those are discussed in other chapters of this book. Some, however, have additional complexities introduced when the intent of a trial is to support multiple-country registrations. These are summarized in Table 5, which may also serve as a final checklist for some key factors for every trial.

Table 5   Special Considerations for International Clinical Trials

Will the clinical trial protocol, including entry criteria and end points, support the ultimate labeled indication, package insert, or summary of product characteristics that is
desired in each country where registration will be sought?

Are there sufficient nonclinical data or preliminary clinical data to support commencing the trial in all countries of interest?

Is a mechanism in place to assure that all adverse events, regardless of where they occur, are collected on a timely basis and reported according to the regulatory requirements of all countries where the trial is being conducted, and that serious adverse
events are reported within statutory time limits?

Obviously, organizing a clinical trial introduces an additional level of complexity. Organizational schemes have been proposed to deal with this (4). Often,
the sponsor will be working with functionally separate corporate affiliates or with
independent development partners or distributors in conducting the international
trial, and issues of overall management, coordination of data collection, and ownership of data must be resolved early in the process.

X. CONCLUSIONS

An international clinical trial offers the opportunity of an expanded patient population, parallel registration in many countries, and early development of market
support on a worldwide basis. To carry out such a program successfully requires
awareness not only of multiple sets of regulatory requirements but also of cultural
and linguistic differences, and differences in style and standards of clinical practice. Logistic problems involving transportation of clinical trial supplies, blood
and tissue samples, and data must be identified and solved. A well-trained monitoring staff must be available. With proper preparation, an international clinical
trial can be both intellectually and financially rewarding.

REFERENCES

1.   European Agency for the Evaluation of Medicinal Products Human Medicines Evalu-
     ation Unit. ICH Topic E 5: Statistical Principles for Clinical Trials. Note for guidance
     on ethnic factors in the acceptability of foreign clinical data, 1997.
2.   Waxman RD, ed. GCPs in the U.S., E.C., and Nordic Council: an International Com-
     parative Report. Cambridge, MA: Parexel International Corporation, 1991: The Bar-
     nett International Education Program, Clinical Research Education Series.

3. European Agency for the Evaluation of Medicinal Products. Human Medicines Evaluation Unit. ICH Topic E 6: Guideline for Good Clinical Practice, 1996.
4. Simmons R. Management and Implementation of Multinational Pharmaceutical Development Programs. In: Simmons R, ed. Multi-Company Multi-Country Clinical Trials: Implementation, Monitoring, and Regulations. Buffalo Grove, IL: Interpharm Press, 1993: 257–278.

20

Uncertainty in Drug Development:
Approval Success Rates for New Drugs

Joseph A. DiMasi
Tufts Center for the Study of Drug Development, Tufts University, Boston, Massachusetts

I. INTRODUCTION

The viability of new drug development is critically dependent on the success rates that pharmaceutical firms face when they decide to pursue promising investigational drugs. Despite the fact that when a new drug enters the development pipeline the expectations of the drug's sponsor are that this particular drug will succeed in development and reach the marketplace, an undeniable axiom of drug development is that only a small percentage of such drugs will actually make it to market. Drug developers are well aware of this reality, but they must make decisions to proceed with clinical testing of investigational drugs on the basis of limited information about what their effects, good and bad, will be in humans. Depending on the type of drug and the condition that the drug is intended to treat, animal models can be more or less useful in making predictions about the effects in humans. In all cases, though, the uncertainty is substantial.

If firms knew in advance which drug candidates will fail in testing, then they certainly would not spend millions of dollars and years of effort on what will turn out to be a futile enterprise. For an individual drug, its ultimate fate is the outcome of a binary process. Either the drug will be approved for marketing or it will not. At any point in development, when considered in isolation, the decision to go further with a particular drug must be made on the basis of an evaluation of the likelihood that the drug will turn out to be scientifically successful and commercially viable. Industry averages may mean much less to this kind of decision than do the data that have already been gathered on the drug. Nonetheless, decisions regarding the management of large portfolios of drug candidates, the relative benefits and costs of allocating R&D dollars to different therapeutic programs, and the allocation of venture capital to start-up firms with limited drug portfolios can be usefully informed by data on industry averages about attrition rates and approval success rates for drugs as a whole and for drugs in various therapeutic categories. Public policies that can affect the drug development process can also be better formed if reliable information about technical risks (i.e., the likelihood of obtaining marketing approval) are made generally available.

Given that quantification of the technical risks in drug development can benefit decision makers in industry and government, it is useful to have gathered in one place what the literature on the new drug development process can tell us about these important risks. This chapter is an effort to fill that need. The chapter surveys the published results on attrition and success rates for new chemical entities (NCEs) and new biopharmaceutical entities (NBEs) and also offers updated information on some of these risks using information in Tufts Center for the Study of Drug Development (CSDD) databases.

II. METHODOLOGIES EMPLOYED IN SUCCESS-RATE STUDIES

Studies of clinical success rates for new drugs have focused on periods following enactment of the 1962 Amendments to the federal Food Drug & Cosmetics Act. This emphasis can be explained by at least two facts. Development data for periods prior to enactment of the Amendments are limited, and the addition of a proof of efficacy requirement introduced by the Amendments substantially altered the new drug development process.

The methods used to determine success rates have ranged from descriptive statistics on the proportions of investigational drugs first tested during a given period that have, up to some point in time, been approved for marketing, to inferential statistical techniques designed to predict the proportion of a group of investigational drugs that will eventually be approved. The ultimate fate of the set of investigational drugs under consideration is what we most want to know. However, useful information can be garnered from observing the pattern of approvals up to the end of the study period, especially if nearly all of the drugs in the group have reached their final outcomes.

A series of studies dating back to the 1970s has documented observed success rates for investigational NCEs contained in a CSDD database (1–6). In particular, these studies use survey information on the development history of NCEs taken into clinical testing in the United States by a large number of pharmaceutical firms. The group of firms included in each study varies somewhat from survey to survey, but, by some measures, these firms have conducted about 90% of U.S. NCE development (6). Cumulative success rates at successive years from investigational new drug application (IND) filing for various IND filing periods are presented in these studies.

The Congressional Office of Technology Assessment (OTA) has also examined success rates in this manner using data obtained from the Food and Drug Administration (FDA) (7). Most recently, using CSDD databases, Gosse et al. (8) have presented cumulative success rates for NBEs with first IND filings in the 1980s and compared them to corresponding success rates for NCEs.

While observed success rates at a given point in time provide useful information, by themselves they do not tell us anything about what will be the fate of the drugs in the group under consideration that are still in active testing or are under review by regulatory authorities. A number of studies have used nonstatistical mathematical modeling to account for the contribution that drugs still active at the time of the study will have on the final approval rate (9–11). These studies apply the experience of drugs whose fate has already been determined to those that are still active. Typically, the assumption is made that the ratio of the number of drugs that have been discontinued in a clinical phase to the total of drugs that were either discontinued in the phase or had moved on to the next phase can be used as the discontinuance rate for those drugs that were still active in the phase at the time of the study. This allows for the calculation of phase transition probabilities and an overall clinical approval rate determined as the product of these transition probabilities. A number of other studies have used this approach to estimate phase attrition rates, but have used other means to determine an approval rate for drugs that enter clinical testing (12–14).

The confidence that one can have in these transition probabilities depends, of course, on the extent of the uncertainty, i.e., the proportion of drugs that are still active at the time of the study. It also depends on whether the uncertain fate of drugs that are still active tend to be mirrored by the experience of drugs that have already attained their ultimate outcome. This can be problematic if, for example, the rate of discontinuance (or approval) varies systematically with the amount of time spent in testing. The drugs that are still active may be predominantly those that have long testing periods. Given that the study periods in these analyses are usually defined in terms of when clinical testing began, the issue is more likely to arise for drugs that are in late-stage clinical testing (i.e., for the late clinical phase transition probabilities).

A number of studies have used statistical techniques to predict clinical approval rates when some of the drugs under consideration are still active. Early formulations of this approach were done by Cox (15) and by Sheck et al. (16). The methods were expanded and refined in a number of later studies (12–14,17). In these analyses the estimation problem is decomposed into two stages. Survival analysis is used to estimate the probability that some outcome will occur a given

Table 1 Success Computations for Hypothetical Portfolio of 100 NCEs

Years from IND	Number abandoned	Number approved	Percent active	Percent completed	Conditional probability of approval	Probability of approval	Cumulative probability of approval
2	25	0	75	25	0	0	0
4	23	2	50	25	.08	.02	.02
6	17	3	30	20	.15	.03	.05
8	6	4	20	10	.40	.04	.09
10	4	4	12	8	.50	.04	.13
12	3	4	5	7	.57	.04	.17
14	2	3	0	5	.60	.03	.20

number of years from the start of clinical testing. A binary regression technique is then applied to the data to estimate the probability that the outcome will be a success (i.e., marketing approval). Combining the estimates yields an estimate of the probability that a drug will be approved a given number of years from the start of clinical testing. A final success rate is then obtained by summing the estimates for each year (more precisely, by integrating over time in the usual continuous formulation of the estimation problem).

The basic approach can be illustrated with a simple example. Table 1 shows the hypothetical outcomes of clinical testing on a group of 100 NCEs. Outcomes are given at 2-year intervals from the date of IND filing. The fate of all drugs in the portfolio is determined at 14 years from IND filing. In this case we know what happens to all the drugs over time, but in a real success rate analysis there would be some uncertainty because some of the data would be censored (i.e., some drugs would still be active at the time of the study). The fifth column of the table (percent completed) gives the probabilities that an outcome will occur in each of the 2-year intervals (survival analysis). The sixth column gives the probability that the outcomes will be successes given that an outcome occurs (binary regression). The seventh column (probability of approval) is the product of the fifth and sixth columns; it gives the probabilities that a success will occur in each of the 2-year intervals. In the last column the probabilities in the sixth column are cumulated. The last element of this column is the final approval success rate.

III. SUCCESS RATES FOR NEW CHEMICAL ENTITIES

DiMasi (17) presents the most recent comprehensive results on clinical approval success rates for NCEs. Both observed and predicted success rates were determined for the NCEs of a large number of pharmaceutical firms by IND filing period. Observed success rates were shown for approvals through the end of 1993. We can extend that analysis and observe approval success rates for the same set of firms through the end of 1995. Figure 1 shows the pattern of approvals over time for self-originated NCEs (i.e., NCEs developed entirely by one firm) for various IND filing periods. For comparative purposes, the 1975–1979 IND filing period results are shown in both parts of the figure. Only 13.7% of the NCEs with INDs filed from 1964 to 1969 have been approved. For the 1970s and the early 1980s IND filings, approval success rates are approaching 20% (18.7%, 19.3%, and 17.7% for 1970–1974, 1975–1979, and 1980–1984, respectively). Further approvals for these groups can be expected, as a number of the NCEs from these periods are still active. Only 8.7% of the NCEs with INDs filed in the late 1980s have been approved, but given the lengths of the drug development and regulatory review processes, many of the drugs from this period should eventually be approved. Some of the drugs in this group have had little more than 6 years from IND filing to reach a final outcome. The approval experience of this group through 1995 shows approval rates that are about 2 percentage points lower than those of NCEs with INDs filed in the 1970s and early 1980s at 6 years from IND filing.

Drugs that have been licensed-in or otherwise acquired tend to have much higher success rates than do self-originated drugs. DiMasi (17) found predicted success rates for acquired drugs that were more than double those of self-originated NCEs for IND filing periods up to the 1980s. The difference in success rates was not as large, but still substantial for NCEs with INDs filed in the early 1980s; the predicted success rate was 48% higher for licensed drugs (30.3% versus 20.5%). A plausible explanation for the much higher approval rates is that acquisition candidates effectively undergo a screening process in which the candidates that are acquired tend to be those with the best prospects. Often some clinical testing experience is available before a decision is made to acquire an investigational drug. Figure 2 shows the success rate patterns for self-originated and acquired NCEs combined. The general pattern of changes over time is similar to those for self-originated drugs, but, as expected, the approval rates are higher when acquired drugs are included in the analysis. Through 1995, 16.2%, 22.7%, 23.3%, 19.9%, and 12.2% of the NCEs with INDs filed during 1964–1969, 1970–1974, 1975–1979, 1980–1984, and 1985–1989, respectively, had been approved.

The two-stage statistical estimation process described above was used in DiMasi (17) to predict success rates by IND filing period. Figure 3 shows these predicted approval success rates for self-originated and for all NCEs. The amount of time available to obtain approvals was too short to make predictions for the 1985–1989 period. Final success rates increased notably after the 1960s, but they have remained relatively stable since then. Since the 1970s, approximately one in five self-originated NCEs that enter clinical testing in the United States will

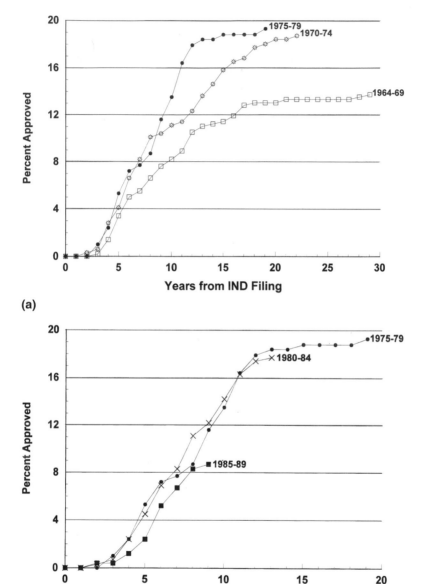

(a)

(b)

Figure 1 Cumulative approval success rates for self-originated NCEs with INDs filed from 1964 to 1989. Success rates are shown for the IND filing periods, 1964–1969, 1970–1974, and 1975–1979 in (a), and for the periods 1975–1979, 1980–1984, and 1985–1989 in (b). Approvals are counted through December 31, 1995.

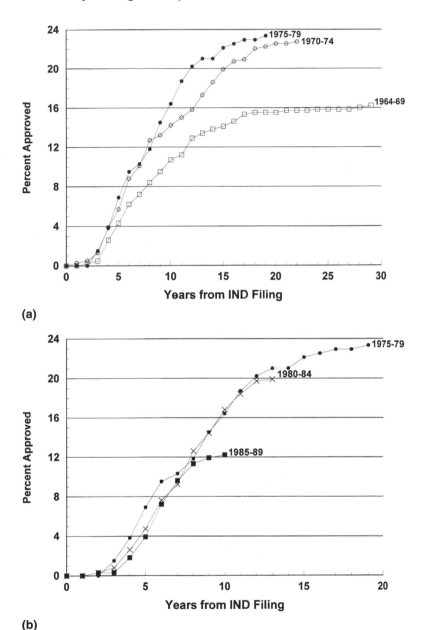

Figure 2 Cumulative approval success rates for all NCEs with INDs filed from 1964 to 1989. Success rates are shown for the IND filing periods, 1964–1969, 1970–1974, and 1975–1979 in (a), and for the periods 1975–1979, 1980 to 1984, and 1985–1989 in Panel (b). Approvals are counted through December 31, 1995.

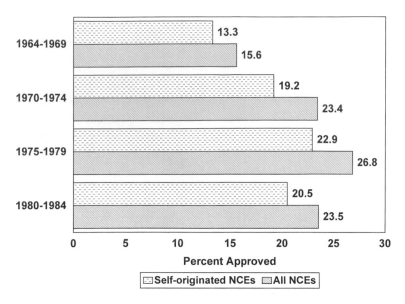

Figure 3 Predicted final approval success rates for self-originated and all NCEs by IND filing period. (Data from Ref. 17.)

be approved. Success rates for all NCEs are about 3%–4% higher than for self-originated NCEs.

The same methodological approach to estimating final approval success rates can also be applied to estimating the likelihood that a new drug application (NDA) will be submitted to the FDA. Figure 4 shows predicted NDA submission success rates for IND filing periods. The pattern of change over time is similar to that for approval success rates. These results can be used with those in Fig. 3 to infer an NDA success rate (i.e., the probability that an NCE with an NDA submitted will eventually obtain marketing approval). These calculations indicate a weak downward trend in NDA success rates, ranging from 86.7% for INDs filed from 1964 to 1969 to 82.2% for INDs filed from 1980 to 1984.

A.   Success Rates by Therapeutic Category

Technical success may be more or less likely for some therapeutic categories. In a study of R&D costs by therapeutic category, DiMasi et al. (13) found different clinical success rates and phase attrition rates for a number of therapeutic categories. A sample of self-originated NCEs first tested in humans from 1970 to 1982 was partitioned into therapeutic classes. Enough data were available to

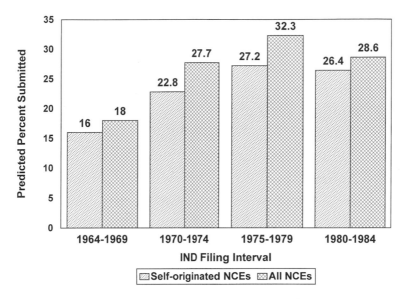

Figure 4 Predicted final NDA submission success rates for self-originated and all NCEs by IND filing period. (Data from Ref. 17.)

determine estimates for R&D costs and attrition rates for four categories. Statistical modeling was used to determine approval success rates for drugs entering clinical testing, and the approach to determining phase transition probabilities described above was used to determine attrition rates for clinical phases. The proportion of drugs in the sample that were still in active testing was relatively small (9.7%).

Figure 5 shows estimated probabilities of marketing approval by therapeutic category for this sample of self-originated NCEs. The probabilities for Phase I are approval success rates for drugs that enter clinical testing. The likelihood of approval for drugs that enter Phase II and Phase III are also shown. The highest overall clinical success rate is for the anti-infective category and the lowest is for the neuropharmacological group. These results likely reflect, to some extent, differences by category in the capacity for preclinical in-vitro and in-vivo testing to predict human efficacy. The risks in neuropharmacological development remain substantial throughout the process. The results indicate that only about one-half of the neuropharmacological drugs that enter Phase III testing will make it to marketing approval. Overall, more than one-third of the NCEs that enter Phase III testing will fail to make to the U.S. market.

The data for this study were also used to examine differences by therapeutic category in dropout rates at various points in the development process. Figure 6

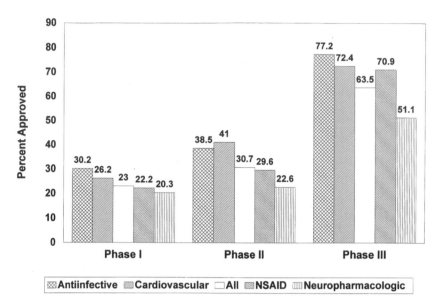

Figure 5 Estimated probabilities of attaining U.S. marketing approval by therapeutic category and clinical phase for a sample of self-originated NCEs first tested in humans anywhere in the world from 1970 to 1982. (*Source:* Ref. 13.)

shows these dropout rates by clinical phase and therapeutic category. Relatively few neuropharmacological failures are screened out in Phase I. Only 10.3% of neuropharmacological NCEs are dropped in Phase I (12.9% of all neuropharmacological failures), compared to 25% for all NCEs (32.5% of all failures). Conversely, a relatively large number of cardiovascular NCEs are dropped in Phase I (36.1%, or 48.9% of all cardiovascular failures). At the other end of the development process, the performance of neuropharmacological NCEs is also noteworthy. Nearly one-fourth of all neuropharmacological failures occur after Phase III, the most expensive of phases, is entered.

B. Reasons for Failure

Aside from submission and approval success rates, the DiMasi (17) study also reports on trends in the distribution of reasons why research is terminated on investigational NCEs. The CSDD database of investigational NCEs that was used to estimate success rates also provides information on the reasons why research was terminated on the drugs that were abandoned. The primary reasons for abandonment were grouped into three broad categories: efficacy (e.g., "activity too

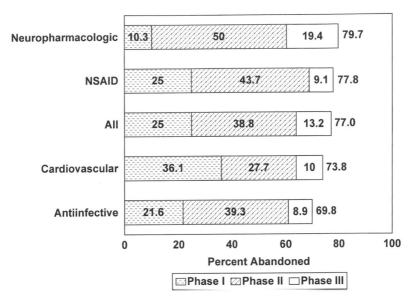

Figure 6 Estimated probabilities of research abandonment by therapeutic category and by clinical phase for a sample of self-originated NCEs first tested in humans anywhere in the world from 1970 to 1982. (Data from Ref. 13.)

weak'' or ''lack of efficacy''), safety (e.g., ''human toxicity'' or ''animal toxicity''), and economics (e.g., ''commercial market too limited'' or ''insufficient return on investment'').

Figure 7 shows two notable trends in these data. First, efficacy's share of the primary reasons for abandonment of research has declined since the 1960s. Second, economics became a relatively more important factor in decisions to terminate research. One qualification to these results is that since the time available for drugs to reach a final outcome is necessarily limited, the termination results are biased in favor of reasons that tend to be discovered relatively early in the process. The bias would be greatest for the later IND filing periods. This caveat, however, serves only to reinforce the evidence for an increasing trend for the economics category. As shown in Fig. 8, decisions to terminate research for economic reasons tend to occur later in the process than do decisions based on safety or efficacy; for all periods, the median time to abandonment was longest for economics. The trend toward abandonment for economic considerations is consistent with a changing marketplace for pharmaceutical products as managed care in the United States and cost-consciousness by foreign reimbursement authorities has grown over time. As purchasers seek ways to control expenditures, fewer development projects will be seen to be commercially viable, especially

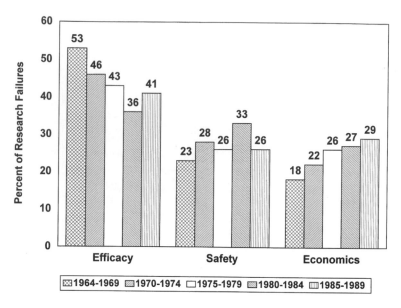

Figure 7 Percentage distribution of the primary reason for abandonment of research on NCEs by IND filing period. A small percentage of terminations in each period could not be unambiguously categorized. (Data from Ref. 17.)

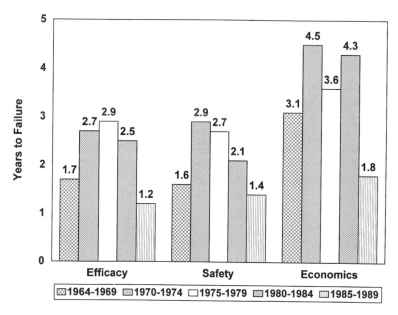

Figure 8 Median time to abandonment of research by primary reason for termination of research and by IND filing period. (Data from Ref. 17.)

products that appear to be therapeutically similar to others that have already made it to market.

IV. SUCCESS RATES FOR NEW BIOPHARMACEUTICAL ENTITIES

The biotechnology revolution has matured to the point where a large number of drugs have entered clinical testing and some have reached the marketplace. Several studies have been conducted in recent years to examine the success rates for biotechnology-derived investigational drugs. Bienz-Tadmor et al. (10) examined success rates for biopharmaceuticals using a database of therapeutic protein drugs that entered clinical testing from 1980 to 1988. Biopharmaceuticals were defined as drugs derived either through recombinant DNA technology or through hybridoma technology (monoclonal antibodies). Given the limited amount of time available for these products to have proceeded through development and regulatory review at the time of the study, Bienz-Tadmor et al. (10) defined success to be the submission of a product license application (PLA) with the FDA. PLA submission success rates were estimated by applying a nonstatistical mathematical approach that used the final outcomes that had occurred at the time of the study to predict what would happen to drugs that were still in testing. Struck (11) succeeded this study with an analysis of phase transition probabilities and approval success rates for biopharmaceuticals that were in development from 1983 to 1991. The data included biologicals derived from nonrecombinant production methods.

Both Bienz-Tadmor et al. (10) and Struck (11) found success rates that are much higher than those that have been found for NCEs. Bienz-Tadmor et al. (10) predicted that the probability of PLA submission for NBEs will be in the range 56%–64%. Multiplying estimated phase transition probabilities, Struck (11) found an approval rate of 71% for biopharmaceuticals that enter clinical testing. For the purpose of estimating success rates, however, both studies used datasets that had strong limitations. For the Bienz-Tadmor et al. (10) analysis, 55% of the drugs in the sample were still active at the time of the study (i.e., they had neither been discontinued nor had a PLA submitted). In the case of Struck (11), 90% of the products were still in development or regulatory review. In addition, using lengthy study periods for a new and evolving technology sector can disguise important changes that occur during the period analyzed. Specifically, implicit in these studies is an assumption that success and attrition rates for biopharmaceuticals would be the same for the early 1980s, when the first investigational drug candidates entered clinical testing, as they would be for the late 1980s or early 1990s.

The most recent study of biopharmaceutical success rates is Gosse et al. (8). This study has the advantage over the earlier ones of being able to use a dataset for which the outcomes of drugs that entered clinical testing in the 1980s were observed over a longer period. The authors obtained information on discontinuations and approvals through the end of 1995. The nature of the data was such that a full statistical modeling to predict future success rates was not feasible. While survival analysis was used to estimate that rate at which drugs drop out of active status (either through abandonment or marketing approval), the data did not fit binary regression models sufficiently well to conduct a second-stage analysis on the conditional probability of approval.

The Gosse et al. (8) study presented cumulative success rates at successive years from IND filing. The first recombinant proteins and therapeutic monoclonal antibodies (TMAbs), which that entered clinical testing during 1980 to 1994, were analyzed. The recombinant proteins were grouped into two categories: new recombinant entities (NREs) and recombinant versions of already-approved products (NRVs). NREs were defined to be proteins derived from recombinant DNA technology that had not previously been tested in humans. The outcomes for NREs and TMAbs through 1995 have been tabulated from results in Gosse et al. (8) and are shown in Table 2. Combining the NREs and TMAbs (arguably the most innovative of the groups of drugs analyzed), we observe that only one

Table 2 Approval and Discontinuance Rates for New Recombinant Entities (NREs) and Therapeutic Monoclonal Antibodies (TMAbs) Entering Clinical Testing in the United States, 1980–1994

IND filing period	Number of INDs	Number of approvals	Number of discontinuations	Percent approval	Maximum percent approved
1980–1984					
NRE	16	6	9	37.5	43.8
TMAbs	4	1	3	25.0	25.0
NREs + TMAbs	20	7	12	35.0	40.0
1985–1989					
NRE	43	3	27	7.0	37.2
TMAs	45	1	32	2.2	28.9
NREs + TMAbs	88	4	59	4.5	33.0
1990–1994					
NREs	65	1	16	1.5	75.4
TMAs	55	0	17	0	69.1
NREs + TMAs	120	1	33	0.8	72.5

Data source: Gosse et. al., *Clin Pharmacol Ther*, 1996; 60:608–618.

of the 20 drugs that had a first IND filed from 1980–1984 had not attained a final outcome by the end of 1995. For the 1985 to 1989 first IND filings, 28% of the drugs were still active at the end of 1995. Relatively few of the NREs and TMAbs with first IND filings during 1990–1994 have reached a final outcome; 71% were still active at the end of 1995.

The results in Gosse et al. (8) reveal a notable change in success rates for biopharmaceuticals over time. While 35% of the NREs and TMAbs with 1980–1984 IND filings have been approved, only 7% of the NREs and 2.2% of the TMAbs with first INDs filed from 1985 to 1989 have approved. The gap in success rates between these two periods will surely narrow, since a much higher percentage of the biopharmaceuticals with IND filings in the late 1980s are still in active testing than is the case for drugs with filings in the early 1980s. However, even if all of the active drugs are eventually approved, the approval rates for the late 1980s would still be lower than for the early 1980s (last column of Table 2). Additionally, the gap is so great at this point in time that it appears very likely that the final approval rates for the late 1980s will fall well short of the maximum approval rates. The approval rate at 6 years from IND filing is nearly three times as large for the 1980–1984 filings than it is for the 1985–1989 filings.

The apparent decline in success rates for biopharmaceuticals is consistent with a theory of the development of new technologies that posits in effect that the low-lying fruit will tend to be picked first. That is, early development will, for the most part, be focused on projects that have the most favorable technical prospects. As biotechnology matures, success rates for biopharmaceuticals may be seen to be similar to those for traditional chemical compounds. In fact, the success rate through 1995 for the NCEs of the firms included in the DiMasi (17) study with INDs filed from 1985 to 1989 is comparable to that of one group of biopharmaceuticals with INDs filed in the same period (8% for the NCEs versus 7% for NREs).

V. CONCLUSIONS

New drug development is unquestionably a risky endeavor. The question of just how risky drug development is in a technical sense (likelihood of reaching the market) has been the focus of a number of studies. Analyses of new drug success rates have consistently shown that the vast majority of investigational drugs will never be approved for marketing. Since the 1962 Amendments to the federal Food Drug & Cosmetics Act, U.S. approval rates for NCEs have risen from the approximately one in seven for testing that began in the 1960s to between approximately one in five and one in four for later periods. Success rates for NCEs appear to have peaked for U.S. clinical testing that began in the late 1970s and declined somewhat for the early 1980s. Limited evidence for the late 1980s suggests a further decline, although a definitive conclusion awaits further study.

Biotechnology continues to hold great promise as a source of new therapeutic drugs and as a tool used in the development of small molecules. Important new therapies have already been brought to market, and undoubtedly, other important discoveries will be made. However, despite an impressive early record of success in reaching the marketplace, biopharmaceuticals that have been taken into clinical testing since the mid-1980s are faring no better than traditional chemical compounds. The evidence, however, is still limited, and so further study of approval success rates for biopharmaceuticals is warranted.

New drug success rates are important determinants of the financial viability of new drug development for pharmaceutical and biotechnology firms. Although the clinical research costs for a drug that makes it to market tend to be greater than the costs for a drug that fails at some point in testing, in aggregate the costs of research failures are substantial (12–14). Managerial and technical innovations that reduce the number of projects tested in humans that will ultimately have to be abandoned or that allow for earlier decisions to terminate research on such projects can have large economic payoffs. In turn, these efficiency gains can increase incentives to discover and develop safe and effective new therapies. In a marketplace in which pressures to contain costs through generic substitution, therapeutic substitution, drug utilization review, and other means have limited profit opportunities, firms may respond not only by seeking ways to improve the efficiency of the drug development process but also by altering their new drug project portfolios. Greater emphasis may be placed on discovering and developing breakthrough products and less emphasis may be given to products for markets that are already well served. A changing market environment and high (and likely rising) R&D costs make examination of approval success rates and of the nature of the drugs that enter the development pipeline worthy topics for continued research.

VI. REFERENCES

1. Wardell WM, Hassar M, Anavekar SN, and Lasagna L. The rate of development of new drugs in the United States 1963 through 1975. Clin Pharmacol Ther 1978; 24:133–145.
2. Wardell WM, DiRaddo J, and Trimble AG. Development of new drugs originated and acquired by United States-owned pharmaceutical firms, 1963–76. Clin Pharmacol Ther 1980; 28:270–277.
3. Wardell WM, May MS, and Trimble AG. New drug development by United States pharmaceutical firms with analyses of trends in the acquisition and origin of drug candidates, 1963–79. Clin Pharmacol Ther 1982; 32:407–417.
4. Mattison N, Trimble AG, and Lasagna L. New drug development in the United States, 1963 through 1984, Clin Pharmacol Ther 1988; 43:290–301.

5. DiMasi JA, Bryant NR, and Lasagna L. New drug development in the United States from 1963 to 1990. Clin Pharmacol Ther 1991; 50:471–486.

6. DiMasi JA, Seibring MA, and Lasagna L. New drug development in the United States from 1963 to 1992, Clin Pharmacol Ther 1994; 55:609–622.

7. Pharmaceutical R&D: Costs, Risks, and Rewards. (OTA-H-522). Washington, DC: U.S. Congress, Office of Technology Assessment, 1993.

8. Gosse ME, DiMasi JA, and Nelson TF. Recombinant proteins and therapeutic monoclonal antibody drug development in the United States: 1980–1994. Clin Pharmacol Ther, 1996; 60:608–618.

9. Tucker SA, Blozan C, and Coppinger P. *The Outcome of Research on New Molecular Entities Commencing Clinical Research in the Years 1976–78.* (OPE Study 77). Rockville, MD: Food and Drug Administration, 1988.

10. B Bienz-Tadmor, DiCerbo PA, Tadmor G, and Lasagna L. Biopharmaceuticals and conventional drugs: clinical success rates. Bio/Technology 1992; 10:521–525.

11. Struck MM. Biopharmaceutical R&D success rates and development times. Bio/Technology 1994; 12:674–677.

12. DiMasi JA, Hansen RW, Grabowski HG, and Lasagna L. Cost of innovation in the pharmaceutical industry. J Health Econ 1991; 10:107–142.

13. DiMasi JA, Hansen RW, Grabowski HG, and Lasagna L. Research and development costs for new drugs by therapeutic category: a study of the US pharmaceutical industry. PharmacoEconomics 1995; 7:152–169.

14. DiMasi JA, Grabowski HG, and Vernon J. R&D costs, innovative output, and firm size in the pharmaceutical industry. Int J Econ Business. 1995; 2:201–219.

15. Cox C. A statistical analysis of the success rates and residence times for the IND, NDA and combined phases. In: Lasagna L, Wardell WM, Hansen RW, eds. *Technological Innovation and Government Regulation of Pharmaceuticals in the United States and Great Britain*. Washington, DC: National Science Foundation, 1978.

16. Sheck L, Cox C, Davis HT, Trimble AG, Wardell WM, and Hansen RW. Success rates in the United States drug-development system. Clin Pharmacol Ther 1984; 36: 574–583.

17. DiMasi JA, Success rates for new drugs entering clinical testing in the United States. Clin Pharmacol Ther. 1995; 58:1–14.

21

Contract Clinical Research:
Value to In-House Drug Development

F. Richard Nichol
Nichol Clinical Technologies Corporation, Newport Beach, California

I. OVERVIEW

The contract clinical research industry had its genesis in the biotechnical contracting industry that was essentially established in the late 1940s, as a result of the application of selected technologies developed during World War II, to the life sciences industry. Organizations such as Battelle, Stanford Research Institute, and others provided services to the pharmaceutical industry in the areas of chemical synthesis subcontracting and related technical services. At about the same time, the contract toxicology laboratory industry was established, and government regulations evolved during the 1950's which aided the growth of that industry. These contract providers grew rapidly after the passage of an updated version of the Pure Food and Drug Act in 1962. This set of regulations required pharmaceutical manufacturers to demonstrate both safety and efficacy as a requirement for approval of the sale of new medications in the United States This milestone provides impetus for what ultimately evolved into the contract clinical research industry, commonly referred to today as the "CRO industry."

During the balance of the 1960s, pharmaceutical companies established medical research departments, biostatistical and regulatory affairs units, and related corporate functions to comply with the relatively new U.S. Food and Drug Administration (FDA) regulations requiring safety and efficacy. By the mid-1970s, it was obvious to some in the industry that additional resources might be needed to complement pharmaceutical company resources, which could supply additional capabilities relative to the requirements of preclinical and clinical development of new pharmaceutical products. At that time, there was both internal resistance and little economic incentive for companies to outsource clinical research functions, and so the infant CRO industry grew slowly between 1975 and 1985.

During the 1980s, the cost of pharmaceutical product discovery and development soared, and parallel increases in annual health care costs were in the double-digit range. By the late 1980s it was apparent that these trends could not continue, and in the early 1990s, particularly with the advent of the managed care industry and the election of President Bill Clinton, it was obvious that significant cost control pressures would be promptly applied to the health care industry during the 1990s. This led to pharmaceutical companies considering strategies involving consolidation, streamlining, outsourcing, and virtual corporation structures. Additional momentum was provided by the rapid emergence of the biotechnology industry, which frequently was more creative and more productive in leveraging resources than traditional pharmaceutical companies.

II. PROFILE OF THE CONTRACT RESEARCH ORGANIZATION INDUSTRY

Today the CRO industry is robust, with annual growth rates in the 20% range and total revenue in the $5.0 billion range. It is not surprising that this rapid growth has attracted many additional service suppliers, many in the niche category. The following are characteristics of the CRO industry.

From a financial perspective, there are approximately 10 CROs with annual revenues of over $60 million, with the largest companies in the market having clinical research revenues of over $6.3 billion per annum. In addition, large, full-service, multinational CROs such as PPD, Quintiles, and Parexel, have expanded via acquisition into vertically positioned service areas. For example, Quintiles provides services in all disciplines required for product registration, including preclinical pathology and toxicology, reference laboratory services, and outcomes research services, and related functions, such as packaging, formulation, and contract sales services. Large CROs will continue to make strategic acquisitions to increase market share, which will be necessary for publicly traded CROs to support their market valuations.

Diversification into genomics, health care database management, and managed care has occurred. Looking at the CRO market as a pyramid, the lower segment is occupied by companies with specialized services. Companies with strength in product registration, strategic planning, and regulatory consultation, such as CATO Research, serve an important segment of the market, particularly for biotech companies, and have reduced emphasis on capital-intensive elements and related labor-intensive services common to large CROs. There are also a number of providers who specialize in physician, medical institution, and patient resources, and they are enjoying rapid growth as they offer niche services to pharmaceutical, biotechnology, and large, full-service, multinational CROs. Networks of physicians in specialty and subspecialty areas—urology, psychiatry, etc—have evolved, as well as providers of potential patient populations utilizing the Internet and other electronic patient identification technologies. These service offerings are expected to expand and increase in popularity in Eastern Europe, South America, and the Far East, as product sponsors and CROs desire larger market share outside the three major pharmaceutical markets of North America, Western Europe, and Japan.

Contract research organizations have traditionally been ''commercial'' in nature, but the intense cost control pressures in the health care market have created a need for medical schools, teaching hospitals, and research institutes to increase their clinical research services as commercial enterprises. A number of such institutions have begun to offer services similar to CROs—for example, Duke, Columbia, the University of Wisconsin, and Penn State's Hershey Medical Center. By developing a user-friendly clinical research resource base, these institutions can provide services to the major customers they serve, e.g., managed care providers, as well as the National Institutes of Health, pharmaceutical, biotechnology, and CROs.

A. Full-Service Multinational CROs

Full-service, multinational CROs have evolved to occupy the central and top portion of the CRO market pyramid, and have been generally highly successful in the public equity market. They are financially sound, experienced, and capable of undertaking ''turnkey'' development projects, worldwide, as well as providing ''unbundled'' services to clients on a stand-alone basis.

Approximately 10–12 firms exist which have fully integrated service offerings under their complete control; alliances of different companies having complimentary service and geographic presence exist, but lack of central control, different financial capabilities, and cultural differences are major problems with such groups.

B. Specialized Service Firms

A wide variety of specialized service contractors have evolved in the industry, and today it is believed that over 3000 firms exist worldwide to offer selected services in all of the areas required for product development and registration.

1. *Preclinical pathology, toxicology, and animal pharmacology compa-nies.* Offering a wide variety of support services for the development

of potentially promising therapeutic entities, these services can be contracted on a free-standing basis or as part of a full-service CRO developmental package.

2. *Analytical chemistry and methods development contractors.* Specialized services in areas of both methods development and related technology, such as stability testing and dissolution studies, are available from such providers. They frequently work in concert with large product development companies, CROs, and Phase I contractors.

3. *Clinical pharmacology companies.* Phase I contractors can be both commercial and academic, and are frequently chosen on the basis of the specific expertise and experience of clinical pharmacologists and clinical specialists in specific therapeutic and disease areas. Some vendors in this area serve primarily generic and branded generic companies.

4. *Contract manufacturing and formulation companies.* Contract manufacturing companies, some of which are primarily generic manufacturers, can provide synthesis of products for both preclinical and clinical evaluation which comply with Good Manufacturing Process (GMP) standards. This may also involve incorporating dosage forms from other subcontractors who provide unique delivery system technology. Selection of such firms should be based on reputation, price, and technical experience. Choosing the contract manufacturer is one of the most important decisions a product company makes in outsourcing of clinical development services. Some of the more complicated and challenging contracts involve the manufacture of polypeptides and vaccines, although commercial synthesis of therapeutic compounds and metabolites can also be very problematic, particularly if they are relatively insoluble, requiring creative formulation approaches.

5. *Contract packaging.* Contract packaging firms can be retained independently or as part of a full-service multinational CRO. Expertise in these areas has benefited from the availability of experienced personnel from large pharmaceutical manufacturers who down-sized and right-sized during the 1990s.

6. *Clinical data management and information technology.* Effective management of clinical data requires significant expertise from clinical data management experts working closely with information technology professionals. This area is one which is often neglected at small pharmaceutical and biotech companies, and service providers in this sector can supply important services to smaller sponsors.

Investment in cost-effective technology in data management has often not kept pace with other advances in clinical research. This is particularly true in the "front-end" data collection function at investigative sites. Successful evolution of the site management organization (SMO) (see Sec. III) industry will be partially dependent on such advances, especially by SMOs that wish to differentiate their service offerings.

7. *Other Services.* The management of clinical studies is the responsibility of the sponsoring firm, but elements of the program can be delegated to CROs or unbundled to specialty service providers and managed on a "modular" basis. A vast array of these specialty companies exist in the marketplace, and one of the significant challenges of pharmaceutical and biotechnology product companies is to assess the likelihood of performance, quality, and price in this highly segmented market prior to vendor selection.

III. THE SITE MANAGEMENT ORGANIZATION (SMO) INDUSTRY

The SMO industry began in early 1975, when the Institute for Biological Research and Development (IBRD) began contracting with Multispecialty Group Practices (MSGP) for exclusive rights for outpatient clinical trials. By 1978, IBRD had exclusive, 5-year sales and clinical research management contracts with 52 MSGPs, primarily in the Western, Midwestern, and Southwestern United States. In 1983 the company began adding CRO services and evolved into the first CRO/SMO in the United States.

During the 1990s, the number of SMOs increased rapidly. In early 1999, nearly 60 commercial SMO organizations existed, from small two- and three-person groups to companies with more than $20 million in annual revenues.

Many SMOs originated as networks of specialists and sub-specialists; the majority of SMOs are in the United States. Many specialty-oriented networks are now expanding into other areas in order to sustain growth, spread financial risk, and benefit from economies of scale.

SMOs have two primary customers: large and middle market pharmaceutical and biotechnology companies (product sponsors), and large CROs. To date, SMOs have avoided ownership or special relations with CROs, since such arrangements may preempt them from being vendors to other large CROs.

In the future, large CROs may buy or affiliate with large national physicians' networks for the purpose of creating their own SMO. Some CROs have begun to provide management services to physician groups, with the interest of capturing exclusivity for their studies at that site. Eventually, SMOs may reach sufficient size and diversity to create a buying opportunity for large CROs.

IV. KEY CONSIDERATIONS IN CLINICAL RESEARCH OUTSOURCING

Product development companies (sponsors) must consider several factors when determining the need for outsourcing of clinical development services. The experience of the internal team in the therapeutic area is important, and if it is available, it can be used to leverage outside resources using a virtual approach to product development. Individuals in key development areas internally who have experience with the type of product being developed can then function as internal project management staff, and manage the identification, evaluation, selection, contracting, and management of various support functions from different contractors, which have been approved by the "gatekeeper."

If internal experience does not exist in the product development area, which may occur in smaller companies, or if capacity is unavailable, then significant consideration must be given to the selection of a full-service multinational CRO. These companies are listed in multiple directories, and most pharmaceutical and biotechnology firms have direct experience with such firms, or have personnel who have had relevant experience dealing with external service providers.

V. METHODOLOGIES FOR SELECTING A CRO

The CRO industry has grown rapidly since the mid-1980s, and several directory services can provide useful information regarding the profiles of large and small contractors. As mentioned, larger sponsors have "gatekeepers," who can be very helpful in matching internal needs with the right CRO in terms of size, price, experience, geography, and interpersonal "chemistry" with the therapeutic team. If the sponsor has contracted with the group previously, and had a positive experience in the same research area, requests for specific vendor personnel to be assigned to the new project may be accommodated by the CRO.

Absent a previous working relationship with the vendor, the following are key elements of due diligence which can lead to a successful relationship.

> *Experience.* The CRO should have experience in the disease area, with a project of similar clinical research complexity. Programs with multiple indications (i.e., duodenal and peptic ulcer disease at the same site), inpatient versus outpatient (e.g., bone marrow transplant studies versus late Phase III outpatient hypertension), and simultaneous multinational registrations offer different challenges, and vendors need to have the capacity and experience to accommodate these different sponsor needs.
> *Capacity.* It is crucial to determine the capacity of the vendor to provide quality services to the sponsor. This is one of the most difficult areas to

assess for a sponsor, as new contracts, in the same therapeutic category or other areas, can impair the quality of the CRO's service. Quality CROs will reserve capacity given commitments by sponsors, and capacity issues are key drivers of CRO–sponsor preferred vendor agreements.

Financial stability. A significant number of CROs are publicly traded, so financial information is available. Nonpublic CROs can provide financial information through bank references and disclose the principal ownership of the company, should financial guarantees be an element of their corporate financial policy. Usually, the degree of financial risk, which may affect the ability of the CRO to remain viable for completion of the contract, decreases with the length of time the CRO has operated successfully. Significant caution needs to be applied to consideration of using a clinical contractor which has over 50% of current revenues and backlog with one study sponsored by one sponsor.

Confidentiality/conflict of interest. It is difficult to assess the level of confidentiality that a CRO maintains. This is one of several instances where client references are valuable. Also, sponsors should be satisfied that the major shareholders of a CRO are not in a position to benefit from confidential clinical data generated by a trial conducted by the contractor.

Reputation. The single most important element of CRO selection is the reputation it has developed with other sponsors, particularly in the disease area where the new clinical trial is to be conducted. It is common for both gatekeepers and therapeutic team leaders to share information on CROs they have engaged, and relocation of product development personnel from one sponsor company to another is also common. A reliable measure of customer satisfaction in the CRO and SMO industries is the percentage of repeat business the vendor has secured with its clients. The competency and quality of CROs has little to do with their size; as in most cases involving service provider selection, careful consideration of experience, quality, and price is the key determinant of value. CRO reputation involves many factors, including regulatory compliance, history, enthusiasm, integrity, experience and the sense of urgency of the personnel, "on time, on budget" performance history, and performance history with investigators, including prompt grant payments, when warranted. It is useful to contact several investigators who have had experience working with the CRO to assess their level of satisfaction with the contractor.

With regard to selection of potential vendors, it is important to conduct thorough site visits to several potential vendors, where a direct comparison of experience, reliability, personnel experience and turnover, and general working conditions are assessed. It is exceptionally important that the sponsor have a well-developed plan of registration, since time and money can be saved if there is a clear set of targets and goals in the clinical plan that is both realistic and achievable. Protocols, case record forms, and clinical brochures should be reviewed by potential vendors prior to bid preparation. It is also important to indicate to potential contractors the budgets relevant to the registration project, and if these are not within the range considered feasible by the contractor, then alternative strategies can be considered.

Once a short list of potential vendors has been established (usually three), site visits need to be scheduled unless a preferred vendor agreement exists. These should be at least one day in length, and should involve presentations from executives and staff in all functional units that will provide services on the project. A checklist of all functions should be prepared by the sponsor, and each presentation graded by quality of presentation, experience of staff, knowledge of the specific area, capacity, and a clear indication from the CRO regarding the percentage of time each participant will charge to the project. This is also important when analyzing budgets for billable-hour expectations and commitments. The sponsor should make clear the deliverables it expects at agreed-upon milestones, and should also commit to a timetable of its own for vendor selection, so the successful vendor can reserve key personnel for the project.

Once site visits are complete and project specifications finalized, a bid consisting of line items of charges and labor rates should be submitted to the sponsors' "team leader" and gatekeeper. Bids should be prepared within 10 working days of final specifications, as this is a routine practice for CROs utilizing computerized bidding formats. If a CRO takes longer than 2 weeks to prepare a bid when specifications are available, this should be viewed as problematic and possibly indicative of future difficulties. Bids submitted to sponsors should be signed off by the senior ranking officer for the CRO's clinical operations unit and chief financial officer, not just the sales or business development manager. Bids should be effective for 60 to 90 calendar days from the date of bid, and include a "change order" provision during the bid process and in the contract.

Project prices can be fixed or based on actual cost plus a percentage of profit for the vendor. There are different views of which is best, but most sponsors prefer a fixed-cost format with a "change order" provision to protect them and vendors from significant changes in the project which affect investigators, patients, protocols, or other important elements of the program. Fixed-cost contracting provides sponsors with an element of comfort regarding the control of the study to ensure improved odds of "on time, on budget" performance by the CRO. The "change order" provision usually provides sufficient flexibility for both sponsor and contractor.

While public corporate status can be valuable to CROs in many ways, clients can benefit from review of quarterly and yearly Securities and Exchange Commission (SEC) information disclosing the financial state of a U.S.-based company. Careful attention should be paid to the operating profit and the sales, general, and administration (SGA) data contained in the financial reports. CROs with SGA exceeding 25% are usually enjoying financial benefits at the expense of their customers, and sponsors can utilize this information to negotiate reduced prices, as margins can be preserved by the vendor by cutting overhead burden and not quality of services. Prices should be negotiated before the contract is finalized, with rates and charges fixed for the duration of the contract, depending on the length of the engagement.

Once the bid is accepted, the contract finalization is critical to the success of the project. If sales personnel are not completely conversant with all elements of the contract and contract language, this is troublesome. While virtually all CROs use a "team sell," the quality of sales personnel can be a reliable barometer of the quality of the organization and its likelihood of success on the project.

Contracts should be clear and straightforward. Clinical research is an imprecise activity at best, and contracts should reflect that reality. Penalty and performance clauses should be avoided, since they can be misconstrued legally should a damage claim arise from subjects or patients in a clinical study. As a service provider, a CRO's most precious asset is its reputation, so rewards and penalties should not be necessary in the contract.

Contracts should include payment language tied to the agreed-upon schedule and quality of deliverables and prices contained in the final bid. An orderly, well-understood mechanism for change orders is essential, in the event they are needed. Contract amendments should be reserved for major changes only, as they often require review by the sponsor's legal department. If "preferred vendor" arrangements exist with several CROs, a master contract usually exists, and amendments can be promptly executed.

Disputes can arise, and in the past usually arose due to some CRO's delaying investigator grant payments that had been made to them by sponsors. Currently, most sponsors pay investigators directly, based on performance milestones provided by the CRO and validated by the sponsor's staff.

VI. SPONSOR/CRO INTERFACE

Once the selection process has been completed, it is essential that timelines with appropriate deliverables be published to all members of the internal and external development team. Assuming all clinical supplies are available and properly packaged, the pre-study meeting represents one of the most important steps in the entire development process. These meetings are usually held at pleasant and relaxing sites with appropriate amenities, ensuring a positive kick-off to the registration process. This meeting will include investigators and their support personnel, members of the sponsor's development team, and all managers from the contracting firm who will have a direct role in project management, field monitoring, data management and analysis, and related functions. Since this meeting is designed to ensure that investigators and their support personnel are clearly oriented toward the objectives of the study and the importance of compliance with federal regulations, it is exceptionally important that competent medical personnel from the sponsor and the contractor play an active role in the pre-study meeting. The protocol should be finalized prior to the pre-study meeting. Also, given the importance of adverse reaction tracking and related regulatory issues, a regulatory presence from both sponsor and contractor is essential.

If at all possible, an agenda for the meeting should be delivered to participants at least one month in advance, and protocols, case record forms, and other pertinent regulatory information need to be part of the preliminary package. Frequently, slight modifications are made to the protocol at this meeting; particularly if the protocol has been reviewed with the FDA, modest adjustments to the study documents can be considered. As mentioned above, it is highly unlikely that major protocol changes can be made, but tips on patient recruitment, co-investigator cooperation, and data collection and quality can be very helpful.

Once the study has been initiated, frequent contacts between the project management staff of the contractor and the responsible parties of the sponsor are paramount. These meetings should be designed to support the partnership development strategy, and should be managed carefully, including specific agenda items which relate to enrollment, adverse reactions, quality of data, and other important deliverables in the project management process. All full-service CROs and most sponsoring companies have well-developed project management software systems, which can be exceptionally valuable in the management and reporting process. Thus, electronic communication can be on a daily basis regarding the study status, and meetings can be both face to face and via electronic teleconferencing. Within well-developed CROs, the project management software systems are integrated into the bidding process, which supports sales, as well as the accounting process, so that payables can be promptly managed in accordance with the performance deliverables specified in the contractual agreement.

The area of clinical data management is one that is exceptionally important to the development process. Significant amounts of investment in technology which can improve both the quality and timeliness of data have been developed over the last few years, and sponsors will have considered this expertise in the CRO selection process. Data management is an area of potentially high labor cost, so efficient control of this function by both vendor and sponsor is essential. Investigative sites are also very important, as delayed or defective data can cause budget and return-on-investment problems.

There are a wide variety of automated clinical data collection methodologies, which utilize fax, Internet, and wireless electronic data transmission. All of these methodologies have positive and negative features, and the expense associated with each data retrieval, transport, and analysis platform is unique. In addition, the compatibility of the data collection technology with the investigative site's resources is exceptionally important, as are issues of confidentiality.

As is the case with virtually all technology, it needs to be carefully integrated into the total process, which includes training of investigative site support personnel. In addition, the human resource aspect of this process is exceptionally important, since availability of personnel, their competence, and their motivation must be considered in the development paradigm. On long-term development projects, especially those involving a multinational registration strategy, the evolution of the clinical data management process is paramount, particularly as technologies move rapidly toward higher levels of efficiency and performance.

Virtually all submissions to regulatory authorities can currently be made in an electronic format. In planning a good relationship with the reviewing group within a regulatory agency, accommodation of their preferences regarding electronic or hard-copy clinical data is crucial. As electronic submissions increase in regularity and their reliability is validated, it is likely that significant hard-copy validation data may be eliminated, particularly if there is a rapid movement toward electronic patient record systems in most investigative environments.

One of the key elements of a constructive relationship between sponsors and CROs is the issue of payments. These are defined in the original contractual agreements, but are frequently affected by changes in development strategies necessitated by a multitude of factors, including drug toxicity, regulatory changes, and even in some cases the approval of competitive therapeutic agents. In the difficult financial environment that health care entered in the early 1990s, strains appeared in the financial relationships between sponsors and some CROs. As the pharmaceutical and biotechnology industries continue to evolve and become more familiar and comfortable with outsourcing, these problems will decrease.

Issues regarding payment schedules and amounts are normally dependent on milestones, sponsor and contractor business practices, and, with regard to multinational trials, currency exchange rates. It is also possible that advanced payments can be part of the developmental package, and are usually negotiated on a customized basis when the original contract is executed.

Once the study has been completed, summary reports, return of study materials, potential regulatory issue follow-up, and CRO performance evaluations are all important. Many vendors will submit questionnaires to members of the development team from the sponsoring company, getting a frank appraisal of their impressions of the vendor's performance during the study. These are quite important to vendors, as they reflect a feedback mechanism which can improve the service offerings of both large and small contractors to their customer base.

VII. MAXIMIZING CRO VALUE TO SPONSOR

The evolution of the CRO industry over the last 25 years has been remarkable, and the industry currently is going through significant metamorphosis as it responds to changes in the health care environment, customer requirements, and the intense competition which exists in the market. Combined with CRO access to public equity, which commenced in 1993, this will ultimately result in significant improvements in quality. CRO businesses will expand and prosper. When combined with progressive attitudes and creativity in the contractor market, which is absolutely essential because of the high level of competition, this may result in innovations and developments that may exceed the financial resources and the core competency of sponsoring companies. This represents a major shift in sponsor philosophy, but in other industries, particularly telecommunications and information technology, interlocking relationships, and alliances between vendors and manufacturers, have been the key to success in highly competitive markets.

As the cost and risk of development of pharmaceutical products increases, and as the impact of 21 CFR part 11 and HIPAA regulations emerge, careful and appropriate reliance on contractors can be the difference between financial success and failure, especially for small companies. Sponsors will learn to recognize and utilize vendors who can produce higher-quality deliverables at a lower cost, and much of this enhancement of the development process will be strongly influenced by capital availability and the vision of management in the CRO sector.

It is also likely that a trend will evolve in the middle-market segment of the CRO industry. Also, niche providers will offer components of the development process which can be integrated into a sponsor's virtual development model, and will probably compete on a very aggressive price and service basis, as large multinational CROs, particularly those that are publicly traded, continue to evolve toward larger multinational contracts with more desirable pricing structures. Middle-market growth has occurred in retailing, information technology, and a host of other highly competitive young but evolving industries, and it is expected to occur in the CRO industry.

Taken together, the combination of highly qualified, experienced, and reliable niche providers in concert with the full-service large multinational CROs gives customers a substantial choice, which will result in lower costs and higher quality deliverables with improved time frames. Overall, the trends in the industry appear to be quite favorable to sponsors, as the natural evolution of this service industry moves toward maturation via investment in cost-effective technology.

22

Package Inserts as Viewed by the Busy Private Practitioner

Jean M. Findlay
Regional Pediatric Associates, Durham, North Carolina

I. PURPOSE OF THE PACKAGE INSERT

Package inserts were originally intended to provide drug information to practicing physicians. Drug labeling regulations began in 1906 with the enactment of the Pure Food and Drug Act and were expanded in 1938 with the passage of the Federal Food, Drug and Cosmetic Act. The latter act required all drugs be dispensed with information regarding method and duration of use, as well as warning information about unsafe dosages. After the thalidomide tragedy in Europe, labeling requirements in the United States were strengthened in 1962 by amendments to the act. The warning labels were required to include information regarding the active ingredients, the indications and directions for use, the mechanism for drug action, and potential adverse effects of the drug. Over the years, these warning labels have expanded in their content and scope, and are commonly referred to as package inserts.

Although originally intended for physician reference, few actual package inserts are handled by physicians, with the exception of drugs dispensed in office settings, such as samples, injectables, and vaccines. Instead, physicians commonly use the *Physicians' Desk Reference* (PDR), a compilation of copies of the actual package inserts. The PDR was first published in 1946 and contained about 300 pages; in 2001, it contained about 3500 pages. Updated editions are published annually, and supplements are distributed as needed.

A. Medical, Informational, and Legal Considerations

The design of the package insert has to take into consideration the concerns and interests of groups whose needs vary greatly. Physicians need basic, concise information that will enable them to make the best decisions regarding the risks and benefits of any given drug. Not only must that information be assimilated by the prescribing physicians, it must also be translated into the writing of each prescription, so that the necessary information is conveyed to the patient in a manner the patient can understand. For pharmaceutical companies, the considerations for package inserts have to weigh strongly in favor of protecting the liability of the company at the same time as promoting a product for as wide a use as possible. The U.S. Food and Drug Administration (FDA) has to protect the patients' welfare and protect itself from liability.

During the last decade, the FDA, with input from the pharmaceutical industry and from medical and pharmaceutical informational professional groups, has done much to adapt the package insert. One objective has been to adapt the insert to communicate more effectively to professional users, especially health care practitioners in clinical practice. The second objective has been to improve patient information by introducing inserts designed specifically for consumers, and the third objective, which has now been initiated, is to improve the labeling for pediatric use.

II. PHYSICIAN USE OF THE PACKAGE INSERT

To understand the primary care practitioner's use of the package insert, it is first useful to review the practitioner's reasons for using the document, as summarized in Table 1. To establish clearly the risk–benefit ratio of the drug, practitioners may review the adverse reaction section of the package insert just before prescribing. At the same time as physicians decide whether the risk–benefit ratio is acceptable, they also decide what risks to describe to the patient. This is clearly

Table 1 Physicians' Purposes for Using Package Inserts

   I. Prescribing a drug
      A. To establish a risk–benefit ratio
      B. To decide what information to convey to the patient
      C. To establish necessary monitoring procedures for the new medication
          1. Frequency of monitoring
          2. Laboratory determinations
      D. To evaluate potential drug interactions
  II. Choosing between various drugs for the same indication
 III. Searching for documentation that a given adverse effect is associated with the drug in question

---

necessary for medico-legal purposes, but it is also a critical transaction in educating patients and allowing them to share responsibility for the decisions about their medical care. As a backdrop in this process of comparing risks and benefits and assessing medico-legal implications, practitioners must constantly weigh the differences between serious and nonserious adverse effects.

In a busy practice, time constraints weigh heavily on these decisions. Pediatricians in our practice see 25 to 45 patients per day, depending on the season. We prescribe medications 10 to 20 times per day and recommend at least as many over-the-counter (OTC) medications. Reviewing the entire package insert for every prescription is clearly impracticable. We rely on prior review of literature, memorization of the important details of each drug, update information provided by individual pharmaceutical companies, and information from pharmaceutical representatives visiting the office. One package insert for a newer antibiotic was 3 ft long and 2.25 in. wide, with fine print on both sides consisting of approximately 1100 lines with 63 characters to the line. That is equivalent to about 24 pages of this book condensed into leaflet form, then folded into a small wedge of paper and attached to the bottle being dispensed. Not even a speed-reader without presbyopia (farsightedness) could assimilate all that information in the time allowed. It is simpler for physicians to refer to a handy guide such as the Harriet Lane Handbook, in which drug information is presented in extremely brief format. In this guide, in usually fewer than 10 lines, and 4 columns, the most critical information is condensed: brand and generic name; how supplied; dose for each age group or weight or dose specific for each usage; general precautions and warnings; and monitoring requirements or suggestions. Additionally, software is now available for handheld electronic devices used by many physicians, for quick reference to this information.

Another factor that must be taken into consideration is the individual concerns of the patient or family member. This person's need for information will be influenced by things such as prior knowledge, anxiety level, input from media, friends and family, as well as personal experience. In one instance, a patient may need the reassurance that the benefits of a medication far outweigh the risks. An example of this would be vaccines, whose adverse events have received intense public scrutiny. Conversely, a physician may have to caution strongly against the use of a drug. For instance, antibiotics or steroids may be requested for a more speedy return to work or daycare, and the effects of indiscriminate use may have to be strongly worded to the patient. Additionally, the patient may read or listen to the information provided, and then ask questions that have already been answered, or simply ask, ''What do you recommend?'' Documenting the fact that information has been provided becomes crucial for medico-legal reasons. This is also the essence of the content of the package insert. It is the legal documentation that the information has been provided to the physician, who, along with the pharmacist dispensing the drug, is then responsible for conveying that information to the patient.

The physician reviewing the package insert information must also determine the monitoring procedures necessary for the new medication. Decisions must be made about the frequency of physician evaluation, and the need for periodic laboratory work to follow potential adverse effects. At the same time, potential drug interactions with medications the patient currently uses can be identified. It should be noted, however, that not all patients give an accurate history of concurrent medications, for various reasons, including embarrassment, use of more than one physician, lack of knowledge, or the notion that OTC medications do not "count." Pharmacists with a computer system or listing of other medications prescribed may be in a better position to detect potential drug interactions.

Physicians often refer to package inserts to choose between various drugs for the same indication. Factors considered in this decision include adverse reactions, cautions for use in certain populations, efficacy, contraindications, cost, and, in the pediatric population, the form in which it is supplied (many young children cannot swallow a pill, or the dosage of the medication may be inappropriate).

A final reason physicians may refer to package inserts is for information to confirm that a patient's reported adverse experience is actually associated with the drug being taken.

III. STANDARDIZING THE FORMAT OF PACKAGE INSERTS

Package inserts are prepared by many different individuals and groups, and may vary considerably in their content. The FDA requires that all labeling include the following information:

1. Description
2. Clinical pharmacology
3. Indications and usage
4. Contraindications
5. Warnings
6. Precautions
7. Adverse reactions
8. Drug abuse and dependence
9. Overdosage
10. Dosage and administration
11. How supplied
12. Animal pharmacology or animal toxicology or both
13. Clinical studies

ADVERSE REACTIONS (Benadryl Parenteral)
The most frequent adverse reactions are underscored.
1. *General:* Urticaria, drug rash, anaphylactic shock, photo-sensitivity, excessive perspiration, chills, dryness of mouth, nose, and throat
2. *Cardiovascular System:* Hypotension, headache, palpitations, tacchycardia, extrasystoles
3. *Hematologic System:* Hemolytic anemia, thrombocytopenia, agranulocytosis
4. *Nervous System:* Sedation, sleepiness, dizziness, disturbed coordination, fatigue, confusion, restlessness, excitation, nervousness, tremor, irritability, insomnia, euphoria, paresthesia, blurred vision, diplopia, vertigo, tinnitus, acute labyrinthitis, neuritis, convulsions
5. *GI System:* Epigastric distress, anorexia, nausea, vomiting, diarrhea, constipation
6. *GU System:* Urinary frequency, difficult urination, urinary retention, early menses
7. *Respiratory System:* Thickening of bronchial secretions, tightness of chest or throat and wheezing, nasal stuffiness

REPORTED ADVERSE EVENTS WITH AN INCIDENCE OF MORE THAN 2%
IN PLACEBO-CONTROLLED ALLERGIC RHINITIS CLINICAL TRIALS
IN PATIENTS 12 YEARS OF AGE AND OLDER
PERCENT OF PATIENTS REPORTING

	LORATADINE 10 mg QD n = 1926	PLACEBO n = 2545	CLEMASTINE 1 mg BID n = 536	TERFENADINE 60 mg BID n = 684
Headache	12	11	8	8
Somnolence	8	6	22	9
Fatigue	4	3	10	2
Dry Mouth	3	2	4	3

ADVERSE REACTIONS
CLARITIN Tablets: Approximately 90,000 patients, aged 12 and older, received CLARITIN Tablets 10 mg once daily in controlled and uncontrolled studies. Placebo-controlled clinical trials at the recommended dose of 10 mg once a day varied from 2 weeks' to 6 months' duration. The rate of premature withdrawal from these trials was approximately 2% in both the treated and placebo groups. [See table above.]
Adverse events reported in placebo-controlled chronic idiopathic urticaria trials were similar to those reported in allergic rhinitis studies.
Adverse event rates did not appear to differ significantly based on age, sex, or race, although the number of nonwhite subjects was relatively small.
In addition to those adverse events reported above (>/= 2%), the following adverse events have been reported in at least one patient in CLARITIN clinical trials in adult and pediatric patients:
Autonomic Nervous System: altered lacrimation, altered salivation, flushing, hypoesthesia, impotence, increased sweating, thirst.
Body as a Whole: angioneurotic edema, asthenia, back pain, blurred vision, chest pain, earache, eye pain, fever, leg cramps, malaise, rigors, tinnitus, weight gain.
Cardiovascular System: hypertension, hypotension, palpitations, supraventricular tachyarrhythmias, syncope, tachycardia.

Central and Peripheral Nervous System: blepharospasm, dizziness, dysphonia, hypertonia, migraine, paresthesia, tremor, vertigo.
Gastrointestinal System: altered taste, anorexia, constipation, diarrhea, dyspepsia, flatulence, gastritis, hiccup, increased appetite, loose stools, nausea, vomiting.
Musculoskeletal System: arthralgia, myalgia.
Psychiatric: agitation, amnesia, anxiety, confusion, decreased libido, depression, impaired concentration, insomnia, irritability, paroniria.
Reproductive System: breast pain, dysmenorrhea, menorrhagia, vaginitis.
Respiratory System: bronchitis, bronchospasm, coughing, dyspnea, hemoptysis, laryngitis, nasal dryness, sinusitis, sneezing.
Skin and Appendages: dermatitis, dry hair, dry skin, photosensitivity reaction, pruritus, purpura, urticaria.
Urinary System: altered micturition, urinary discoloration, urinary incontinence, urinary retention.
In addition, the following spontaneous adverse events have been reported rarely during the marketing of loratadine: abnormal hepatic function, including jaundice, hepatitis, and hepatic necrosis; alopecia; anaphylaxis; breast enlargement; erythema multiforme; peripheral edema; thrombocytopenia; and seizures.

Figure 1 Comparison of adverse reaction sections for a drug approved more than 25 years ago with one recently approved.

Although the FDA requires these standard categories of information to be included in the package insert, a standardized method of gathering and presenting the information does not currently exist. The information for the insert may be gathered in scientifically different ways, and then presented in formats that vary from one label to another. For instance, one package insert may list adverse reactions by body system category, another by relative frequency of the side effect, and still another by comparison to other drugs in the same class or to drugs having the same therapeutic effect. The format for the presentation of this information may be descriptive or in table form, with numerical frequency rates or percentages. Important information and warnings may be capitalized or framed in a box.

The amount of information contained in the package insert may vary according to the age of the drug and how much information was required by the FDA before approval of the drug for each indication. Data on adverse effects may be collected in different ways. Data may represent a specific premarketing clinical trial experience, or they may include postmarketing data. They may be with or without comparison to placebo or active drug. In Fig. 1, the adverse reaction section of an antihistamine approved more than 25 years ago is contrasted with one more recently approved. The adverse reaction section of the more recently approved drug specifies that the adverse events described were from both controlled and uncontrolled clinical trials. It gives the range of drug exposure before the adverse reaction report and describes the usual dose prescribed. It includes a comparison of placebo with active control, and separates adverse events reported in *controlled* studies from *all* clinical studies. The adverse reaction section from the drug approved more than 25 years ago does not describe the frequency of any of the reported adverse effects, nor does it quantify the duration of exposure to the drug before the report.

IV. CHANGING THE PACKAGE INSERT
FOR PHYSICIAN USE

Considerable recent interest has arisen in providing drug labeling that is easier for busy practicing physicians to use. Research has shown that most physicians use the PDR or package insert primarily as a reference tool. The results of a physician survey conducted by the FDA were presented at a public meeting on October 30, 1995 (*Federal Register*, Vol. 65, No. 247, December 22, 2000, p. 81084). In addition to presenting the survey data, information and input were solicited from interested parties regarding professional labeling for practicing physicians. Of 204 primary care physicians and 200 specialists who responded to questionnaires, only 5% used the package insert directly, and 88% used the

PDR. Reference to labeling was made at least once a week by 95% of primary care providers and by 83% of specialists. Table 2 shows the frequency of referral to the PDR and the relative importance placed on each section.

Of the respondents, 106 physicians offered the following suggestions for items to be omitted: clinical pharmacology (44%), chemical composition/formula structure/pharmacokinetics (10%), and common adverse events (9%). Fifteen percent indicated the information should be condensed. Of 190 physicians who suggested changes, the following new sections were recommended: cost or cost comparisons (23%), drug interactions (15%), adverse event occurrence rates (9%), generic availability (8%), pediatric information (6%), and pregnancy/lactation information (5%).

The three factors most likely to trigger referral to labeling were (a) new drug, (b) patient overdoses or severe adverse event, and (c) patient adverse events. Factors least likely to trigger a referral were (a) seeing an advertisement for the drug, (b) manufacturer representative mentioning the drug, and (c) drug appearing ineffective.

Suggestions for format changes included increasing the type size used, highlighting the most important information, adding an abstract of the most important information, and using more tables, graphs, and lists. Highlighting important information was preferred over providing an abstract by 62%; increased type size was preferred by 77%; and tables, graphs, and lists were preferred by 83%. Abstracts were preferred over increased type size by 65%, and over tables, graphs, and lists by 72%. Thus, it appears that most practicing physicians are asking for a more concise document in a more easily consulted format.

Table 2 Referral Frequency and Relative Importance of PDR Sections[a]

Section	Referral	Importance
Dosage and Administration	3.4	3.8
Contraindications	3.2	3.7
Warnings	3.1	3.7
Adverse Reactions	3.0	3.6
Precautions	3.0	3.5
Indications and Usage	2.7	3.4
How Supplied	2.7	3.3
Overdose	2.1	3.0
Clinical Pharmacology	2.0	2.9
Drug Abuse and Dependence	2.0	2.8

[a] PDR = Physicians' Desk Reference.

V. FUTURE RECOMMENDATIONS FOR THE PACKAGE INSERT

As previously described, rapid access to the most important information is critical to busy physicians. They must make fast, careful decisions about prescribing, including assessing the risks of a particular drug and weighing the consequences of not treating. Because such a burden of responsibility rests on the physician, it seems reasonable to demand a format for the package insert that could realistically be assimilated in the time available. Table 3 lists some suggestions for improving the writing of such a document.

Review of the survey of practicing physicians is very helpful in making suggestions for writing the package insert. Generally, it seems to be agreed that the original labeling should not be superseded by a shorter form. This is largely because health professionals need a reliable source to answer any specific questions regarding a particular drug's use. It is also of great importance to the pharmaceutical manufacturer to disseminate enough information, especially regarding adverse effects. The survey indicated that physicians would continue to refer to the larger insert for specific issues, even if a brief summary were made available, and that they would continue their present use of the insert as a reference guide. However, they would include the most important features requiring the most urgent attention in the proposed brief summary.

At another public meeting in February 1995, representatives from the FDA presented a proposal for a brief summary. Figure 2 shows a prototype for one

Table 3 Suggestions for Writing Package Inserts

   I. Format suggestions.
       A. Separate serious from nonserious adverse effects.
       B. Highlight the adverse effect in the text.
       C. Provide tables of dosages for specific indications.
  II. Quantitation of adverse effects.
       A. Provide the relative frequency of adverse effects, and explain how data was gathered.
       B. Compare the frequency and occurrence of adverse effects from long-term vs. short-term therapy.
 III. Additional sections or subsections to include.
       A. Provide more information regarding use in specific populations.
       B. List drug interactions.
       C. Give information on drug abuse and dependence.
       D. Supply patient counseling information.
       E. Add a separate section specifying recommendations for baseline and periodic laboratory work.

SUMMARY OF PRESCRIBING INFORMATION
CAPOTEN® TABLETS   ℞
(captopril tablets)

WARNING REGARDING USE IN PREGNANCY
Can cause injury and death to developing fetus when used in second and third trimesters. When pregnancy detected, discontinue use as soon as possible. (1, 7.5)

• • • • • • • • • • • • • • •NEW INFORMATION• • • • • • • • • • • • • • • •

• • • • • • • • • • • •INDICATIONS AND USAGE• • • • • • • • • • • • • • •
• Hypertension (caution in renally-impaired patients) (3.1)
• Congestive Heart Failure (3.2)
• Left Ventricular (LV) Dysfunction after Myocardial Infarction (LV ejection fraction ≤ 40% (3.3)
• Diabetic Nephropathy (Type I IDD with proteinuria > 500 mg/day and retinopathy) (3.4)
• • • • • • • • • •DOSAGE AND ADMINISTRATION• • • • • • • • • • • • • •

General: Take 1 hour before meals. Individualize dosage.

Indication	Initiation of Therapy	Usual Daily Dose	Do Not Exceed
Hypertension	25 mg bid or tid	25-150 mg bid or tid*	450 mg/day
Heart Failure	25 mg tid	50-100 mg tid	450 mg/day
LV Dysfunction after MI	12.5 mg tid †	50 mg tid	
Diabetic Nephropathy		25 mg tid	

* Usual daily dosing does not exceed 50 mg BID or TID. Consider adding a thiazide-type diuretic. (4.2)
† A single dose of 6.25 mg should precede initiation of 12.5 mg therapy. (4.4)

Dosage adjustment in renal impairment is required. (4.6, 7.7)

COMPLETE PRESCRIBING INFORMATION: CONTENTS

• • • • • • • • • • • • • •HOW SUPPLIED• • • • • • • • • • • • • • • • • •
Tablets: 12.5, 25, 50, 100 mg; scored (5)
• • • • • • • • • • • •CONTRAINDICATIONS• • • • • • • • • • • • • • • • •
Known hypersensitivity (e.g., angioedema) to any ACE inhibitor.
• • • • • • • • • • • •WARNINGS/PRECAUTIONS• • • • • • • • • • • • • •
HYPERSENSITIVITY REACTIONS
• Angioedema with possibility of airway obstruction (7.1)
MAJOR TOXICITIES
• Neutropenia (<1000/mm³) with myeloid hypoplasia (7.2)
• Excessive hypotension (7.4)
• Fetal/Neonatal Morbidity and Mortality (7.5)
• Hepatic failure (7.6)
GENERAL PRECAUTIONS
• Use with caution in renal impairment. (4.6, 7.7)
MOST COMMON SIDE EFFECTS (≥1/100) (11)
• rash (sometimes with arthralgia and eosinophilia), taste impairment (diminution or loss), cough, pruritus, chest pain, palpitations, tachycardia, proteinuria
• • • • • • • • • • • • •DRUG INTERACTIONS• • • • • • • • • • • • • •
• Diuretics (9.1)
• Other vasodilators (9.2)
• Agents Causing Renin Release (9.3)
• Beta-Blockers (9.4)
• Agents Increasing Serum Potassium (9.5)
• Lithium (9.7)
• • • • • • • • • • • • •SPECIFIC POPULATIONS• • • • • • • • • • • •
• Pregnancy Category C (first trimester) and D (second and third trimesters) (7.5, 10.1)
• Nursing Women: Potential for serious adverse reactions in nursing infants (10.2)
• Pediatric Use: Safety and effectiveness not established. Use only if other measures ineffective. (10.3)
• Renal Impairment: Use with caution. (4.6, 7.7)
• • • • • See 17 for PATIENT COUNSELING INFORMATION• • • • •

PROTOTYPE

Figure 2 Prototype of a proposed package insert summary.

drug's brief package insert. It lists, in very concise form, with capitalized headings, tables, and bulleted listings, the following sections:

Indications and Usage
Dosage and Administration
How Supplied
Contraindications
Warnings/Precautions
Drug Interactions
Specific Populations

This summary is then followed by a table of contents for the package insert that is organized by section and number (3.1, 9.4, etc.).

Although this format was greeted favorably by physician groups, representatives from the pharmaceutical industry raised objections based both on the extra cost of production and the increased medication packaging size needed to enclose the even greater bulk of the revised package insert.

Other package insert areas under review are the patient information leaflet and changes in labeling for pediatric use. The first of these is still under consideration, and although some companies have already initiated their own patient information package in easy-reading lay language, the issue of regulation versus recommendation is still being studied. The second area was addressed in a final rule by the FDA issued in May 1996, (Guidance for Industry, Content and Format for Pediatric Use Supplements, May 1996. http://www.fda.gov/cber/gdlns/ GDEPED.pdf). This rule revised the current "pediatric use" subsection. It continues to permit a pediatric indication for a particular drug (e.g., desmopressin for childhood enuresis), but also allows labeling for pediatric use based on adequate and well-controlled trials in adults, together with other information regarding pediatric use. This is of particular importance to pediatricians who prescribe medications that, although commonly used in the pediatric age group, have not been officially approved for pediatric use. The rule also requires dosage instructions for each age group, including adolescents, who were previously grouped with adults in dosage recommendations.

VI. CONCLUSIONS

Designing package inserts for use by busy practicing physicians involves several conflicting issues. Physicians must rapidly make decisions regarding use of a particular drug by gathering as much information as possible. The more easily available the information, the better. Patients have a right to know what their choices are when trying to make responsible decisions about their health. Pharmaceutical companies are interested in promoting products in which they have invested a large amount of time and money, and at the same time protecting themselves from liability due to untoward effect or inappropriate use of the product. Lastly, the FDA has a responsibility to the public in general, both to allow the use of a drug that may significantly reduce the morbidity and mortality from a particular disease, while also protecting the same public from harm caused by such a drug. The sooner a suitable solution can be reached, the sooner patients will benefit.

23

New Directions in Pharmaceutical Promotion:

Regulatory Concerns and Contrivances

Louis A. Morris
Louis A. Morris & Associates, Dix Hills, New York

Peter H. Rheinstein
Cell Works Inc., Baltimore, Maryland

I. INTRODUCTION

Since the 1962 amendments to the Federal Food, Drug, and Cosmetic Act (the Act), overseeing pharmaceutical promotion has been under the jurisdiction of the Food and Drug Administration (FDA). Under the Act, the FDA regulates pharmaceutical advertising and labeling to assure that promotional materials are not false or misleading and that they provide adequate risk disclosures.

During the initial years of FDA regulation, pharmaceutical marketers provided a continuous flow of materials to health care providers. For the most part, these materials described the results of scientific studies and the clinical impact of pharmaceutical products. The materials were directed primarily at health care providers, particularly prescribing professionals. FDA staff reviewed promotional materials for compliance with the Act and regulations and provided feedback to the industry, primarily in the form of letters noting marketing claims and practices considered to be false or misleading, lacking in fair balance, or otherwise in violation of the Act.

Over the past two decades, the FDA has continued to review promotional materials and provide regulatory feedback regarding observed violations. However, in our view, much has changed in the nature and type of promotion. Innovation in the development of new pharmaceutical products and an explosion in the number of distribution channels for advertising information have dramatically changed the face of pharmaceutical promotion. Our speculation is that two fundamental changes in the pharmaceutical marketplace—the increase in generic competition and the movement to managed care insurance coverage—have produced profound changes in pharmaceutical marketing. We further speculate that numerous technological, demographic, and economic changes have also played significant parts in dramatically shifting the focus, means, and desired endpoints of pharmaceutical promotion.

It is difficult, if not impossible, to prove causal relationships for broad, societal change. However, one is free to conjure up presumed explanations. Our belief is that in the late 1970s and early 1980s pharmaceutical brand managers, for the first time, faced the prospect of losing the majority of their market share within a few years of patent expiration. Generic competition placed a great burden on marketers to recover developmental costs in ever-briefer time frames. Marketing managers reacted with early and aggressive marketing for their products. During the late 1980s and early 1990s, pharmaceutical marketers began to compete on the basis of economic value, sometimes attempting to demonstrate product benefits in direct comparison to market competitors. Proving that a drug was safe and effective was necessary for regulatory approval but no longer sufficient for marketplace acceptance. In crowded therapeutic markets, being cheaper than competitors, bundling products or otherwise increasing ''market value,'' or demonstrating cost effectiveness, became a necessary precondition for success. Power in the pharmaceutical distribution channel shifted to large purchasing groups that could move volumes of product and effectuate changes in market share. These groups demanded value as a purchasing requirement.

Changes in medical marketing have also served as a background for rapid transformations in pharmaceutical promotion. New informational technologies have produced many new promotional outlets. New audiences for pharmaceutical messages have led to the development of a portfolio of information, not only for the traditional dispensers and prescribers, but also for the users and the payers.

There are also new messages used to promote drugs. Driven by vertical integration (such as the merging of drug manufacturers with mail-order pharmacies), new ''informational products'' are being developed. These promotions combine the traditional descriptions of clinical effects with information about comparative resource effects and ''value-added'' aspects of the product. These aspects of the ''extended product'' include patient education programs, formulary management incentives, disease management algorithms, drug utilization review information, provider incentives, and other information-based interventions. New messages often seek to persuade purchasers of the product's value through cost-effectiveness or quality-of-life analyses.

The FDA has adapted to these dramatic shifts in pharmaceutical promotion, seeking to apply the regulatory concepts developed during the 1960s and 1970s to modern marketing interventions. Rules prohibiting false or misleading promotion and required disclosure of balancing information remain a solid cornerstone of regulatory philosophy and legal enforcement. However, questions about the application of these principles to certain messages, certain audiences, certain channels of communication, and under certain conditions have been raised in legal proceedings, in public forums, and in direct response to the FDA's invitation to make presentations in formal hearings.

The purpose of this chapter is to review some of the current controversies regarding pharmaceutical promotion. We organize this review by focusing on the five structural communication elements: message, channel, audience, source, and effects. For many of the elements we discuss, regulatory philosophy and policy are under review. Therefore, much of this chapter focuses on the controversies and the issues facing the FDA and the pharmaceutical industry.

Before prior to reviewing these issues, we first discuss the basis of the FDA's authority and responsibility as described in portions of the Act and in advertising and labeling regulations.

II. REGULATION OF MARKETING PRACTICES

The Act specifies that a drug is considered misbranded (a prohibited act) if its labeling or advertising is false or misleading. Labeling is defined as written, printed, or graphic material that accompanies the drug. Advertising is described as being composed of various examples including print advertisements in journals and broadcast through television and radio. As a general principle, labeling and advertising material distributed by drug companies must be consistent with, and not contrary to, the approved product labeling. In addition, there must be adequate risk disclosures to assure that the audience is not misled and that recipients of the promotional intervention have adequate access to prescribing information. The false or misleading provisions of the Act not only cover what is stated, but failure to reveal material facts in light of what is stated is also considered misbranding a drug.

To avoid being misbranded, both labeling and advertising pieces must contain adequate information about drug usage, effects, and risks, to permit safe and effective use of the product. This information is in the form of ''full disclosure'' (i.e., reprinting the entire package insert) for labeling pieces and ''brief summary'' disclosure (i.e., reprinting most of the major sections of the label except indications, clinical trials, and dosage and administration) for advertisements.

For broadcast materials, advertisements must contain a brief summary, and important product risks must be summarized in a ''major statement'' included in the advertisement. Alternatively, companies may include the major statement and make "adequate provision" for the dissemination of full product labeling. Recently, the FDA announced that a multiple-component distribution system (e.g., toll-free telephone number, concurrent print advertisements, Internet address, reference to health professionals) would be considered an acceptable method of distributing prescribing information.

Although most advertising material must conform to the disclosure requirements of the Act and regulations, there are a few significant exceptions. Reminder advertisements, which mention the drug name but make no suggestions or representations about the product, do not require brief summary disclosures. Similarly, price advertisements, which make no suggestions or representations except price information (or general claims of being less costly) do not require brief summaries. Also, "institutional" advertisements, which seek to promote the drug company or which seek to stimulate help seeking for medical conditions, are not considered advertisements for prescription drugs and, therefore, do not require risk disclosures.

III. NEW ISSUES

With changing themes and distributional vehicles, the industry presents promotional information that constantly tests the limits of the FDA's interpretations of the Act and its regulations. For the remainder of this chapter, we review some of these changes and the FDA's regulatory responses. We start with some of the newer messages that the industry seeks to deliver.

IV. NEW MESSAGES

Prescription drugs are approved on the basis of their safety and effectiveness. When innovative new products are approved in classes in which no competition exists, communication of the mere presence of a product to treat an otherwise untreated (or poorly treated) condition is often sufficient to market a product successfully. However, when products are introduced into crowded markets, a comparative advantage is important to differentiate the new product from the competition.

Comparative claims representing direct, head-to-head studies of competing products can provide audiences with highly informative and persuasive information. Accordingly, the scientific basis for such claims must be firmly established. FDA regulations require "substantial evidence" for comparative claims, generally defined as two adequate and well-controlled clinical trials.

Comparative claims denoting clinical improvement can be met by head-to-head clinical trials. The FDA reviews such evidence to assure that the trials are fair or unbiased (e.g., the dosages of competing products are equivalent). More complicated claims are derived from "equivalency" trials, in which an innovative product is compared to an existing product to enable claims of "no difference" among competing products. Such studies are reviewed to guard against such methodological pitfalls as insufficient power, insensitive measurements, and equivalence due to no effect (i.e., all of the examined products are ineffective in the particular study, thus necessitating the inclusion of a third-arm placebo control in the trial to assure that at least one of the investigated products is effective).

Other types of comparative claims have evolved in recent years as companies have become more interested in making claims about products' comparative economic value (e.g., cost-effectiveness claims) and humanistic value (e.g., quality-of-life claims). The FDA's position has been to view claims of comparative economic value as being composed of two parts, a statement of comparative safety or effectiveness (e.g., clinical outcomes) and a statement of economic valuation (e.g., dollars expended). Historically, the FDA has asked for disclosure of the economic valuation portion of a claim and substantiation for the clinical outcome portion of the claim. For example, claims based on the assumption of equal clinical outcomes but differences in economic valuation (e.g., cost-minimization claims) such as, "we're cheaper" or "a good value," are common in pharmaceutical promotion. For such claims, FDA asks that the claims be truthful and that the source of the economic claims be disclosed.

However, for claims based on presumed differences in clinical outcomes (e.g., fewer physician visits are needed because of a less pronounced side-effect profile), the FDA has sought substantiation of the claims based on evidence from adequate and well-controlled studies. This position has remained controversial because critics have maintained that such evidence is not needed for cost-effectiveness claims, and that data-based evaluations or single clinical trials could be used for substantiation.

It must be noted that although there has been much discussion about comparative claims, relatively few studies have been submitted to the FDA for review. One may speculate that this is because of the difficulty of the necessary methodology, the extra costs incurred in doing these studies, and the probability that it is extremely difficult to demonstrate difference among therapeutically similar products.

Differences among products on noncomparative humanistic outcomes, such as the influence of a pharmaceutical product on the patient's health-related quality of life (HRQL), have grown in importance for pharmaceutical companies. HRQL is measured by a number of scales that seek to assess outcomes along a variety of dimensions. Single-dimension utility scales are often used as part of broader pharmacoeconomic evaluations (e.g., cost–utility analyses using a standard gamble technique) and are usually not considered to be primary HRQL outcome measures. Multidimensional HRQL scales focus on either general health status (e.g., the SF36 scale) or on disease-specific outcomes (e.g., asthma, epilepsy, or migraine-specific quality-of-life scales). For the most part, pharmaceutical companies have begun to concentrate on disease-specific quality-of-life measures because these measures are generally more sensitive (i.e., they are more likely to discern real difference among products).

The FDA has expressed concern about the measurement and analysis of HRQL. The psychometric qualities, especially the validity, of such scales are often questioned. Examination of some claims has resulted in the FDA determining that the scales were not sufficiently well validated and that the claims were not substantiated. For example, in one case the manufacturer selected only a few items from an existing multi-item scale, profoundly influencing the validity or meaning of the measured concept. Other concerns, such as the selective reporting of data (reporting outcomes on some dimensions but not on others), failure to account for multiple analyses (inflating alpha levels), and other biases, have been expressed by its review of HRQL data.

V. NEW CHANNELS

Examination of recent enforcement letters sent by the FDA's Division of Drug Marketing, Advertising, and Communications (DDMAC) indicates the incredible diversity of source documents (i.e., promotional channels and materials) that served as vehicles for violative promotional messages. Violative messages were sent through traditional sources such as journal advertisements and letters to health professionals, contemporary sources, such as television and telephone communications, and newly evolving sources, such as Internet communications. It is clear from such an examination that pharmaceutical marketing involves an increasingly broad array of communications channels for message delivery.

The Internet: Technology has continued to modify the way promotional messages are delivered. Perhaps the most dramatic new information channel is the use of the Internet to provide a large variety of messages. Many pharmaceutical manufacturers have developed home pages and/or specific product/disease-oriented Web sites. These sites offer Web users the opportunity to obtain a variety of communications regarding the company, as well as information about services, products, and selected health conditions.

The FDA held Part 15 hearings about Promotion on the Internet in October 1996. At those hearings, the FDA posed several questions. These included the following:

> Should products that are listed on the Internet as "in the pipeline" be considered institutional statements or preapproval promotion?

To what extent should pharmaceutical companies be held responsible for chat rooms, news groups, and linkages?

How should FDA regulate international messages?

Comments submitted in response to a *Federal Register* announcement as well as comments made at the meeting ranged from a request for the FDA to carefully consider restricting information flow, to suggesting that technological solutions were preferred over regulatory solutions. Although some advocated no federal government involvement, others suggested the need for regulatory oversight.

The DDMAC has taken several regulatory actions through enforcement letters to companies that have posted information on their Web sites that was considered violative of the Act. In several cases, news releases have been the focus of the FDA's actions. In all cases, false or misleading promotion claims have triggered the regulatory actions. Web messages are reviewed by the FDA for compliance with the Act and regulations just as if they were delivered through more traditional communications channels. It is also clear that some contentious issues await resolution. The international implications of Internet communications present some of the most challenging regulatory problems. What is considered violative in one country may be perfectly acceptable in another country. In May 1997, the World Health Organization passed a resolution calling for the formation of a working group to collect information and present recommendations for international regulation of Internet communications now available.

The FDA also uses the Internet and views it as an important communications tool. Through its own Web site, the FDA's Center for Drug Evaluation and Research (CDER) posts its newly issued regulations, guidances, and internal operating procedures or MaPPs (Manual of Policies and Procedures). Further, since the fall of 1996, the CDER has posted copies of enforcement letters on its Web site. This provides the industry and other interested parties easy access to letters regarding recent regulatory actions.

VI. NEW AUDIENCES

A. Consumers

Although direct-to-consumer (DTC) promotion has been a popular form of communication for pharmaceutical manufacturers for many years, 1996 was the first year in which the amount of money spent advertising products to consumers surpassed the amount spent on advertising to physicians. It is estimated that approximately $600 million was spent on DTC promotion in 1996. Much of this money has been spent on magazine or newspaper advertisements that inform readers about the product's uses, benefits, and side effects. Magazine and newspaper advertisements contain sizable labeling disclosures (called "brief summaries") that often entail an extra half to a full page for the advertisement.

In addition to print advertisements, manufacturers have also used television advertisements to promote the use of prescription products. Television advertisements have remained primarily in the form of help-seeking or reminder advertisements, neither of which requires brief summary disclosures.

Full product advertisements have recently appeared on network television after the FDA announced a change in its interpretation of requirements for "adequate provision" for the distribution of labeling information. According to FDA regulations, if brief summary information is not made available in conjunction with the advertisements, then "adequate provision" must be made for the distribution of labeling information to the audience that views the broadcast advertisement.

In October 1995, the FDA held a Part 15 hearing to gather public perceptions about DTC advertising. While a variety of opinions was expressed about DTC, the majority of those presenting viewed some disclosure requirements as overly burdensome.

In addition to these administrative actions, a lawsuit was filed in December 1995 questioning the FDA's authority to regulate DTC advertising under the current regulations and alleging that the inferred requirements were overly burdensome. The FDA filed a motion to dismiss the action in March 1996, citing the lack of "standing" of those bringing the suit (three consumers and two health professionals) and the lack of "ripeness" for the case in light of the FDA's continuing administrative actions. In May 1997, a federal judge granted the FDA's motion to dismiss the case.

B. Formularies

Another new audience for pharmaceutical companies is the formulary committees of managed care organizations (MCOs). Formularies have existed for many years in hospitals and at MCOs. However, MCOs have recently begun to use formularies more aggressively as a means of controlling the cost of operations. By limiting the purchase of medicines to a few members of drugs in a class, the MCO can engage in bulk purchasing and selection of less costly medications. Since formulary members are usually charged with reviewing drugs to determine the most cost-effective products in the therapeutic class, they have, in some instances, been a prime target for pharmaceutical marketers.

VII. NEW SOURCES

Not only has the audience for pharmaceutical messages changed, the source of those messages has also changed. Horizontal and vertical integration in the pharmaceutical industry has changed the face of medical marketing. Drug companies have begun to integrate physical distribution and disease management strategies into their basic marketing focus.

The development of new chemical entities has always been the primary method through which pharmaceutical companies innovate. However, some companies have begun to view their offerings as "disease treatment" programs rather than merely as chemical entities. Thus, some companies have created "extended products" that include a range of "informational products" in addition to the prescription drug chemical. These information products include informational services necessary to treat the diseases for which the prescription drug is indicated. For example, disease treatment protocols have been offered that specify algorithms to treat different diseases. The marketing of extended products has transformed the drug company's focuses beyond their own products. To serve the needs of MCOs more fully, pharmaceutical companies may suggest the use of competing products to treat certain aspects of the disease (e.g., early stages or less serious forms of the ailment), reserving its more potent medication for more serious disease states.

The promoted effects of a drug are no longer limited to the safety and effectiveness of the product. Rather, pharmaceutical companies conduct analyses that seek to demonstrate cost-effectiveness, especially in the environment in which the drug will be used. While the concept of "moving market share" often entails the promotion of pharmaceutical products to MCOs, pharmaceutical marketers have not abandoned the individual prescriber or user of the product as a promotional target. Even if a MCO purchases a product, a physician must prescribe it and a patient must use it. This "elongated" focus of marketing messages recognizes the importance of understanding the process of drug-usage decision making and the roles of a variety of individuals in diverse roles. Pharmaceutical marketing has become increasingly complex as these new audiences for marketing messages become a focus of marketing interventions.

VIII. CONCLUSION

Although pharmaceutical marketing has gone through an explosion of new audiences, new channels, and new messages, the basic premise of the Act, that advertising must provide truthful, nonmisleading, and balanced communications, remains the goal of FDA regulation. Clear, substantiated, and balanced messages remain the cornerstone of FDA regulatory actions, regardless of whether the message is delivered through a hand-printed sign or an Internet Web site; whether it is delivered to a formulary chair or a consumer; or whether it involves the pharmacokinetics or the pharmacoeconomics of the product. As the relationship between the pharmaceutical industry and MCOs continues to evolve, and as technology changes, the role of the FDA will also evolve.

ACKNOWLEDGMENTS

We would like to express appreciation to our colleagues at the Food and Drug Administration who made helpful comments on earlier versions of this manuscript. The views expressed are solely those of the authors and do not reflect the policy of the Food and Drug Administration. The authors prepared this manuscript in 1997.

24

The Campus Researcher and Industry:
Issues of Intellectual Property and Technology Transfer

Todd S. Keiller
Healthcare Business Development, Inc., Hopkinton, Massachusetts

I. INTRODUCTION

An often-overlooked source of potential new drugs is the academic research lab. This chapter discusses how technology from these labs is accessed and how the intellectual property process works in academia. In addition, because funding this early-stage technology can be a major problem, this chapter looks at various funding alternatives.

II. ACADEMIC TECHNOLOGY OVERVIEW

A. Public Benefits

In 1996, the Massachusetts Institute of Technology (MIT) released the results of a study showing that 45 biotechnology companies nationwide either had founders associated with MIT or had licensed technology patented by MIT (1). These companies employed nearly 10,000 people and produced aggregate annual revenues of $3 billion. Overall, the academic sector has had a huge economic effect on research. According to the Association of University Technology Managers (AUTM) Licensing Survey for Fiscal Year (FY) 1999 (2), the 190 universities surveyed reported that academic discoveries licensed to industry generated over

$40 billion in economic activity and supported 270,000 jobs during that fiscal year. According to the survey, since 1980, almost 3000 new companies have been formed based on licenses granted from the academic community.

This collaboration between academia and business began with the passing of the Bayh-Dole Act in 1980. The objective of this act was to encourage academic institutions receiving federal funding for research to take an active role in patenting and licensing their intellectual property. The federal government recognized that universities were not capable of aggressively transferring ideas from basic research to tangible products in an efficient manner. The Bayh-Dole Act allows these academic institutions to seek patents, market these patents to commercial entities, and receive royalties that will be distributed to the inventor and the institution.

Many products resulting from the patenting and licensing of intellectual property have had tremendous public benefit. According to the AUTM FY 99 Licensing Survey (2), some recent examples are as follows:

> Natura™ hearing aids (Brigham Young University)—hearing aid that is customized to correct each customer's particular impairment and can selectively suppress noises.
>
> Periostat® (State University of New York at Stony Brook)—a nonantibiotic dental treatment to protect bone and gums from collagen-destroying bacteria in our mouths.
>
> Cohn Cardiac Stabilizer™ (Beth Israel Deaconess Medical Center)—a device that assists surgeons performing beating-heart, open-heart surgery.
>
> Green Steel (University of Pittsburgh)—a lead-free, machinable steel that frees factories from the need to protect their workers from lead fumes and from the lead-containing scrap produced when the steel is machined into parts.
>
> NiAl (Carnegie Mellon University)—new thin-film magnetic disk drive memory medium that allows increased density for laptop hard drives.

In previous years, products have included a topical treatment for Kaposi's sarcoma, an aid in wound healing, and a product that provides replacement skin for burn victims (3). These are only a few of the many available products based on academic research.

B. Technology Transfer Offices

At the heart of patenting and licensing intellectual property resulting from academic research is the Technology Transfer Office (TTO). Most major universities have invested in a TTO to oversee this process. The TTO manager is responsible for evaluating invention disclosures made by principal investigators (PIs) at the institution. The TTO manager often assists the PI in obtaining industry-sponsored research to augment federal funding and thereby helps progress the science or provides proof of concept.

After evaluating the invention disclosure, the TTO manager must decide whether to invest in a patent application. Because patent expenses can quickly escalate, the TTO manager must be able to evaluate commercial potential at a very early stage of the development of the invention and identify appropriate corporate sponsors and licensees. The TTO manager must efficiently and diligently direct the marketing activities to appropriate sources so the scientific idea can advance. In this way, the science progresses, and the financial responsibilities of the institution for patent expenses are minimized.

The TTO negotiates licensing terms, monitors the transactions, and follows up the terms of the agreement. Throughout the academic world, the number of agreements is growing. In FY 1999, nearly 4000 licenses and options were executed at academic institutions—a 7% increase over the previous year and a three-fold increase over FY 1991, when the AUTM conducted its first survey (2).

It is also important, however, to understand what the academic institutions and their TTOs do not do. TTOs are involved in discovery research, but are not product-development or regulatory experts. Commercial partners who expect product-development or regulatory expertise will quickly experience the cultural differences between business and academic research and likely will be disappointed in the performance of university researchers. The academic institution's philosophy of advancing science by promoting the open and free exchange of ideas among peers who have the freedom to publish the results is often in conflict with corporate philosophies. Survival in the corporate world may mandate keeping quiet, waiting, and announcing the idea to the competition when the company is ready. In the university world, however, success is measured by the number of publications and by the length of a researcher's CV rather than by return on investment.

This is not to say that would-be entrepreneurs do not exist in the university research community. Many of the 3914 licenses signed in 1999 were nurtured, expedited, and even negotiated by university scientists eager to experience the best of both worlds—that is, the shelter of academia and the financial upside of licenses. Such licensing is usually done in an ethical, sincere manner; however, temptations exist that academic scientists may not be able to resist. The problem of scientists taking the proverbial bite of Eden's apple has led to stricter oversight of licensing practices and PI behavior. Therefore, the prospective licensee must understand the academic institution's policies and procedures and work directly with the TTO at the very beginning of the process. Horror stories can be told about industry negotiating deals directly with a PI, only to have the terms invalidated by the PI's institution and conflict-of-interest violations brought forth.

C. Conflict-of-Interest Policies

To avoid such unfortunate incidents, most academic institutions have conflict-of-interest or conflict-of-commitment policies that all staff members must follow. In fact, certain types of federal funding sources require that these policies be in place. Such policies define the amount of time an investigator is allowed to spend on projects outside the academic appointment. The amount of time allowed for outside projects varies from institution to institution, but generally averages 20% of the work week or 1 day per week, as long as the time is approved by the appropriate authority within the institution and the details of the finances associated with the project are fully disclosed. The conflict-of-interest policy will often describe the types of relationships allowed, including statements about equity ownership, board participation, and consulting arrangements. Any corporate sponsor should become familiar with institutional conflict-of-interest and conflict-of-commitment policies to avoid placing the investigator in conflict.

In spite of best intentions and progress made, however, academia may still have many details to work out in their use of these policies. A recent study [4] found that conflict-of-interest policies at many U.S. research institutions are so general in their terms and varied in their enforcement that confusion is quite likely among potential industrial partners. In addition, the vaguely worded or differentially followed policies may not provide the support and foundation for the traditional academic standards as competition is generated among universities vying for corporate sponsorship.

III. ACADEMIC PATENT PROCESS

A. Current Practice

A patent is awarded when the idea presented is useful, unique, and nonobvious to one skilled in the art. Changes in U.S. patent law in 1995 now provide for a 20-year time frame to file a patent, issue that patent, and then provide exclusive protection of the idea. Previous law permitted an unlimited amount of time to file and prosecute the patent application, then granted a 17-year protection period. This could result in what is known as "submarine patents," in which a company would keep a patent application alive through a series of amendments for long periods of time until it was commercially useful to complete the prosecution and allow the issuance of the patent. The patent would then surface at a competitively useful time, catching the competitor off guard because the contents of the patent application had been kept confidential by the U.S. Patent Office. Current law safeguards against this possibility.

In academia, the inventor often is motivated to file a patent because of the need to publish results. Publication of results without filing for a patent will result in the information becoming public domain. If this occurs, the published information can be used to disqualify the idea as being unique or nonobvious and therefore disallow a patent.

The TTO often works within a very tight budget and is pressured to hold down patent expenses by not filing until a licensee is found or sometimes by prematurely terminating patent prosecution. The AUTM FY 99 licensing survey showed that 12,324 invention disclosures were received that fiscal year, and 5545 new U.S. patents were filed (2). During this time, $121 million was expended on legal fees for these patents and patents in prosecution, although survey respondents were ultimately reimbursed $52 million for patent expenses. The TTO has a huge incentive to license such patents quickly and to have the licensee reimbursed for past expenses as well as paid for future expenses.

B. Differences from Industry

Academic researchers often have a strong incentive to publish their work in peer-reviewed journals. Publication is fundamental to their work and often to their advancement within the university community. This academic policy differs from most in scientific industry, because industry must keep information confidential to remain competitive. In fact, the patent process often conflicts with the academic publishing incentive. The TTO must ensure that the PI understands the patent process and communicates efficiently with the TTO about the potential intellectual property. The TTO should in no way impede the publication process. Therefore, the office must make sure the PI works closely with patent counsel to both protect the intellectual property and allow a free flow of information to the academic community. The awareness among academic scientists has grown since TTOs were first instituted in 1980, and some of the changes in U.S. patent law in 1995 make it easier to file a ''provisional application'' to preserve the property while a complete application is prepared.

Companies licensing from academic institutions must be aware of this basic difference between the university and the corporate environments. Although most academic institutions will allow a short period for review of licensed technology information, they will stand firm about defending the right of their scientists to publish results.

A corporate sponsor can seem to be a hero by stepping in with financial backing for the licensee. Reimbursing past patent expenses may initially amount to $10,000 to $20,000. Even when the cost of future expenses for that licensee is added in, such backing could be an especially wise investment for the corporate sponsor if the rights to the invention are obtained. However, almost all academic institutions have patent policies in place dictating that all rights to inventions discovered at the institution will be assigned to that institution. The TTO will pay patent expenses until a licensee is found. The institution will have a royalty-sharing plan for the inventor and possibly for the inventor's lab. The balance of the royalties will go to the institution and possibly to the inventor's department. This plan is more lucrative than that for the corporate inventor, whose reward comes in salary and possibly a bonus. As an example, the more successful drug compounds may yield corporate sales in excess of $500 million. If such compounds are invented at an academic institution, a royalty of between 1% and 4% would be reasonable. A 2% royalty would yield $20 million in royalties, and the inventor would receive between $2 million and $5 million.

A downside for enthusiastic potential inventors in academic research is that the chance for such success is similar to the chance for an amateur or collegiate athlete making a high-paying professional sports team. For all those making millions playing for the National Basketball Association, thousands are shooting baskets in playgrounds. In 1999, academic units received $862 million in license income (i.e., running royalties, cashed-in equity, and all other types of income) on 8308 licenses (2).

Another important difference between academia and industry is the nature of research. Companies often are frustrated by the seeming slowness of academic research. That the funding for academic research is equivalent to the budget for a corporate division is a common industry misconception. Despite what can be sizable amounts of industry-sponsored research, the academic scientist usually has numerous responsibilities within the institution, and may have priorities different from those of the company.

IV. TTO COMMERCIALIZATION STRATEGY

A. Process

Academic institutions often have difficulty deciding whether to market a new technology before filing, after filing, or after patent issuance. Marketing before filing is often difficult because of concern over confidentiality. This difficulty may not be the case for a new algorithm or a new protein, but it is often the case for new devices. Most institutions cannot afford to delay marketing until after the patent issues, but their case for the patent is certainly strengthened if this delay is possible. The most common time for marketing is after the patent application has been filed, and a confidentiality agreement is required to allow review of the patent application.

The information available to a company for evaluation of a technology from an academic institution will vary widely from institution to institution and from inventor to inventor. Some institutions are able to develop a sophisticated technology brochure that is, in essence, a miniature business plan for the invention. Other institutions can provide nothing more substantial than a hastily written "back-of-the-envelope" description. In either case, it is critical for the key scientific decision makers in both the company and the university to communicate with each other both about the inventor's ideas and about the company's areas of interest. The TTO should facilitate this communication and should understand the business requirements of the company as they relate to the invention.

Often, a TTO will develop an inventory of inventions available containing brief and nonconfidential descriptions of the inventions. Companies interested in investing can quickly scan the inventory and target areas of interest. A company can also follow academic publications relating to its field of interest. Upon finding a relevant publication, the company may work with the author's TTO to evaluate and transfer technology more efficiently.

B. Financing Alternatives

Sometimes corporate sponsorship of academic research is not possible because the academic discovery research is not at a stage to justify a company's investment. Overall pressures to reduce health care spending have squeezed funding for corporate research and development, which, in turn, has squeezed available funding for academic research. However, from the company's perspective, properly managed academic research may in fact be a less expensive alternative when compared with the costs of the company's own research. Industry often balks at the overhead rates a university places on its direct costs. However, those in industry who review these budgets often are not aware of their own company's corporate overhead rate, which is often much higher than the academic rate. In many instances, the company can collaborate with a university to create a research program that suits the company's needs and can pay for the academic scientists to perform the targeted work. The company does not need to hire personnel on a full-time basis, and the existing university laboratories can efficiently meet the company's needs. Once the research is over, the company has no further responsibility for the personnel and the laboratories.

In addition, corporate sponsorship usually results in a license or an option to license intellectual property either currently available or discovered during a sponsored research program. To follow good business sense, a company must consider numerous factors before licensing academic technology, including the following:

> Exclusive or nonexclusive rights
> Length of time for development
> Royalty or compensation for the license
> Field of use
> Territory
> Infringement
> Sublicensing rights

Due diligence
Indemnification
Payment timing and late penalties
Termination conditions

Without direct corporate sponsorship and a licensing arrangement, academia often turns to alternative funding sources, such as various government sources, joint ventures, or venture capital. Examples of alternative governmental funding sources fostering good scientific ideas in university research include the following:

Small Business Innovation Research
Small Business Technology Transfer
Advanced Technology Program
Technology Reinvestment Program
Cooperative Research and Development Agreement

In dealing with such financing alternatives, the university often must consider timing and the size of available funds.

Establishing a joint venture between an academic institution and a commercial entity can be useful for both parties. The company may need the academic institution for the basic research function, and the academic institution may need the company for other areas of expertise such as distribution, manufacturing, development, or strategic planning. In a joint venture, both parties share the risks, and the idea may be advanced to another level before achieving its full potential.

The venture capital community has invested close to $500 million in the biotechnology industry. Academic-based intellectual property can be an important part of this investment.

V. CONCLUSION

Partnerships between campus researchers and industry offer lucrative, mutual benefits. Researchers and their institutions receive financing to continue their research efforts, they gain peer recognition through publication of their work, and they can receive royalties from their marketed products. Corporations can meet their business objectives of developing new products, and they do not have to worry about hiring and housing research personnel. Certainly such liaisons are attractive to both parties involved, but ultimately, it is the public who benefits because the new drugs and devices are available to those needing them much sooner than if they had been developed without external funding.

REFERENCES

1. Campbell KD. Study examines impact of MIT biotech research. MIT Tech Talk. January 24, 1996. Available at: http://web.mit.edu/newsoffice/tt/1996/jan24/41460.html. Accessed January 2, 2001.
2. The Association of University Technology Managers. The AUTM Licensing Survey: FY 1999. Available at: http://www.autm.net/surveys/99/survey99A.pdf. Accessed January 2, 2001.
3. The Association of University Technology Managers. The AUTM Licensing Survey: FY 1998. Available at: http://www.autm.net/pubs/surgey/menu.html. Accessed October 5, 2000.
4. Cho MK, Shohara R, Schissel A, Rennie D. Policies on faculty conflicts of interest at US universities. JAMA 2000; 284:2203–2208.

25

Anatomy of Drug Withdrawals in the United States

Marion J. Finkel
Pharmaceutical and Regulatory Consultant, Morristown, New Jersey

I. BACKGROUND

Each year approximately 20 to 30 drugs constituting new chemical entities enter the U.S. market. In addition, new salts or esters, combinations of already marketed drugs, and trade and generic versions of marketed drugs enter the commercial arena.

The U.S. Food and Drug Administration (FDA) must give prior approval in order for a prescription drug to be marketed (except for new generic versions of drugs originally marketed prior to 1938). The FDA also controls withdrawals from the market for safety or effectiveness reasons; companies may, however, withdraw a drug for these reasons on their own initiative.

The FDA's control of both marketing and drug withdrawal is exerted through the instrument of a New Drug Application (NDA), which a company submits when it feels that it has accumulated sufficient data to support marketing of its product. Such applications have been required to be submitted since 1938, when Congress amended the Food, Drug and Cosmetic Act to require a manufacturer to make a showing of safety before a drug can be marketed. In 1962, the act was again amended to require a showing of effectiveness. In addition, the 1962 amendments required that all clinical investigations prior to marketing approval be monitored by the FDA. These changes in the act were triggered by two tragedies. First, in the elixir of sulfanilamide episode, a U.S. manufacturer solubilized sulfanilamide for the pediatric market by using diethylene glycol, the major component of antifreeze. More than 100 patients died, mainly children. The second tragedy occurred primarily but not exclusively outside the United States and involved the sedative-hypnotic, thalidomide. Administration of this drug to pregnant women resulted in limb deformities in a significant percentage of their offspring.

II. REASONS FOR DRUG WITHDRAWAL

A drug can be withdrawn from clinical study while it is in the investigational phase for reasons of toxicity, inadequate effectiveness, or lack of advantage over competitive products. The overwhelming majority of discontinuances in the premarketing stage are based on decisions made by the manufacturer. After a drug has entered the market, the primary reason for withdrawal, since 1962, other than obsolescence, has been one of safety. Because, since 1962, the law has required evidence of effectiveness based on well-controlled studies, once such evidence has been accepted by the FDA, effectiveness is no longer an issue unless the data are subsequently shown to be fraudulent.

Safety concerns derive from manufacturing problems or other matters leading to a defective product, from new animal studies suggesting a carcinogenic or teratogenic potential of a drug, and from adverse reactions to the drug, including the human experience of teratogenesis or tumorigenesis. The human findings may be newly discovered after marketing or may have been suspected or identified prior to marketing but better defined following marketing.

Drug companies and the FDA maintain a continuing surveillance for adverse drug information. Months or years after introduction into the market, the benefit/risk ratio of a drug may be altered to the point where withdrawal is considered mandatory. In the vast majority of cases, however, new adverse information, whether animal or clinical, results in labeling changes that cite the findings. In the more severe cases, labeling changes provide warnings or precautions and, in the most serious situations, limit the use of the drug to certain subpopulations of patients.

Less than 2% of drugs representing new chemical entities have been withdrawn from the U.S. market because of adverse effects inherent in the drug (i.e., not due to its method of extraction or manufactured of the final dosage form). Almost all of these were based on adverse reactions occurring in patients. Animal findings usually have been handled by the labeling changes described above.

Bakke and associates, using certain defined criteria, found that between 1964 and 1983, only 14 drugs were withdrawn because of safety concerns (1). Almost all of the withdrawals were initiated by the FDA. Five of these drugs (three analgesics, an anti-infective, and an antihistamine) were introduced to the market between 1900 and 1947, but the remainder appeared after 1956. Of the 14 drugs, two were withdrawn because of animal tumors. Five drugs were withdrawn by manufacturers for safety reasons between 1984 and 1994. During this 10-year period, more than 260 new chemical entities were approved for marketing. The small number of withdrawals constitutes a remarkable safety record for pharmaceuticals.

III. MECHANISMS OF WITHDRAWAL

When the FDA initiates an action to remove a drug from the market for safety concerns, it does so by proposing to withdraw approval of the company's New Drug Application. The Food, Drug and Cosmetic Act requires the FDA to permit the holder of the application an opportunity to present its views at a hearing. Such hearings may be public or may be held before an administrative law judge in closed session. Often the FDA elects to present the matter to one of its advisory committees with the dual purpose of (a) obtaining the opinion of a group of experts following presentations of both sides of the issue and (b) hoping to obviate a formal hearing if the committee recommends withdrawal. In the latter case, a company may still pursue the route of a formal hearing, but that route becomes less desirable when an eminent group of experts has recommended removal of a drug form the market, a recommendation not lost on the medical and lay press and financial circles because of the open nature of the FDA's advisory committee meetings. As will be seen below, a recommendation by a committee against withdrawal also carries great weight with the FDA.

This chapter is devoted to case histories of certain drug withdrawals or withdrawal of one of the indications for a drug, and in one instance an aborted withdrawal, that were based, with two exceptions, on scientifically documented adverse clinical experience. The cases are illustrative of the diversity of forces that play a role or come into play before or after a decision to withdraw a drug has been made. These forces include, in addition to FDA staff, FDA advisory committees and consultants, drug companies and their consultants, the medical profession, the public, consumer organizations, the media, and Congress. In recent years, litigation has played an increasing role in company decisions to remove a drug (or medical device) from the market, and in the future one can expect that even the specter of such litigation may be enough to cause a precipitate withdrawal.

IV. TICRYNAFEN

Ticrynafen (trade name Selacryn) was marketed in May 1979 as a diuretic and antihypertensive agent by Smith Kline and French Laboratories (SKF). The drug had, in addition, a uricosuric effect, a property that distinguished it from the thiazides and that rendered it of particular interest for patients who developed hyperuricemia from the thiazides or who had concomitant gout.

During the investigational drug studies conducted in the United States prior to marketing, a small cluster of patients with hepatic abnormalities were reported by two investigators. Some patients had jaundice and others only elevated transaminase levels. In one cluster (six patients), the majority were considered to have viral hepatitis or abnormalities due to alcoholism based on serological evidence, history, and the prominence of viral hepatitis in the community at that time. In the other cluster (two patients), one was considered to have viral hepatitis. Hypersensitivity to ticrynafen, however, could not be ruled out in several cases. Because there were no other cases of hepatic injury in more than 500 patients studied in the United States prior to marketing, the FDA approved the drug with the requirement that the labeling alert physicians to the potential for hepatic abnormalities and jaundice, although no causal relationship to ticrynafen had been established.

Ticrynafen had an eventful history almost from the inception of marketing. The first event consisted of reports of several cases of acute renal failure, attributed to probable deposition of uric acid crystals in the kidneys. The manufacturer notified physicians that patients must be well hydrated before the administration of ticrynafen.

In November 1979, after 6 months of marketing, SKF reported 11 cases of hepatic injury. The FDA became aware of five more cases, and in January 1980, the FDA met with the manufacturer (2). By that time, the firm had received reports of a total of 52 cases of significant hepatic injury. The majority of patients had jaundice as well as elevated serum transaminase levels. A few patients were rechallenged and again developed increased transaminase levels. Death occurred in five patients, in only three of whom viral or alcoholic hepatitis could be considered causal. By that time, approximately 300,000 patients in the United States had received the drug, with an estimated incidence of hepatic injury of about 1 in 5000.

At the meeting, a representative of the French company that had been marketing ticrynafen in France for about 4 years reported that more than 1 million patients had taken the drug in that country and that 22 cases of hepatic injury had been reported, several of which showed positive rechallenge. Although there was some initial discussion on the part of SKF of leaving the drug on the market for a limited patient population, the meeting participants concluded that the drug should be immediately withdrawn from the market. On the following day SKF mailed a letter to all physicians informing them of the adverse reactions and of a recall of the drug from all wholesalers and retail and hospital pharmacies (3). A press release was issued jointly by the FDA and SKF announcing the recall and advising patients to contact their physicians for alternative therapy. In addition, the FDA informed the World Health Organization and drug regulatory agencies in Canada, the United Kingdom, and Germany of the action taken with respect to ticrynafen.

V. BENDECTIN

Bendectin, manufactured by the William S. Merrell Company (subsequently Merrell National Laboratories and Merrell-Dow), was a combination drug product first marketed in the United States in 1956 for the treatment of nausea and vomiting of pregnancy. Approval occurred prior to the period when proof of effectiveness became a requirement for marketing. The drug product originally consisted of three ingredients: dicyclomine, doxylamine, and pyridoxine. It was subsequently reformulated to remove the dicyclomine component after controlled clinical trials performed at the request of the FDA revealed that dicyclomine provided no additional effectiveness beyond what could be achieved with the other two ingredients.

Bendectin was widely marketed. By 1979, about 20 million women had taken it worldwide, including about 5 million in the United States. Because it was specifically labeled for nausea and vomiting of pregnancy, and the only product so labeled, it was the most commonly used antiemetic in pregnant women. The thalidomide disaster in the early 1960s had heightened scientific awareness of drugs as a potential cause of congenital abnormalities. Epidemiological studies of drug use during pregnancy and of prevalence of congenital abnormalities were conducted. The widespread use of Bendectin made it a logical candidate for such studies. At the same time, the horror of the thalidomide-related limb deformities was firmly etched in the minds of the public. In its spontaneous adverse reaction reporting system, the FDA began to find a disproportionate number of limb deformities reported in the offspring of mothers who had taken Bendectin compared with other congenital abnormalities in Bendectin users. The FDA followed these reports closely, but their uncontrolled nature made them of little use. There was no way of knowing whether the disproportionate incidence in the FDA Bendectin reports was due to the thalidomide legacy.

By 1968, of 39 reports of congenital anomalies in offspring of Bendectin users received by the FDA, 38% (15) described major limb defects with or without other anomalies. (The incidence of limb deformities in the general population is 3% of congenital abnormalities.) In some cases, Bendectin was given too late in pregnancy to have affected limb development; in other cases, other drugs, including thalidomide, had been ingested (4).

Also in 1968, the FDA undertook a re-review of the animal reproduction studies that had been performed in rats and rabbits with the combination drug and with dicyclomine and doxylamine alone. It was concluded that there was no evidence of drug-related teratogenesis in these studies (5). Subsequent studies in rats and rabbits given doxylamine plus pyridoxine in doses up to 90 times the maximum human dose were judged as providing no suggestion of a teratogenic effect (6,7).

In the 1970s, Bendectin became the object of press inquiries because of a publicized trial in which a parent sued the manufacturer, alleging that the drug caused a limb deformity in her child. In 1979 the FDA prepared a ''Talk Paper'' to be used for responses to press inquiries in which it stated that animal studies and several large epidemiological studies in women who received Bendectin during pregnancy provided ''no evidence that Bendectin is associated with an increased risk of birth defects'' (8).

A small settlement was awarded to the plaintiff by the jury that participated in the aforementioned trial. This award was overturned by the judge on the grounds that the jury did not follow his instructions to decide whether or not the defendant was guilty. A new trial was ordered. Meanwhile the plaintiff organized a group to help persons desirous of filing lawsuits against the manufacturer, and another couple filed a suit in the same state as the original plaintiff.

The FDA decided to present all available data bearing on the issue of the safety of Bendectin to its Fertility and Maternal Health Drugs Advisory Committee. The presentations to the committee occurred over a 2-day period in September 1980. The meeting was public, and the audience included many representatives of newspapers, magazines (domestic and foreign), television, and Wall Street brokerage houses, as well as laypersons from pertinent organizations, Congressional staff, and interested scientists.

The committee listened to presentations by epidemiologists, obstetricians, and pharmacologists and reviewed data from 13 epidemiological studies and from the animal reproduction studies. Of the 13 studies, 11 concluded that Bendectin did not appear to be associated with an increased risk of congenital defects, including limb defects. In a hypothesis-generating case-control study, a slightly increased risk of cleft palate was reported (the investigator considered the results equivocal), and in another study of this nature, an increased risk of cardiac anomalies was noted. Cleft palate and heart defects were examined specifically in many of the other studies, and no increased in risk was noted in Bendectin offspring.

The committee concluded that the data did not demonstrate an association between Bendectin usage and birth defects; however, it felt that some residual uncertainty existed because of the findings from the two hypothesis-generating studies and the fact that although the epidemiological studies were large enough to rule out a relatively small increase in defects (i.e., a doubling of the overall malformation rate), they did not have the power to rule out a doubling of a specific malformation (9). The committee concluded that the safety of Bendectin had been evaluated to a much greater extent and was therefore preferable to other antiemetics for nausea and vomiting of pregnancy. There was some concern on its part that Bendectin may be prescribed more often than necessary. Therefore, the committee recommended the issuance of labeling addressed to patients and some changes in the physician labeling to narrow the indications for use. The manufacturer complied with FDA requests for labeling changes (10–12).

The matter did not end there, however. Newspaper reports continued to question the safety of Bendectin. One article mentioned an increase in incidence of diaphragmatic hernias in rats given near-toxic doses of the doxylamine component of Bendectin. The FDA also received data from a small, uncontrolled study in Bendectin-treated pregnant monkeys in which an interventricular septal defect was noted in offspring examined prior to delivery but not in those examined after normal delivery. The manufacturer was asked by the FDA to conduct a controlled trial in monkeys, but the FDA stated, in a ''Talk Paper'' in 1982, that the significance of the recent rat and monkey studies, even if the findings could be reproduced, was ''debatable in view of the more pertinent human epidemiologic data that have not, to date, provided convincing evidence of . . . birth defects'' (13).

In May 1983, a jury awarded $750,000 to a child with a limb defect whose mother had taken Bendectin during pregnancy. Faced with about 300 other lawsuits pending in federal and state courts, the manufacturer notified the FDA that it was ending its production and worldwide distribution of Bendectin on June 9, 1983 (14,15).

With the withdrawal of Bendectin from the market, there remained no drug that had been studied and approved by the FDA as safe and effective for nausea and vomiting of pregnancy.

VI. PHENFORMIN

Phenformin (trade name DBI), an oral hypoglycemic agent for the treatment of non-insulin-dependent adult-onset diabetes mellitus, was approved for marketing in the United States in 1959. Shortly thereafter, reports began to appear in the medical literature of lactic acidosis in association with use of phenformin. This resulted in a precautionary statement in the labeling for the drug. Reports became more numerous in the early 1970s. The high mortality rate (about 50%) in patients who experience lactic acidosis resulted in considerable concern regarding the phenformin-associated phenomenon.

In 1973, the FDA reviewed the subject with its Endocrinology and Metabolism Advisory Committee. At that time, 4 million retail prescriptions of phenformin per year were being filled in the United States. The committee concluded that various predisposing factors, such as myocardial infarction or renal disease, were required in order to precipitate lactic acidosis in phenformin users, and if patients with such predisposing factors were eliminated from phenformin usage, adequate benefit/risk ratio existed to support continued marketing of the drug (16).

The labeling of the drug was strengthened and eventually included a black-box warning concerning fatal metabolic acidosis. Continuing accumulation of case reports of lactic acidosis, however, resulted in further consultation with the Advisory Committee in October 1976. At that time, prescriptions were still numerous, about 3.5 million per year. The risk of developing lactic acidosis could not be defined precisely but was felt to be about 0.25 to 4 per 1000 users per year. The committee recommended removal of the drug from the market and indicated that there was evidence that not all patients at risk may be identifiable. The committee did, however, feel that in a small patient population, the benefits of the drug outweighed the risks, but it could not clearly define this subpopulation (16).

Shortly afterwards, the labeling of phenformin was again changed in indicated that the drug should be considered only as a last resort when other oral agents were ineffective and insulin could not be used. This labeling change was a temporary measure until the drug could be withdrawn from the market (17).

If a manufacturer does not voluntarily discontinue distribution of a drug, the process by which the FDA can withdraw approval for marketing is a protracted one. The law requires that the manufacturer be given an opportunity for a hearing on the grounds that evidence amassed following approval for marketing shows that the drug is not longer safe for use (18). The only method by which a drug can be removed immediately from the market by the government is a declaration by the Secretary of Health and Human Services (formerly Health, Education and Welfare) that the drug represents an "imminent hazard" to health (19).

In April 1977, the Secretary of Health, Education and Welfare received a petition from the Health Research Group, a private organization that monitors drug safety, demanding an immediate ban of phenformin as an "imminent hazard" to health (17). As a result, the FDA published a Notice in the *Federal Register* in April 1977 that a hearing would be held in May on the issue of whether the "imminent hazard" provision of the Food, Drug and Cosmetic Act should be invoked. However, the conditions for drug withdrawal on the ground of imminent hazard did not exist, since phenformin had been marketed for 18 years and the risk of lactic acidosis had been known for almost that long. Therefore, any attempt to withdraw the drug as an "imminent hazard" would likely be met with a challenge in court. Accordingly, in May 1977, the FDA published a Notice that a formal evidentiary hearing would be held on a yet unspecified date on the question of withdrawal of approval for the marketing of phenformin (16). This Notice was independent of the imminent hazard issue and was based on the recommendations of the FDA's Advisory Committee.

However, as a result of the evidence considered at the imminent hazard hearing in May 1977, consultation with health officials in other countries, and interpretation by FDA attorneys that recent court decisions might now permit immediate withdrawal of a drug on the ground of a "substantial likelihood of serious public harm," the FDA recommended to the Secretary of Health, Education and Welfare that he suspend marketing approval of phenformin (20). Such suspension occurred in July 1977, but a 90-day transition period was allowed to permit patients to be changed to other therapy (17,20). This marked the first time in the history of the FDA that the "imminent hazard" provision of the Food, Drug and Cosmetic Act had been invoked.

In addition, a court challenge against suspension was mounted by the Committee on the Care of the Diabetic, a group of diabetologists and patients. This challenge was not, as had been expected, based on the "imminent hazard" suspension of the drug due to a risk of lactic acidosis. Rather, it was founded largely on a belief that the FDA had erred in accepting the findings of a controlled clinical trial published some years earlier that noted an increase in cardiovascular mortality in patients receiving phenformin or another hypoglycemic agent (tolbutamide) when compared to those receiving insulin or diet alone. (The findings led to an FDA attempt to change the labeling for these drugs and were viewed by the Committee on the Care of the Diabetic as contributing to the FDA's desire in 1977 to withdraw phenformin from the market.) The challenge was subsequently withdrawn by the plaintiff (21).

In November 1978, the FDA issued a final order withdrawing approval of the marketing applications. The Committee for the Care of the Diabetic, which had testified at the formal hearing, petitioned the Commissioner of the FDA to reconsider his withdrawal on the basis of "new facts." The Commissioner denied the petition after finding those facts not pertinent to the central issue (22).

The formal hearing dealt with the issue of whether phenformin should continue to be available under general marketing conditions. Withdrawal of approval for marketing did not preclude distribution under controlled conditions to a very limited patient population. On the basis of testimony from experts, the FDA concluded that phenformin should continue to remain available to a very small number of patients for whom diabetologists considered the drug to be mandatory. It found that no acceptable plan could be devised to permit such distribution through retail pharmacies. Therefore, with the cooperation of the primary manufacturer, the FDA developed a system that would allow distribution under a master Investigational Drug Application prepared by the FDA for that purpose. Physicians with patients who met certain criteria were permitted to submit an application to the FDA for each patient, asserting that the patient met all of the specified criteria; written informed patient consent was required (23,24). The manufacturer, Ciba-Geigy, agreed to ship drug to physicians whose applications were approved by the FDA.

In the early years of this distribution, about 1000 patients continued to received the drug. (Approximately 350,000 patients were receiving phenformin when general marketing was suspended in July 1977) (25). The number of patients receiving the drug dwindled further. Distribution was discontinued in 1994; however, at that time, an investigational application was available for a related drug, metformin, permitting the switch of patients, if deemed advisable.

VII. ERYTHROMYCIN ESTOLATE

Erythromycin estolate (trade name Ilosone), an antibiotic manufactured by the Eli Lilly Co., has been known for decades to be associated with the risk of toxic hepatitis, predominantly in adults. This adverse effect was added to the labeling in 1962 and was strengthened by a black-box warning in 1973 after the FDA asked its Anti-Infective Agents Advisory Committee to review the question of whether the drug should be removed from the market. At that time, the committee recommended that the drug remain on the market because it might be therapeutically superior in certain situations to other erythromycins, due to the higher blood levels achieved with the estolate.

Other erythromycins are also known to pose some risk of toxic hepatitis, but it was generally felt at the time that the estolate had a greater potential in this regard.

The FDA continuously reviewed the adverse reaction reports for the estolate and found that, between 1969 and 1978, 93% of hepatoxicity reported for the erythromycins occurred in those taking the estolate. To some extent, this figure represented reporting bias because of the known risk of the estolate, but the overall evidence supported the general assumption of increased adverse hepatic effects with the estolate. This was particularly so in view of the fact that practicing physicians, recognizing the risk, prescribed the estolate for adults to a significantly lesser extent than they did other erythromycins.

Techniques developed since the 1973 Advisory Committee meeting permitted measurement in the blood of the active moiety of the erythromycins, viz., erythromycin base. Previous techniques had been able to measure only erythromycin estolate, a procedure that measured the base plus the inactive ester. New studies showed that a single dose of erythromycin estolate produced only 45% of the blood level of active base produced by erythromycin stearate. With multiple dosing, five doses of estolate were required to achieve an acceptable blood level of the active moiety when compared to administration of erythromycin base. The FDA did find that, when taken with food, the estolate produced less variable blood levels than did the base, but this fact was not considered sufficient to overcome the perceived hepatic risk.

The FDA proposed in November 1979 to remove the solid dosage form of the estolate from the market, because the published literature failed to reveal any therapeutic advantage for the estolate. No decision was made at that time on whether any action would be taken relative to the pediatric dosage form (26). In addition, the pediatric suspension was found to produce satisfactory and even superior blood levels, depending on the erythromycin product to which it was compared.

The FDA convened an Ad Hoc Erythromycin Estolate Advisory Committee in April 1981 to consider the bioavailability data, reports of clinical trials in various infections, and adverse reaction reports. The manufacturer and its consultants argued that erythromycin estolate did not pose a greater threat to the liver than other erythromycins or, at most, the increased risk was too small to outweigh the benefits of the drug; that greater reliability of blood levels after food (at least in comparison with erythromycin base) constituted an important advantage, and that preliminary data from ongoing clinical trials suggested that the estolate might be more effective than other erythromycin products in Legionnaire's disease. In addition, although the pediatric formulation was not under discussion, unpublished results were presented that showed the superiority of the estolate to erythromycin ethylsuccinate in streptococcal pharyngitis in children. These findings were postulated to be due to superior tissue levels of the estolate.

The Ad Hoc Committee concluded that erythromycin estolate did pose a greater risk of hepatoxicity in adults, but that data were inadequate to determine the relative risk of the estolate versus other forms of erythromycin. In addition, it noted the improved bioavailabilty when taken with food as compared with erythromycin base and the possibility of superior activity within tissues. It recommended that the solid dosage form of the estolate continue to remain on the market. It advised physicians to exercise clinical judgement in evaluating the benefit/risk ratio in an individual patient (27). The FDA accepted the advice of the committee and withdrew its proposal to remove the drug from the market (28).

As noted earlier, and as always the case with drugs known to pose a special risk, physicians had been exercising considerable judgment in the use of erythromycin estolate in adults, although not to a sufficient extent to reduce the risk to an absolute minimum. For the year ending December 1981, the year of the Advisory Committee review, only 35% of physician prescribing of the estolate consisted of the solid dosage form and only 34% of total estolate use was in patients over 9 years of age (29). Similar figures can be found for the year ending March 1986. By contrast, for the latter period, 76% of physician prescribing for erythromycin ethylsuccinate constituted the solid dosage form and 76% of total ethylsuccinate use was in patients over 9 years of age (30). Physicians continued to exercise discretion in use of erythromycin estolate. In 1995, only 11% of prescriptions were written for the solid dosage form (31).

VIII. NONIFENSINE

Nonifensine (trade name Merital) is an antidepressant drug that was introduced in Europe in the mid-1970s. It was first marketed in the United States in 1985, by which time it was known that rare instances of hemolytic anemia occurred in association with use of nonifensine.

Not long after its appearance in the United States, an increasing number
of cases of hemolytic anemia were reported in Great Britain, triggering a review
by that country's Committee on the Safety of Medicines. In addition, this increase
raised the concern of the manufacturer, Hoechst Group AG. The firm decided to
suspend sales worldwide in January 1986 (32). At the time of the suspension,
the drug had been taken by more than 14 million patients in 80 countries. Fifteen
deaths in the previous decade had been attributed to hemolytic anemia in patients
taking nonifensine. The reason for the increase in reports of hemolytic anemia
in Great Britain was not known.

The withdrawal of the drug from the market produced mixed feelings at
the time, even among regulatory agencies, because of the paucity of available
antidepressant drugs. There are no plans to reintroduce the drug into the market.
The extent to which withdrawal was based on the financial drain of possible
liability claims in comparison with volume of sales can only be conjectured.

IX. BROMOCRIPTINE

Bromocriptine (trade name Parlodel), is a synthetic ergot derivative with potent
dopamine receptor agonist activity. Such activity is responsible for its effectiveness in the control of motor function in Parkinson's disease and for its inhibition
of prolactin secretion from the anterior pituitary with resultant suppression of
postpartum lactation and of galactorrhea secondary to prolactin-secreting adenomas. In addition, its suppression of excessive growth hormone levels makes it
useful in the treatment of acromegaly.

In 1994, after years of contention with the FDA on the safety of bromocriptine for the prevention of postpartum lactation in women who choose not to breast
feed, the U.S. manufacturer voluntarily acceded to the FDA's request for removal
of the indication from the labeling of the drug. Bromocriptine remains available
for its other uses.

The fact that it is an ergot derivative has undoubtedly played a significant
part in FDA perceptions of its possible risk for postpartum women. Ergot derivatives are typically regarded as having vasospastic properties, e.g., the ergotamines
that are used for the treatment of migraine, and ergonovine for the facilitation of
labor. Under certain circumstances, the ergot derivatives with potent vasospastic
activity can cause precordial pain, electrocardiogram changes, hypertension,
stroke, and gangrene.

Bromocriptine, on the other hand, is a vasodilator. It uniformly lowers
blood pressure in animal models of hypertension and was once considered for
development as a treatment for hypertension. Therapy with bromocriptine is initiated with a low dose to avoid the risk of a hypotensive episode. In addition, the

drug has been shown to have anticonvulsant properties, and was considered for possible use in epilepsy.

Bromocriptine was marked in the United States in 1978 for treatment of galactorrhea and amenorrhea in patients with prolactin-secreting adenomas. In 1980, the FDA approved the drug for prevention of postpartum lactation in women who choose not to breast feed. The other indications in the labeling appeared later. There was considerable interest on the part of the FDA and its advisors, and of practicing obstetricians, in the availability of an alternative to estrogens for prevention of postpartum lactation, because the doses of estrogens used in the postpartum period pose a risk of thromboembolism. Bromocriptine became the drug of choice for postpartum use. About 30% of the women in the United States who chose not to breast feed received the drug, and most of the remainder used conventional breast binders, ice pads, and analgesics to relieve the pain and congestion that occur when lactation is not prevented.

Hypertension occurs frequently in the pre- and postpartum period. The postpartum period is also associated with other serious but, fortunately, uncommon risks. These include seizures, strokes, and myocardial infarction, which occur in incidences of 1 per 5000 to 1 per 20,000 patients. Not surprisingly, therefore, since about 600,000 postpartum women per year were receiving bromocriptine in the United States, the manufacturer began to receive reports of these events in women who at the time were taking bromocriptine. The FDA requested the manufacturer to list these adverse events in the labeling for bromocriptine. The company objected on the grounds that the anecdotal reports did not constitute scientific evidence of causality. The company finally yielded, however; the FDA did permit it to add a statement to the labeling that the relationship of the adverse reactions to the administration of the drug was not certain. Subsequently, at the FDA's request, warnings and contraindications were added to the labeling proscribing use of bromocriptine in uncontrolled hypertension and severe unremitting headache, which is a common prodrome of stroke.

The manufacturer conducted a case-control study on the association of seizures and strokes and use of bromocriptine in postpartum women. The study showed that the drug had a protective effect against postpartum seizures, providing a nice confirmation of its anticonvulsant effect in animals. No useful information was obtained with respect to stroke because bromocriptine use in the control group was only a fraction of the expected use as measured in the entire population, thus preventing any meaningful analysis of the data.

In 1988, the FDA asked an advisory committee to comment on the safety of bromocriptine for postpartum women. The committee concluded that the available data provided no evidence of a causal relationship to stroke and seizures. The FDA also asked whether drugs should be used to prevent postpartum lactation, an indication which, in contrast to its views in 1980, the FDA characterized as "trivial.'' The committee stated that these drugs should not be used "routinely," but should be available for special situations, such as after stillbirth (33).

In 1989, the FDA asked its advisory committee a somewhat different question, namely, whether there was a *need* for drugs to prevent postpartum lactation. The committee concluded that there was no need—that patients could use conventional methods for suppressing lactation (34). This view allowed the FDA to state that where there was no need, any potential risk of a drug was not justified.

The FDA asked estrogen and androgen manufacturers and the manufacturer of bromocriptine to remove the indication from their labeling. The other manufacturers complied, but the bromocriptine manufacturer did not. Instead, it gathered support from eminent obstetrician/gynecologists who indicated that there was a need for drugs to prevent lactation, and that there was no evidence that bromocriptine was unsafe.

The FDA took no formal action between 1990 and 1994. However, in 1994 it received the second petition from the Health Research Group, a voluntary organization that monitors the safety of drugs in the marketplace, requesting it to take steps to rescind approval of the indication for bromocriptine in postpartum lactation. The FDA then announced that it would do so.

Between 1989 and 1994 the media (newspaper and magazine articles, television programs) reported on the potential risks to women. Lawsuits arose from women who had experienced postpartum stroke and myocardial infarction. In 1994, the manufacturer decided that it would no longer devote a significant proportion of its resources to the defense of the safety of bromocriptine for postpartum women; it voluntarily withdrew the indication from its labeling. The indication was also withdrawn in a number of other countries at the request of government agencies.

Through the years the FDA's scientists held differing views on the safety of the drug in postpartum women. Some contended that there was clearly a risk, although of unmeasured magnitude, some that the risk was very small, and some felt that evidence of a risk had not been shown but the indication for use was not important enough to warrant a possible risk.

X. CONCLUSIONS

The aforementioned case histories are illustrative of the highly individualized circumstances surrounding an action to withdraw a drug from the market. This is appropriate because of the diversity of adverse drug effect, the severity and frequency of the risks, the therapeutic indications of the drugs, and the degrees of benefit they provide. What is evident is that a decision by the FDA to seek withdrawal of a drug from the market is preceded and accompanied by considerable study and consultation. This conclusion is supported by other cases not described here, including certain oral contraceptives and azaribine for psoriasis.

XI. REFERENCES

1. Bakke OM, Wardell WM, and Lasagna L. Drug discontinuation in the United Kingdom and the United States, 1964–1983: Issues of safety. Clin Pharmacol Ther 1984; 35:559.
2. FDA. Minutes of meeting with Smith Kline and French Laboratories, January 15, 1980.
3. Recall letter issued by Smith Kline and French Laboratories, January 16, 1980.
4. FDA. Summary of supplement to NDA 10–588, July 9, 1968.
5. FDA. Pharmacology summary in NDA 10–588, October 24, 1968.
6. FDA. Pharmacology review in NDA 10–598, May 23, 1977.
7. FDA. Letter to Merrell-National Laboratories, December 27, 1977.
8. FDA. Talk Paper on Bendectin, October 1, 1979.
9. Summary of September 15 and 16, 1980, FDA Fertility and Maternal Health Drugs Advisory Committee meeting.
10. FDA. Letter to Merrell-Dow, January 9, 1981.
11. FDA. Drug Bull 1981, (March):1–2.
12. FDA. Drug Bull 1982 (April):6.
13. FDA. Talk Paper on Bendectin, June 29, 1982.
14. FDA. Talk Paper, "Bendectin Production Ended," June 9, 1983.
15. FDA Consumer, September 1983.
16. Phenformin hydrochloride: opportunity for hearing on proposal to withdraw approval of New Drug Application. Fed Reg 1977 (May 6); 42(88).
17. FDA. Drug Bull 1977 (August): 14–16.
18. Federal Food, Drug and Cosmetic Act, Sec. 505(e).
19. Ibid.
20. FDA. Talk Proper, "Phenformin," May 18, 1977.
21. Neil Chalet, personal communication.
22. Phenformin hydrochloride; denial of petition for reconsideration. Fed Reg 1979 (April 6); 44(68).
23. FDA Physician Sponsor Application and Order Form for Phenformin Under IND 14,000.
24. FDA Instruction for Physician Sponsors Under IND 14,000.
25. Ciba-Geigy Pharmaceutical Co., personal communication.
26. FDA. Drug Bull 1979 (November): 26–27.
27. Summary of Ad Hoc Erythromycin Estolate Advisory Committee meeting, April 16 and 17, 1981.
28. FDA. Drug Bull 1982 (August): 14.
29. National Disease and Therapeutic Index Drug Book, Year Ending December 1981.
30. National Disease and Therapeutic Index Drug Book, Year ending March 1986.

31. IMS National Prescription Audit.
32. FDA. Talk Paper, ''Withdrawal of Nomifensine (Merital),'' January 28, 1986.
33. FDA Fertility and Maternal Health Drugs Advisory Committee Meeting, June 2,
     1988.
34. FDA Fertility and Maternal Health Drugs Advisory Committee Meeting, June 1&
     2, 1989.

Appendices: Routine Clinical Analyte Test Results

Appendix A

First and 99th percentiles of routine clinical analyte test results in 20,102 adults applying for participation in clinical trials (2). Delta limits are the 1st and 99th percentiles of the differences between two samples obtained one to two weeks apart.

Analyte	Age in years: Units	Male Caucasian <50	Male Caucasian ≥50	Male Non-Caucasian <50	Male Non-Caucasian ≥50	Female Caucasian <50	Female Caucasian ≥50	Female Non-Caucasian <50	Female Non-Caucasian ≥50	Delta Limits Low	Delta Limits High
Liver											
ALT	U/L	7-125	5-95	5-121	4-84	5-80	5-80	4-82	4-82	-27	28
AST	U/L	11-79	10-78	11-122	8-84	9-62	9-67	9-66	9-65	-25	22
GT	U/L	6-194	6-193	7-320	5-274	5-127	5-201	5-161	5-190	-30	29
Alk. Phosphatase	U/L	30-153	28-163	32-151	27-174	28-131	31-168	31-138	33-174	-44	28
Bilirubin	µmol/L	3-31	3-29	3-29	3-22	3-22	3-19	2-21	2-19	-10	10
Muscle											
Creatine Kinase	U/L	17-640	11-426	27-1105	15-940	19-265	0-267	20-453	10-463	-277	236
Kidney											
Creatinine	µmol/L	62-141	71-168	71-168	71-186	53-124	53-150	53-124	53-150	-35	35
Urea	mmol/L	2.5-8.9	2.9-11.1	2.1-8.9	2.1-12.5	1.8-7.9	2.5-11.4	1.8-7.5	2.5-10.7	-3.2	3.2
Uric Acid	µmol/L	167-547	161-583	184-595	208-625	89-470	113-535	107-482	143-619	-125	119
Phosphate (i)	mmol/L	0.72-1.61	0.68-1.49	0.77-1.65	0.68-1.58	0.74-1.65	0.74-1.58	0.74-1.52	0.74-1.61	-0.45	0.42
Calcium	mmol/L	2.07-2.64	2.02-2.62	2.05-2.64	2.05-2.64	2.02-2.62	2.05-2.64	2.02-2.64	2.02-2.69	-0.30	0.30
Electrolytes											
Sodium	mmol/L	135-147	133-148	135-150	134-149	135-147	134-150	135-150	134-152	-8	8
Potassium	mmol/L	3.5-5.5	3.3-5.4	3.0-5.5	3.0-5.4	3.4-5.3	3.3-5.5	3.1-5.3	3.0-5.3	-1.1	1.0
Chloride	mmol/L	96-113	95-112	96-110	95-112	96-114	94-113	96-112	93-111	-9	8
Bicarbonate	mmol/L	21-35	21-35	21-36	21-36	20-33	21-36	20-35	21-36	-7	8

	Units										
Nutritionals											
Glucose, fasting	mmol/L	37-10.8	3.9-14.2	3.8-9.5	3.9-16.8	3.7-9.2	3.7-15.0	3.8-15.3	3.9-20.3	-3.1	3.2
Glucose, nonfasting	mmol/L	3.4-9.8	3.8-14.4	3.4-10.8	4.2-20.3	3.6-11.2	4.3-15.2	3.8-14.7	4.2-18.4	-4.8	4.2
Albumin	g/L	36-52	32-50	34-53	32-49	34-50	32-49	33-49	32-50	-7	6
Protein	g/L	62-83	60-82	63-89	61-87	61-82	60-82	63-86	63-86	-11	10
Cholesterol	mmol/L	2.84-8.56	3.41-8.51	2.77-8.45	2.84-8.95	3.10-7.73	3.65-9.10	3.10-7.73	3.78-9.36	-1.78	1.73
HDL Cholesterol	mmol/L	0.44-2.02	0.47-2.17	0.47-2.48	0.41-2.48	0.59-2.64	0.57-2.56	0.52-2.51	0.52-2.64	-0.85	0.72
LDL Cholesterol	mmol/L	1.50-6.13	1.68-6.08	1.22-6.26	1.42-6.43	1.37-5.46	1.78-6.23	1.16-5.82	1.81-6.83	-1.97	1.78
Triglycerides	mmol/L	0.50-9.53	0.53-8.69	0.45-8.99	0.51-5.05	0.38-6.93	0.58-6.21	0.44-5.59	0.52-4.41	-3.01	2.88
Erythrocytes											
Hemoglobin (Fe)	mmol/L	7.90-11.29	7.10-11.36	6.83-11.23	6.60-11.00	6.80-10.18	6.60-10.36	6.14-10.10	6.21-10.10	-1.20	1.20
Erythrocytes	T/L	4.2-6.2	3.9-6.2	3.9-6.4	3.7-6.4	3.7-5.5	3.5-5.7	3.6-5.7	3.5-5.9	-0.7	0.7
Hematocrit	1	0.38-0.55	0.35-0.55	0.35-0.55	0.33-0.54	0.33-0.49	0.33-0.51	0.31-0.49	0.33-0.49	-0.07	0.06
MCV	fL	78-105	77-107	71-104	74-104	76-103	77-105	67-102	73-102	-9	8
MCH (Fe)	fmol	1.60-2.17	1.60-2.20	1.40-2.17	1.40-2.11	1.50-2.10	1.60-2.11	1.30-2.05	1.40-2.05	-0.19	0.20
MCHC (Fe)	mmol/L	19-23	19-23	18-23	18-22	19-23	19-23	18-22	18-22	-2	2
Leukocytes											
Leukocytes	GI/L	3.6-13.8	3.4-12.8	3.0-13.0	2.9-11.6	3.5-13.4	3.6-12.4	3.2-13.6	3.1-11.4	-4.0	3.7
Bands	GI/L	0-0.62	0-0.54	0-0.27	0-0.32	0-0.75	0-0.55	0-0.37	0-0.20	-0.29	0.26
Neutrophils	GI/L	1.83-9.29	1.82-8.74	1.17-9.24	1.29-7.81	1.70-8.99	1.79-8.52	1.19-8.66	1.31-7.87	-3.38	3.18
Lymphocytes	GI/L	0.88-4.49	0.81-4.32	0.93-4.95	0.82-4.28	0.97-4.20	0.90-4.30	0.94-4.51	0.95-4.47	-1.57	1.54
Monocytes	GI/L	0-0.89	0-0.96	0-0.81	0-0.85	0-0.82	0-0.85	0-0.83	0-0.75	-0.44	0.46
Eosinophils	GI/L	0-0.65	0-0.66	0-0.74	0-0.59	0-0.65	0-0.58	0-0.62	0-0.55	-0.38	0.37
Basophils	GI/L	0-0.18	0-0.18	0-0.15	0-0.14	0-0.17	0-0.17	0-0.16	0-0.17	-0.13	0.13
Platelets	GI/L	136-425	130-483	131-486	123-518	151-501	141-513	144-541	114-559	-93	107
Urine											
Specific Gravity	-	1.006-1.037	1.006-1.035	1.007-1.036	1.006-1.036	1.004-1.036	1.005-1.036	1.005-1.038	1.006-1.037	-0.018	0.017
pH	-	5.0-8.0	5.0-8.0	5.0-8.0	5.0-8.0	5.0-8.0	5.0-8.0	5.0-8.0	5.0-8.0	-2.0	2.0

Appendix B

First and 99th percentiles of routine clinical analyte test results in 4801 adults who denied smoking or drinking ethanol (2).

Analyte	Age in years: Units	Male Caucasian <50	Caucasian ≥50	Non-Caucasian <50	Non-Caucasian ≥50	Female Caucasian <50	Caucasian ≥50	Non-Caucasian <50	Non-Caucasian ≥50	Delta Limits Low	Delta Limits High
Liver											
ALT	U/L	9-97	6-79	4-109	6-68	5-94	5-77	4-89	4-82	-27	28
AST	U/L	11-67	10-55	11-88	9-60	10-64	9-62	8-64	10-65	-25	22
GT	U/L	6-117	5-190	7-148	6-135	5-137	5-148	6-130	5-123	-30	29
Alk. Phosphatase	U/L	29-136	26-162	29-149	29-146	29-136	23-156	24-138	34-171	-44	28
Bilirubin	µmol/L	5-32	3-36	3-29	3-24	3-22	3-19	2-19	2-21	-10	10
Muscle											
Creatine Kinase	U/L	17-667	15-419	15-717	14-1043	10-269	0-235	13-407	11-610	-277	236
Kidney											
Creatinine	µmol/L	62-141	62-168	71-159	71-194	53-124	53-150	53-133	44-150	-35	35
Urea	mmol/L	2.5-9.3	2.9-10.7	1.8-8.6	2.5-11.4	1.8-8.6	2.5-11.1	1.8-7.5	2.9-10.7	-3.2	3.2
Uric Acid	µmol/L	155-547	178-601	184-589	244-601	95-500	113-517	125-476	155-519	-125	119
Phosphate (i)	mmol/L	0.81-1.52	0.68-1.45	0.77-1.68	0.68-1.55	0.77-1.55	0.74-1.58	0.77-1.52	0.84-1.58	-0.45	0.42
Calcium	mmol/L	2.07-2.64	2.05-2.59	2.05-2.64	2.05-2.59	2.02-2.59	2.05-2.64	2.02-2.64	2.10-2.59	-0.30	0.30
Electrolytes											
Sodium	mmol/L	132-148	134-148	135-157	135-150	129-145	134-150	135-150	135-152	-8	8
Potassium	mmol/L	3.5-5.5	3.3-5.5	2.8-7.4	2.8-5.4	3.3-5.3	3.4-5.5	3.0-5.0	3.0-5.2	-1.1	1.0
Chloride	mmol/L	96-112	96-111	93-112	96-111	96-110	95-112	97-110	95-111	-9	8
Bicarbonate	mmol/L	22-36	22-35	21-36	21-36	20-34	21.35	19-36	21-36	-7	8

	Units										
Nutritionals											
Glucose, fasting	mmol/L	3.6-13.2	3.8-16.6	3.9-9.5	3.6-17.5	3.8-12.1	3.8-15.2	3.8-16.0	2.7-21.7	-3.1	3.2
Glucose, nonfasting	mmol/L	4.3-12.6	4.7-14.4	3.4-8.3	4.5-17.3	4.3-9.8	3.5-29.2	4.1-15.8	3.9-22.8	-4.8	4.2
Albumin	g/L	37-51	34-49	34-53	30-48	34-50	33-49	32-49	33-49	-7	6
Protein	g/L	63-84	60-82	61-86	59-86	61-83	62-83	64-85	63-86	-11	10
Cholesterol	mmol/L	3.06-7.81	3.44-8.51	2.79-8.24	3.21-9.05	3.18-8.33	3.70-8.82	3.36-8.51	3.80-9.31	-1.78	1.73
HDL Cholesterol	mmol/L	0.42-2.07	0.55-2.12	0.28-2.43	0.36-2.16	0.49-2.22	0.54-2.53	0.47-2.25	0.52-2.61	-0.85	0.72
LDL Cholesterol	mmol/L	1.48-5.77	1.84-5.48	1.42-6.30	1.32-6.43	0.91-5.28	1.63-6.23	1.66-5.82	2.20-6.57	-1.97	1.78
Triglycerides	mmol/L	0.54-11.02	0.52-8.85	0.44-16.81	0.50-4.19	0.40-9.06	0.67-7.77	0.55-5.59	0.52-4.44	-3.01	2.88
Erythrocytes											
Hemoglobin (Fe)	mmol/L	7.80-11.30	7.50-11.20	6.30-11.00	6.80-10.92	6.64-9.90	6.90-10.24	5.00-10.43	6.30-9.99	-1.20	1.20
Erythrocytes	T/L	4.2-6.3	4.0-6.2	4.0-6.4	3.7-6.2	3.7-5.6	3.7-5.6	3.6-5.9	3.6-5.8	-0.7	0.7
Hematocrit	1	0.37-0.54	0.36-0.54	0.31-0.54	0.33-0.54	0.33-0.48	0.34-0.51	0.27-0.51	0.33-0.49	-0.07	0.06
MCV	fL	77-99	78-103	68-100	74-103	75-101	76-101	66-100	72-100	-9	8
MCH (Fe)	fmol	1.60-2.05	1.60-2.11	1.40-2.00	1.40-2.10	1.49-2.05	1.55-2.10	1.24-2.05	1.40-2.05	-0.19	0.20
MCHC (Fe)	mmol/L	19-23	19-23	18-23	18-22	19-23	19-23	18-22	18-22	-2	2
Leukocytes											
Leukocytes	G/L	3.6-11.5	3.6-12.6	3.1-12.8	2.8-10.9	3.4-13.0	3.7-11.8	3.0-11.5	3.0-10.6	-4.0	3.7
Bands	G/L	0-0.32	0-0.38	0-0.15	0-0.28	0-0.57	0-0.40	0-0.20	0-0.20	-0.29	0.26
Neutrophils	G/L	1.86-7.31	1.89-8.61	1.19-9.06	1.33-7.50	1.63-8.78	1.88-7.83	1.13-8.24	1.33-7.31	-3.38	3.18
Lymphocytes	G/L	0.80-3.92	0.88-4.29	0.84-4.26	0.75-4.15	1.03-4.12	0.96-4.17	0.84-4.03	1.02-4.14	-1.57	1.54
Monocytes	G/L	0-0.85	0-0.90	0-0.78	0-0.82	0-0.80	0-0.88	0-0.83	0-0.71	-0.44	0.46
Eosinophils	G/L	0-0.48	0-0.64	0-0.68	0-0.54	0-0.62	0-0.59	0-0.81	0-0.55	-0.38	0.37
Basophils	G/L	0-0.19	0-0.16	0-0.14	0-0.13	0-0.16	0-0.16	0-0.16	0-0.14	-0.13	0.13
Platelets	G/L	152-420	127-483	156-476	150-443	160-530	157-486	164-541	149-559	-93	107
Urine											
Specific Gravity	--	1.006-1.037	1.006-1.036	1.011-1.040	1.006-1.036	1.005-1.037	1.005-1.036	1.006-1.040	1.006-1.038	-0.018	0.017
pH	--	5.0-8.0	5.0-8.0	5.0-7.0	5.0-8.0	5.0-8.0	5.0-8.0	5.0-8.0	5.0-8.0	-2.0	2.0

Appendix C

First and 99th percentiles of routine clinical analyte test results in 2037 adults who smoked, but denied drinking ethanol (2).

Analyte	Age in years: Units	Male				Female				Delta Limits	
		Caucasian		Non-Caucasian		Caucasian		Non-Caucasian			
		<50	≥50	<50	≥50	<50	≥50	<50	≥50	Low	High
Liver											
ALT	U/L	5-93	4-72	5-95	3-96	4-63	5-61	3-228	4-92	-27	28
AST	U/L	10-60	9-48	11-60	7-84	8-55	10-60	9-139	10-71	-25	22
GT	U/L	8-194	6-94	8-207	6-101	4-252	7-189	5-181	5-190	-30	29
Alk. Phosphatase	U/L	34-136	38-166	36-144	27-194	30-133	39-211	32-121	39-174	-44	28
Bilirubin	μmol/L	3-24	3-21	3-22	3-21	3-17	3-15	2-22	3-15	-10	10
Muscle											
Creatine Kinase	U/L	18-670	15-281	30-1481	17-786	0-218	0-297	15-246	0-328	-277	236
Kidney											
Creatinine	μmol/L	53-141	62-150	53-141	71-194	53-115	53-133	53-124	62-124	-35	35
Urea	mmol/L	2.5-9.6	2.5-10.7	2.1-9.3	2.5-12.9	1.8-7.5	2.1-9.6	1.8-7.1	2.5-9.3	-3.2	3.2
Uric Acid	μmol/L	167-512	119-541	206-571	190-630	83-470	119-547	59-494	155-529	-125	119
Phosphate (i)	mmol/L	0.68-1.58	0.68-1.49	0.81-1.58	0.61-1.58	0.77-1.58	0.90-1.52	0.77-1.49	0.81-1.52	-0.45	0.42
Calcium	mmol/L	2.10-2.67	2.02-2.64	2.05-2.70	2.10-2.72	2.05-2.60	2.10-2.64	2.05-2.64	1.67-2.64	-0.30	0.30
Electrolytes											
Sodium	mmol/L	135-148	134-146	135-148	125-149	135-150	134-153	134-151	135-149	-8	8
Potassium	mmol/L	3.3-5.3	3.1-5.2	3.0-5.3	3.1-5.2	3.4-5.4	2.8-5.7	3.2-4.9	3.1-5.3	-1.1	1.0
Chloride	mmol/L	94-108	96-112	96-109	94-111	96-113	93-112	99-112	95-107	-9	8
Bicarbonate	mmol/L	19-36	22-34	21-35	22-34	19-31	21-34	21-35	22-34	-7	8

Test	Units										
Nutritionals											
Glucose, fasting	mmol/L	3.4-8.3	4.2-15.4	2.8-18.9	3.7-25.1	3.6-9.4	3.7-14.4	4.1-10.3	3.9-20.3	-3.1	3.2
Glucose, nonfasting	mmol/L	4.2-9.0	4.3-22.2	0.7-16.5	4.0-16.7	3.9-21.6	4.5-18.8	3.8-10.7	4.8-13.1	-4.8	4.2
Albumin	g/L	34-53	32-49	36-51	34-47	34-51	33-49	35-49	33-50	-7	6
Protein	g/L	61-83	61-81	63-86	63-80	61-81	59-81	62-84	62-85	-11	10
Cholesterol	mmol/L	2.87-8.77	3.54-8.56	2.74-8.74	2.43-8.90	3.21-7.60	4.03-9.39	3.28-7.32	3.70-9.31	-1.78	1.73
HDL Cholesterol	mmol/L	0.26-1.78	0.36-2.02	0.52-1.76	0.41-2.80	0.47-2.22	0.54-2.30	0.54-2.30	0.67-2.69	-0.85	0.72
LDL Cholesterol	mmol/L	1.81-5.72	1.94-6.71	1.22-5.99	0.70-5.38	1.89-8.04	1.97-6.15	1.16-5.48	2.25-6.83	-1.97	1.78
Triglycerides	mmol/L	0.72-12.78	0.63-9.03	0.43-3.62	0.45-11.49	0.53-6.25	0.87-15.72	0.53-3.82	0.75-4.30	-3.01	2.88
Erythrocytes											
Hemoglobin (Fe)	mmol/L	8.10-11.61	7.00-11.36	7.57-11.23	6.27-11.61	7.10-10.60	6.90-10.43	6.45-10.80	6.60-10.18	-1.20	1.20
Erythrocytes	T/L	4.3-6.4	3.9-6.2	4.0-6.4	3.9-6.6	3.6-5.7	3.8-5.9	3.5-6.0	3.8-5.8	-0.7	0.7
Hematocrit	1	0.39-0.56	0.35-0.55	0.37-0.56	0.33-0.56	0.34-0.56	0.36-0.52	0.32-0.54	0.33-0.50	-0.07	0.06
MCV	fL	78-104	75-106	74-99	73-107	78-105	81-105	70-104	79-103	-9	8
MCH (Fe)	fmol	1.60-2.10	1.40-2.11	1.60-2.05	1.30-2.10	1.60-2.20	1.70-2.11	1.40-2.17	1.49-2.20	-0.19	0.20
MCHC (Fe)	mmol/L	19-23	19-23	18-22	19-23	19-23	19-22	18-22	18-22	-2	2
Leukocytes											
Leukocytes	G/L	4.1-14.9	3.5-13.5	3.1-15.5	2.9-13.1	4.3-14.1	3.9-13.6	3.5-14.8	3.1-12.5	-4.0	3.7
Bands	G/L	0-1.03	0-0.71	0-0.54	0-0.38	0-0.78	0-0.58	0-0.39	0-0.20	-0.29	0.26
Neutrophils	G/L	2.18-10.35	2.05-9.05	1.21-9.66	1.25-8.97	1.96-9.84	1.95-9.80	1.31-10.50	1.85-7.60	-3.38	3.18
Lymphocytes	G/L	1.09-4.84	1.02-4.54	1.06-6.01	0.84-4.37	1.22-4.71	1.06-4.75	1.22-4.87	0.43-4.72	-1.57	1.54
Monocytes	G/L	0-0.83	0-0.92	0-1.04	0-0.85	0-0.85	0-0.87	0-0.93	0-0.75	-0.44	0.46
Eosinophils	G/L	0-0.78	0-0.71	0-0.86	0-0.60	0-0.84	0-0.59	0-0.63	0-0.58	-0.38	0.37
Basophils	G/L	0-0.23	0-0.19	0-0.14	0-0.14	0-0.19	0-0.21	0-0.15	0-0.15	-0.13	0.13
Platelets	G/L	136-457	149-586	116-394	158-486	154-499	127-476	184-550	101-480	-93	107
Urine											
Specific Gravity	–	1.006-1.036	1.006-1.034	1.005-1.036	1.006-1.036	1.005-1.036	1.005-1.043	1.005-1.039	1.005-1.032	-0.018	0.017
pH	–	5.0-7.0	5.0-9.0	5.0-8.0	5.0-7.0	5.0-8.0	5.0-8.0	5.0-7.0	5.0-7.0	-2.0	2.0

Appendix D

First and 99th percentiles of routine clinical analyte test results in 4265 adults who drank ethanol, but denied smoking (2).

Analyte	Age in years: Units	Male				Female				Delta Limits	
		Caucasian		Non-Caucasian		Caucasian		Non-Caucasian			
		<50	≥50	<50	≥50	<50	≥50	<50	≥50	Low	High
Liver											
ALT	U/L	9-102	8-10	6-125	7-101	6-81	7-90	5-52	2-114	-27	28
AST	U/L	11-67	11-83	12-131	12-132	10-70	11-87	8-52	12-106	-25	22
GT	U/L	6-160	6-200	7-207	9-152	5-117	5-201	5-121	5-113	-30	29
Alk. Phosphatase	U/L	25-125	22-124	33-119	22-132	25-115	31-158	29-131	32-192	-44	28
Bilirubin	μmol/L	3-36	3-31	3-29	3-27	3-22	3-22	3-22	3-15	-10	10
Muscle											
Creatine Kinase	U/L	20-563	0-427	35-1070	17-2124	25-273	11-275	34-420	10-361	-277	236
Kidney											
Creatinine	μmol/L	71-141	71-159	71-177	71-150	53-124	53-133	53-133	44-133	-35	35
Urea	mmol/L	2.5-9.6	3.2-10.4	2.5-9.3	2.1-10.4	1.8-7.5	2.5-10.4	1.8-7.9	2.9-10.4	-3.2	3.2
Uric Acid	μmol/L	178-583	178-583	202-607	190-613	89-446	113-547	131-541	83-613	-125	119
Phosphate (i)	mmol/L	0.71-1.52	0.68-1.49	0.77-1.58	0.65-1.45	0.74-1.58	0.74-1.61	0.74-1.55	0.90-1.68	-0.45	0.42
Calcium	mmol/L	2.10-2.62	2.05-2.62	2.10-2.69	2.10-2.69	2.02-2.62	2.00-2.59	2.05-2.59	1.90-2.64	-0.30	0.30
Electrolytes											
Sodium	mmol/L	134-147	135-148	135-150	133-148	135-146	134-147	136-145	137-153	-8	8
Potassium	mmol/L	3.5-5.5	3.3-5.4	3.0-5.5	3.0-6.0	3.2-5.2	3.3-5.3	3.3-5.9	3.1-5.1	-1.1	1.0
Chloride	mmol/L	96-112	97-111	96-110	97-110	95-114	95-113	99-110	99-115	-9	8
Bicarbonate	mmol/L	22-35	22-35	23-36	20-44	21-35	22-36	22-33	22-35	-7	8

	Units										
Nutritionals											
Glucose, fasting	mmol/L	3.7-8.8	4.2-12.5	4.1-8.7	2.9-12.4	3.8-8.1	3.7-18.0	0.9-16.3	2.6-16.6	-3.1	3.2
Glucose, nonfasting	mmol/L	3.4-7.7	1.7-12.1	3.5-13.7	4.8-10.5	4.7-7.7	4.6-13.7	4.8-6.3	4.7-12.0	-4.8	4.2
Albumin	g/L	37-53	36-50	37-53	32-50	34-50	34-50	34-48	33-49	-7	6
Protein	g/L	62-83	61-82	64-86	61-83	62-82	62-83	63-88	59-82	-11	10
Cholesterol	mmol/L	2.95-8.48	3.49-8.43	3.23-8.46	3.41-8.87	3.21-7.47	3.93-9.13	3.59-7.37	3.67-9.36	-1.78	1.73
HDL Cholesterol	mmol/L	0.47-2.17	0.47-2.22	0.44-3.03	0.28-2.53	0.72-2.95	0.65-2.74	0.75-2.87	0.78-2.61	-0.85	0.72
LDL Cholesterol	mmol/L	1.89-5.96	1.68-6.06	1.55-6.26	1.50-6.49	1.37-5.43	1.84-6.54	1.68-4.76	1.24-7.68	-1.97	1.78
Triglycerides	mmol/L	0.47-10.21	0.53-7.81	0.65-8.99	0.54-8.79	0.29-4.44	0.53-4.90	0.38-6.42	0.52-6.51	-3.01	2.88
Erythrocytes											
Hemoglobin (Fe)	mmol/L	7.88-10.96	7.32-11.23	7.50-11.11	5.83-10.67	6.83-9.70	7.00-10.18	6.30-9.62	6.33-10.05	-1.20	1.20
Erythrocytes	T/L	4.2-6.0	4.0-6.1	4.4-6.4	3.2-6.4	3.7-5.4	3.7-5.6	3.8-5.6	3.5-5.7	-0.7	0.7
Hematocrit	1	0.38-0.53	0.36-0.54	0.38-0.54	0.29-0.52	0.33-0.48	0.34-0.50	0.32-0.47	0.33-0.49	-0.07	0.06
MCV	fL	77-102	77-105	74-104	69-102	78-101	78-103	65-100	71-103	-9	8
MCH (Fe)	fmol	1.60-2.11	1.60-2.20	1.40-2.11	1.31-2.05	1.60-2.10	1.60-2.11	1.20-2.00	1.43-2.17	-0.19	0.20
MCHC (Fe)	mmol/L	19-23	19-23	19-23	19-22	19-23	19-23	18-22	18-24	-2	2
Leukocytes											
Leukocytes	G/L	3.4-10.8	3.3-11.8	2.9-9.4	2.9-10.2	3.4-11.8	3.3-10.8	3.0-12.5	3.0-9.4	-4.0	3.7
Bands	G/L	0-0.29	0-0.26	0-0.16	0-0.20	0-0.34	0-0.21	0-0.06	0-0.30	-0.29	0.26
Neutrophils	G/L	1.72-7.67	1.63-7.79	1.06-6.12	0.75-6.28	1.67-8.38	1.39-8.36	1.09-8.54	0.87-5.45	-3.38	3.18
Lymphocytes	G/L	0.87-3.76	0.75-4.42	0.96-4.10	0.82-4.17	0.91-3.65	0.85-3.64	0.94-3.95	0.95-3.96	-1.57	1.54
Monocytes	G/L	0-0.79	0-0.96	0-0.75	0-0.72	0-0.76	0-0.78	0-0.78	0-1.00	-0.44	0.46
Eosinophils	G/L	0-0.53	0-0.68	0-0.59	0-0.50	0-0.50	0-0.59	0-0.48	0-0.54	-0.38	0.37
Basophils	G/L	0-0.15	0-0.17	0-0.15	0-0.19	0-0.17	0-0.17	0-0.20	0-0.19	-0.13	0.13
Platelets	G/L	147-399	131-429	152-506	123-397	168-474	155-514	165-448	145-409	-93	107
Urine											
Specific Gravity	–	1.006-1.037	1.005-1.036	1.007-1.035	1.005-1.036	1.004-1.036	1.005-1.035	1.006-1.036	1.006-1.034	-0.018	0.017
pH	–	5.0-8.0	5.0-8.0	5.0-8.0	5.0-9.0	5.0-8.0	5.0-8.0	5.0-7.0	5.0-7.0	-2.0	2.0

Appendix E

First and 99th percentiles of routine clinical analyte test results in 2974 adults who smoked and drank ethanol (2).

Analyte	Age in years: Units	Male Caucasian <50	≥50	Male Non-Caucasian <50	≥50	Female Caucasian <50	≥50	Female Non-Caucasian <50	≥50	Delta Limits Low	High
Liver											
ALT	U/L	5-143	6-114	6-109	3-77	5-63	7-62	4-112	6-57	-27	28
AST	U/L	11-111	9-104	11-140	11-114	9-55	10-80	8-81	9-62	-25	22
GT	U/L	8-230	5-167	7-390	6-460	6-168	5-148	7-111	7-96	-30	29
Alk. Phosphatase	U/L	31-144	32-137	35-140	36-155	27-136	36-142	35-145	31-235	-44	28
Bilirubin	µmol/L	3-29	3-26	3-29	3-22	3-19	2-17	2-17	2-19	-10	10
Muscle											
Creatine Kinase	U/L	16-615	12-474	27-2770	18-600	20-218	0-308	26-316	0-389	-277	236
Kidney											
Creatinine	µmol/L	62-133	71-141	71-168	62-186	53-124	53-115	53-115	53-159	-35	35
Urea	mmol/L	2.1-8.9	2.5-9.6	2.1-8.6	1.4-12.5	1.4-7.5	1.8-8.6	2.0-7.9	2.1-8.2	-3.2	3.2
Uric Acid	µmol/L	172-547	167-553	178-607	220-571	95-440	143-476	143-476	143-648	-125	119
Phosphate (i)	mmol/L	0.74-1.58	0.78-1.45	0.77-1.61	0.71-1.71	0.81-1.65	0.84-1.58	0.81-1.65	0.61-1.71	-0.45	0.42
Calcium	mmol/L	2.07-2.62	2.05-2.57	2.05-2.64	2.10-2.69	2.02-2.62	2.05-2.64	2.07-2.62	1.90-2.60	-0.30	0.30
Electrolytes											
Sodium	mmol/L	135-147	134-146	136-149	135-153	135-150	134-151	135-150	128-149	-8	8
Potassium	mmol/L	3.6-5.7	3.4-5.4	3.5-5.3	2.8-5.4	3.5-5.3	3.4-5.5	3.4-6.8	2.9-4.7	-1.1	1.0
Chloride	mmol/L	97-115	96-112	96-110	97-114	96-116	95-117	99-112	90-109	-9	8
Bicarbonate	mmol/L	20-34	21-35	21-32	22-38	19-32	22-36	19-35	20-35	-7	8

	Units										
Nutritionals											
Glucose, fasting	mmol/L	3.6-9.9	3.8-12.1	3.6-8.4	4.1-15.1	3.7-8.0	3.8-8.2	3.9-7.8	4.4-23.3	-3.1	3.2
Glucose, nonfasting	mmol/L	2.2-9.8	2.8-11.9	4.1-8.0	4.2-14.5	0.5-11.2	4.4-13.7	0.9-7.4	4.6-18.4	-4.8	4.2
Albumin	g/L	35-52	33-50	33-51	33-51	34-51	35-50	33-53	32-52	-7	6
Protein	g/L	62-84	61-83	63-88	59-87	60-82	61-80	64-93	60-88	-11	10
Cholesterol	mmol/L	2.97-8.84	3.59-8.56	2.61-8.67	2.92-8.61	3.03-8.25	3.70-9.00	3.54-8.84	3.82-11.12	-1.78	1.73
HDL Cholesterol	mmol/L	0.52-2.02	0.42-2.17	0.59-2.64	0.44-2.48	0.70-2.38	0.44-3.10	0.52-2.35	0.06-2.64	-0.85	0.72
LDL Cholesterol	mmol/L	1.45-6.15	1.63-6.10	0.75-6.80	1.42-7.16	1.27-5.46	1.60-5.59	1.06-6.13	2.15-6.15	-1.97	1.78
Triglycerides	mmol/L	0.58-8.24	0.52-8.74	0.53-7.95	0.51-4.14	0.42-5.61	0.51-9.04	0.41-7.69	0.44-3.51	-3.01	2.88
Erythrocytes											
Hemoglobin (Fe)	mmol/L	8.10-11.61	7.60-11.79	6.80-11.42	6.95-11.48	7.02-10.40	7.50-10.98	6.39-10.30	5.80-11.11	-1.20	1.20
Erythrocytes	T/L	4.2-6.1	3.6-6.1	3.6-6.2	3.4-6.9	3.7-5.5	4.0-5.9	3.7-5.6	3.6-6.0	-0.7	0.7
Hematocrit	1	0.39-0.58	0.37-0.56	0.33-0.56	0.34-0.57	0.34-0.50	0.35-0.53	0.33-0.52	0.31-0.53	-0.07	0.06
MCV	fL	75-109	80-111	72-109	75-107	76-105	79-107	71-102	78-104	-9	8
MCH (Fe)	fmol	1.60-2.23	1.68-2.40	1.40-2.23	1.49-2.17	1.60-2.20	1.70-2.17	1.37-2.05	1.49-2.11	-0.19	0.20
MCHC (Fe)	mmol/L	19-23	19-23	19-23	13-23	19-23	19-22	19-23	19-22	-2	2
Leukocytes											
Leukocytes	G/L	3.9-14.3	3.6-12.9	3.0-12.9	3.2-11.5	3.6-14.6	4.4-13.3	3.3-14.4	3.1-11.4	-4.0	3.7
Bands	G/L	0-0.78	0-0.78	0-0.44	0-0.19	0-1.15	0-1.71	0-0.72	0-0.14	-0.29	0.26
Neutrophils	G/L	1.96-9.91	1.84-9.05	0.90-9.15	1.44-8.01	1.71-10.34	2.26-8.79	1.41-8.66	1.60-8.59	-3.38	3.18
Lymphocytes	G/L	0.89-4.80	0.85-4.15	0.93-4.66	0.75-4.65	0.97-4.47	0.90-4.79	1.01-4.88	0.78-4.79	-1.57	1.54
Monocytes	G/L	0-0.95	0-1.13	0-0.81	0-1.00	0-0.83	0-0.93	0-0.84	0-0.65	-0.44	0.46
Eosinophils	G/L	0-0.77	0-0.66	0-0.61	0-0.83	0-0.69	0-0.49	0-0.47	0-0.54	-0.38	0.37
Basophils	G/L	0-0.18	0-0.18	0-0.14	0-0.16	0-0.18	0-0.19	0-0.18	0-0.18	-0.13	0.13
Platelets	G/L	142-424	149-432	148-377	105-574	159-490	121-475	109-489	114-450	-93	107
Urine											
Specific Gravity	--	1.006-1.035	1.005-1.034	1.007-1.036	1.005-1.037	1.004-1.035	1.004-1.036	1.005-1.034	1.005-1.038	-0.018	0.017
pH	--	5.0-9.0	5.0-8.0	5.0-9.0	5.0-7.0	5.0-8.0	5.0-8.0	5.0-7.0	5.0-7.0	-2.0	2.0

Index